MIND MAPS
FOR MEDICINE

Student reviewers

Our medical textbooks are assessed and reviewed by the following medical students:

University of Aberdeen School of Medicine and Dentistry: Dylan McClurg
Barts and The London School of Medicine and Dentistry: Jay Singh
University of Birmingham College of Medical and Dental Sciences: Hannah Morgan
Cardiff University School of Medicine: Chloe Chia
The University of Edinburgh Medical School: Tanith Bain
University of Exeter Medical School: Zoe Foster
Hull York Medical School: Maalik Imtiaz
King's College London GKT School of Medical Education: Karan Sagoo
University of Liverpool School of Medicine: Sophie Gunter
University of Manchester Medical School: Holly Egan
Newcastle University School of Medical Education: Jenita Jona James
Norwich Medical School: Aneesa Khan
University of Nottingham School of Medicine: Tom Charles
University of Sheffield Medical School: Rebecca Nutt
St George's, University of London: Nawshin Basit
Swansea University Medical School: Jack Bartlett
University of Central Lancashire School of Medicine: Katie Chi Kei Cheung
University College London Medical School: Camila Nicklewicz

We are grateful for their essential feedback.

Additional student reviewers wanted

We are keen to recruit more student reviewers, particularly at UK medical schools where we don't currently have anyone in post. If you would like to apply for the position, please contact Simon Watkins (simon.watkins@scionpublishing.com) and explain why you would be suitable for the role.

Feedback, errors and omissions

We are always pleased to receive feedback (good and bad) about our books – if you would like to comment on any of our books, please email info@scionpublishing.com.

We've worked really hard with the authors to ensure that everything in the book is correct. However, errors and ambiguities can still slip through in books as complex as this. If you spot anything you think might be wrong, please email us and we will look into it straight away. If an error has occurred, we will correct it for future printings and post a note about it on our website so that other readers of the book are alerted to this.

Thank you for your help.

MIND MAPS
FOR MEDICINE

Mohsin Azam, MBChB, BSc, MRCGP

General Practitioner, North London

Scion

© **Scion Publishing Ltd, 2021**

First published 2021

A CIP catalogue record for this book is available from the British Library.

ISBN 9781911510369

Scion Publishing Limited

The Old Hayloft, Vantage Business Park, Bloxham Road, Banbury OX16 9UX, UK

www.scionpublishing.com

Important Note from the Publisher

The information contained within this book was obtained by Scion Publishing Ltd from sources believed by us to be reliable. However, while every effort has been made to ensure its accuracy, no responsibility for loss or injury whatsoever occasioned to any person acting or refraining from action as a result of information contained herein can be accepted by the authors or publishers.

Readers are reminded that medicine is a constantly evolving science and while the authors and publishers have ensured that all dosages, applications and practices are based on current indications, there may be specific practices which differ between communities. You should always follow the guidelines laid down by the manufacturers of specific products and the relevant authorities in the country in which you are practising.

Although every effort has been made to ensure that all owners of copyright material have been acknowledged in this publication, we would be pleased to acknowledge in subsequent reprints or editions any omissions brought to our attention.

Registered names, trademarks, etc. used in this book, even when not marked as such, are not to be considered unprotected by law.

Typeset by Medlar Publishing Solutions Pvt Ltd, India

Printed in the UK

Last digit is the print number: 10 9 8 7 6 5

Contents

Chapter 6: Neurology   **181**

Chapter 7: Rheumatology   **227**

Chapter 8: Infectious diseases   **267**

Preface

Mind maps (or similar concepts) have been used for centuries, for learning, brainstorming, visual thinking and problem solving amongst educators, psychologists and people in general. They are particularly helpful for visual learners and help with memorisation and retention, and are a more engaging form of learning, helping to improve productivity, efficiency and creativity. Studies on medical students have shown that using mind maps may yield better pass rates than traditional note-taking.

It was during my second year of medical school that I first really appreciated the value of mind maps after having a go at constructing some myself for the first time. It was certainly a game-changer for me. It enabled me to digest and retain a large amount of information in a structured manner, and therefore resulted in a more efficient learning style. Prior to this I had spent much more time making lengthy notes which I found far less productive and rather tedious. It was at that point that the phrase 'work smarter, not harder' hit home. During medical school, using mind maps helped me with recall in written examinations, but I also found that they enabled me to provide more structured and cogent answers in an OSCE setting, and examiners seemed to prefer this to simply regurgitating lists of unstructured and undifferentiated information.

A few years ago I recognised the need for a medical revision guide set out in a mind map format – existing books seemed to oversimplify their mind maps and not provide sufficient detail. They also failed to supplement the written information with drawings and photos, which I feel is vital in a visual memory aid.

This book takes a systems-based approach and for each of over 100 conditions presents a detailed mind map, taking readers consistently through definition, pathophysiology, causes, clinical features, investigations, management, complications and more. The book is primarily aimed at medical students, but it should also be useful for junior doctors and general practitioners.

Chapters are largely laid out in alphabetical order to allow for readers to easily locate medical conditions. There are a few exceptions, however, where it was felt that some conditions should be grouped together in terms of a spectrum from less to more severe, such as the sections covering angina pectoris and acute coronary syndrome, and also the sections on TIA and stroke.

For substantial topics where all the relevant and important information cannot feasibly fit onto one mind map, additional supplementary information is provided on a *Notes* page overleaf, in an easy to read bullet point format.

Additional memory aids in the form of mnemonics are also included alongside photographs and illustrations to further enhance retention and visualisation.

It is important to note that this book is not intended as a replacement for larger textbooks but should be seen as a companion to them, giving you a more innovative and fun way of learning.

I hope that readers not only find this book enjoyable and useful in providing medical knowledge but that it also inspires you to create your own medical mind maps.

Finally, I wish all readers the best with your medical exams and future careers.

Mohsin Azam

Acknowledgements

I would like to thank the student reviewers for their valuable feedback on the content of some of the chapters.

I am extremely grateful to the team at Scion Publishing Ltd, particularly Dr Jonathan Ray for his advice, encouragement and, above all, patience.

Dedications

To my beloved parents for all the unconditional love and support they have given me throughout my life.

To my sweetheart Sevda for the continued love and patience you have for me.

A special mention goes to my adorable baby daughter, Elanur, you have made me a happy and proud father!

Abbreviations

ABC	Airway, breathing, circulation		COPD	Chronic obstructive pulmonary disease
ABG	Arterial blood gas		CPAP	Continuous positive airway pressure
ABPM	Ambulatory blood pressure monitoring		CRH	Corticotropin-releasing hormone
ACE	Angiotensin-converting enzyme		CRP	C-reactive protein
ACR	Albumin : creatinine ratio		CSF	Cerebrospinal fluid
ACS	Acute coronary syndrome		CT	Computed tomography
ACTH	Adrenocorticotropic hormone		CTPA	Computed tomography pulmonary angiogram
ADH	Antidiuretic hormone		CV	Cardiovascular
ADL	Activities of daily living		CVA	Cerebrovascular accident
AF	Atrial fibrillation		CVD	Cardiovascular disease
AIDS	Acquired immune deficiency syndrome		CWP	Coal worker's pneumoconiosis
AKI	Acute kidney injury		CXR	Chest X-ray
ALP	Alkaline phosphatase		DEXA	Dual energy X-ray absorptiometry
ALT	Alanine transaminase		DI	Diabetes insipidus
AMA	Anti-mitochondrial antibody		DIDMOAD	Diabetes insipidus, diabetes mellitus, optic atrophy, and deafness
AMTS	Abbreviated mental test score		DIP	Distal interphalangeal
ANA	Anti-nuclear antibody		DKA	Diabetic ketoacidosis
ANCA	Anti-neutrophil cytoplasmic antibody		DMARD	Disease-modifying anti-rheumatic drug
Anti-CCP	Anti-cyclic citrullinated peptide		DOAC	Direct oral anticoagulant
APTT	Activated partial thromboplastin time		DVLA	Driver and Vehicle Licensing Agency
ARB	Angiotensin II receptor blocker		DVT	Deep vein thrombosis
ARDS	Acute respiratory distress syndrome		EBV	Epstein–Barr virus
AS	Ankylosing spondylitis		ECG	Electrocardiogram
ASMA	Anti-smooth muscle antibodies		ECHO	Echocardiogram
AST	Aspartate transaminase		EEG	Electroencephalogram
ATP	Adenosine triphosphate		eGFR	Estimated glomerular filtration rate
AV	Atrioventricular		ELISA	Enzyme-linked immunosorbent assay
AVP	Arginine vasopressin		EMG	Electromyography
AXR	Abdominal X-ray		ERCP	Endoscopic retrograde cholangiopancreatography
BE	Base excess		ESR	Erythrocyte sedimentation rate
BIPAP	Bilevel positive airway pressure		FBC	Full blood count
BNP	Brain natriuretic peptide		FEV	Forced expiratory volume
BP	Blood pressure		FSH	Follicle-stimulating hormone
CABG	Coronary artery bypass grafting		FVC	Forced vital capacity
CBT	Cognitive behavioural therapy		G6PD	Glucose-6-phosphate dehydrogenase
CCF	Congestive cardiac failure		GBS	Guillain–Barré syndrome
CK	Creatine kinase		GCA	Giant cell arteritis
CKD	Chronic kidney disease		GCS	Glasgow Coma Scale
CMV	Cytomegalovirus		GFR	Glomerular filtration rate
CNS	Central nervous system			
COCP	Combined oral contraceptive pill			

GI	Gastrointestinal	MI	Myocardial infarction
GLP	Glucagon-like peptide	MND	Motor neurone disease
GORD	Gastro-oesophageal reflux disease	MPTP	1-methyl-4-phenyl-1,2,3,6-tetrahydropyridine
GRA	Glucocorticoid-remediable aldosteronism	MRA	Magnetic resonance angiogram
GTN	Glyceryl trinitrate	MRCP	Magnetic resonance cholangiopancreatography
GU	Genitourinary	MRI	Magnetic resonance image
HAART	Highly active antiretroviral therapy	MS	Multiple sclerosis
HAV	Hepatitis A virus	MSK	Musculoskeletal
HBA1c	Haemoglobin A1c	MSM	Men who have sex with men
HBPM	Home blood pressure monitoring	MTP	Metatarsophalangeal
HDU	High dependency unit	NAC	N-acetyl cysteine
HDV	Hepatitis D virus	NBM	Nil by mouth
HELLP	Haemolysis, elevated liver enzymes and low platelet count	NG	Nasogastric
		NICE	National Institute for Health and Care Excellence
HEV	Hepatitis E virus	NSAID	Non-steroidal anti-inflammatory drug
HF	Heart failure	NSCLC	Non-small cell lung carcinoma
HH	Hereditary haemochromatosis	NSTEMI	Non-ST elevation myocardial infarction
HHS	Hyperosmolar hyperglycaemic state	OA	Osteoarthritis
HIV	Human immunodeficiency virus	OD	Omnie die (once a day)
HLA	Human leucocyte antigen	OGTT	Oral glucose tolerance test
HOCM	Hypertrophic obstructive cardiomyopathy	ON	Omni nocte
HRT	Hormone replacement therapy	OSA	Obstructive sleep apnoea
HSP	Henoch–Schönlein purpura	PBC	Primary biliary cholangitis
HTN	Hypertension	PCI	Percutaneous coronary intervention
IBD	Inflammatory bowel disease	PCOS	Polycystic ovary syndrome
IBS	Irritable bowel syndrome	PD	Parkinson's disease
ICD	Implantable cardioverter-defibrillator	PE	Pulmonary embolism
ICP	Intracranial pressure	PEF	Peak expiratory flow
ICS	Inhaled corticosteroid	PEFR	Peak expiratory flow rate
ICU	Intensive care unit	PENS	Percutaneous electrical nerve stimulation
IDDM	Insulin-dependent diabetes mellitus	PET	Positron emission tomography
IE	Infective endocarditis	PIP	Proximal interphalangeal
IGF	Insulin-like growth factor	PM	Polymyositis
IHD	Ischaemic heart disease	PMR	Polymyalgia rheumatica
INR	International normalised ratio	PPI	Proton pump inhibitor
IPF	Idiopathic pulmonary fibrosis	PSC	Primary sclerosing cholangitis
ITU	Intensive treatment unit	PT	Prothrombin time
IV	Intravenous	PTH	Parathyroid hormone
JVP	Jugular venous pressure	PVD	Peripheral vascular disease
KUB	Kidneys, ureter, bladder	RA	Rheumatoid arthritis
LABA	Long-acting beta agonist	RAAS	Renin–angiotensin–aldosterone system
LAD	Left anterior descending	RBBB	Right bundle branch block
LBBB	Left bundle branch block	RCA	Right coronary artery
LCx	Left circumflex	RF	Rheumatoid factor
LDH	Lactate dehydrogenase	RR	Respiratory rate
LFTs	Liver function tests	RV	Right ventricular
LMWH	Low molecular weight heparin	SABA	Short-acting beta agonist
LOS	Lower oesophageal sphincter	SAH	Subarachnoid haemorrhage
LTRA	Leukotriene receptor antagonist	SALT	Speech and language therapy
LVEF	Left ventricular ejection fraction	SAMA	Short-acting muscarinic antagonist
LVH	Left ventricular hypertrophy	SBP	Systolic blood pressure
MART	Maintenance and reliever therapy	SC	Subcutaneous
MCP	Metacarpophalangeal	SCC	Squamous cell carcinoma
MEN	Multiple endocrine neoplasia	SCLC	Small cell lung carcinoma

SDH	Subdural haematoma	**TED**	Thrombo-embolus deterrent
SHBG	Sex hormone binding globulin	**TENS**	Transcutaneous electrical nerve stimulation
SIADH	Syndrome of inappropriate ADH secretion	**TFTs**	Thyroid function tests
SLE	Systemic lupus erythematosus	**TIA**	Transient ischaemic attack
SMA	Smooth muscle antibody	**TNM**	Tumour, node, metastasis
SNRI	Serotonin and noradrenaline reuptake inhibitor	**TRH**	Thyrotropin-releasing hormone
SNS	Sympathetic nervous system	**TSH**	Thyroid-stimulating hormone
SOB	Shortness of breath	**TTG**	Tissue transglutaminase
SPECT	Single photon emission computed tomography	**U&Es**	Urea and electrolytes
SS	Sjögren syndrome	**UC**	Ulcerative colitis
SSRI	Selective serotonin reuptake inhibitor	**UGIB**	Upper gastrointestinal bleeding
STEMI	ST elevation myocardial infarction	**US**	Ultrasound
STI	Sexually transmitted infection	**UTI**	Urinary tract infection
T1DM	Type 1 diabetes mellitus	**VF**	Ventricular fibrillation
T2DM	Type 2 diabetes mellitus	**VT**	Ventricular tachycardia
TB	Tuberculosis	**VTE**	Venous thromboembolism
TCA	Tricyclic antidepressant	**WCC**	White cell count

Chapter 1

Cardiology

Angina refers to pain in the chest, neck, shoulders, jaw or arms caused by an insufficient blood supply to the myocardium.

Definition

Risk factors

Non-modifiable risk factors

- Increasing age
- Male sex
- Family history of premature coronary heart disease
- Premature menopause

Modifiable risk factors

- Smoking
- Diabetes mellitus (and impaired glucose tolerance)
- Hypertension
- Dyslipidaemia
- Obesity
- Sedentary lifestyle

Angina pectoris

Management

Conservative

Mainly based on modifying risk factors:

- Smoking cessation
- Healthy diet
- Exercise
- Weight loss
- Controlling diabetes, hypertension and raised cholesterol

Pharmacological (**ABC N**ow **S**imply **N**ote **I**t **R**ight away)

- **Aspirin** All patients should receive aspirin 75mg OD for secondary prevention
- **Beta blocker** e.g. Atenolol or **Calcium channel blocker*** depending on comorbidities, contraindications and the person's preference
- **Nitrates** Sublingual glyceryl trinitrate (GTN) for acute symptomatic relief; a long-acting nitrate can also be used 2nd line, e.g. isosorbide mononitrate
- **Statin** e.g. Atorvastatin in the absence of any contraindication
- **Nicorandil** Dual properties of a nitrate and ATP-sensitive K^+ channel agonist; used as 2nd-line agent
- **Ivabradine** A selective inhibitor of sinus node pacemaker activity, used as 2nd-line agent
- **Ranolazine** Reduces myocardial ischaemia by acting on intracellular Na^+ currents, also used as 2nd-line agent

*If a calcium channel blocker is used as monotherapy then a rate-limiting one, e.g. verapamil or diltiazem, should be used; if used in combination with a beta blocker then a long-acting dihydropyridine calcium channel blocker should be used, e.g. nifedipine; beta blockers should not be co-prescribed with verapamil (due to risk of complete heart block).

Revascularisation

Coronary revascularisation is required in those at high risk and those who fail to be controlled by medical therapy. The choice of coronary artery bypass grafting (CABG) or percutaneous coronary intervention (PCI) depends on the distribution of the coronary artery disease, comorbidities and patient preference.

PCI

Generally for patients with isolated coronary artery disease; localised atheromatous lesions are dilated using small inflatable balloons and then a stent is placed; complications include death, acute MI, the need for urgent CABG and restenosis.

CABG

The internal mammary artery or small saphenous vein is used to bypass the stenosis. It is particularly undertaken for left main stem obstruction or triple vessel disease. The main complication is re-occurrence of angina due to accelerated atherosclerosis in the graft.

Symptoms

Classical presentation:

Central crushing, retrosternal chest pain on exertion and relieved by rest within a few minutes. It may also be exacerbated by anger, excitement and cold weather, and frequently radiates to the arms and neck

Other variants:

- **Decubitus angina** Occurs when the patient lies down
- **Nocturnal angina** Occurs at night and often wakes a patient from sleep

- **Variant (Prinzmetal's) angina** Caused by coronary artery spasm (of normal coronary arteries on angiogram) and usually occurs at rest without any provocation.
- **Unstable angina** Recurrent episodes of angina on minimal effort or at rest (see *Ch1: Acute coronary syndrome*)
- **Cardiac syndrome X** Describes patients with combination of angina-like chest pain, positive objective evidence of myocardial ischaemia (e.g. positive exercise stress test) with a normal coronary angiogram

Signs

- Examination is usually normal but important to assess for risk factors such as hypertension and signs of hyperlipidaemia (e.g. corneal arcus and xanthelasma) and underlying causes e.g. aortic stenosis

Clinical features

Notes

Angina pectoris

Investigations

ECG

- **12-lead ECG** May show some ischaemic changes but a normal ECG does not rule out a diagnosis of angina
- **Exercise ECG** Typically ST segment depression after exercising usually diagnostic but normal test does not exclude diagnosis

Bloods

FBC, U&Es, glucose/HbA1c, lipid profile, LFTs, TFTs, troponin

ECHO

- **Resting ECHO** To assess cardiac function, or if hypertrophic cardiomyopathy or aortic valve disease is suspected
- **Stress ECHO** To assess for ischaemic regional wall changes while the patient is subjected to stress in the form of exercise or chemically (if unable to exercise) with dobutamine

Coronary angiography

- Gold standard for assessing coronary artery disease and exact coronary artery anatomy before coronary intervention

Cardiovascular MR/CT angiography

- Non-invasive investigation to assess coronary artery disease

Acute coronary syndrome (ACS) encompasses a spectrum of unstable coronary artery diseases. It covers the following diagnoses:

- **Unstable angina** Symptoms at rest with ECG changes; the myocardial ischaemia is not sufficient to cause myocardial damage and therefore there is no rise in serum markers of myocardial injury e.g. troponin
- **Non-ST elevation myocardial infarction (NSTEMI)** As above but with myocardial ischaemia sufficient to cause myocardial damage and therefore elevation in serum markers of myocardial injury
- **ST elevation myocardial infarction (STEMI)** Symptoms with ST elevation on ECG due to complete occlusion of the coronary artery

The underlying cause of coronary artery disease is atherosclerosis which has several stages:

- **Endothelial cell injury and inflammation** Lipids deposited in the intima layer of coronary arteries together with vascular injury (e.g. from hypertension) cause inflammation, increased permeability and recruitment of white cells; over time inflammatory cells, particularly macrophages, take up the lipid and become foam cells
- **Plaque formation** Foam cells accumulate and smooth muscle cells proliferate resulting in the growth of the plaque
- **Plaque rupture** Activates the clotting cascade and thrombosis which might be sufficient to cause partial occlusion (resulting in myocardial ischaemia and angina) or total occlusion (resulting in myocardial necrosis and myocardial infarction, MI)

Pathophysiology

Definition

Acute coronary syndrome

Complications

Management

Complications of ACS (DARTH VADER)

- **D**eath/cardiac arrest Most commonly occurs due to patients developing ventricular fibrillation
- **A**rrhythmias Tachyarrhythmias (e.g. VF and VT) or bradyarrhythmias (atrioventricular block is more common following inferior myocardial infarctions)
- **R**upture Free ventricular wall/ventricular septum/papillary muscles
- **T**amponade and cardiogenic shock
- **H**eart failure Acute or chronic
- **V**entricular Free wall or interVentricular septum rupture
- **A**neurysm Of the left ventricle
- **D**ressler syndrome Tends to occur around 2–6 weeks following a MI (thought to be autoimmune)
- thrombo**E**mbolism Mural thrombus
- **R**upture Of the papillary muscle and mitral valve **R**egurgitation

Acute

Initial* treatment for all patients (MONA)

- **M**orphine Oral or IV diamorphine, e.g. 2.5–5mg, can be given for pain relief; an anti-emetic such as metoclopramide should be co-prescribed
- **O**xygen Should only be given if hypoxic, or evidence of pulmonary oedema, or continuing myocardial ischaemia
- **N**itrates To relieve ischaemic pain (initially sublingual, e.g. two sprays of GTN); if not effective, IV or buccal GTN or IV isosorbide dinitrate can be given
- **A**spirin All patients should receive 300mg aspirin crushed or chewed ASAP

*Subsequent management depends on whether the patient has unstable angina/NSTEMI or STEMI (see flow chart on Notes page overleaf)

Chronic

See Notes page overleaf.

Non-modifiable

- Increasing age
- Male sex
- Family history of premature coronary heart disease
- Premature menopause

Modifiable

- Smoking
- Diabetes mellitus (and impaired glucose tolerance)
- Hypertension
- Dyslipidaemia
- Obesity
- Sedentary lifestyle

Risk factors

Clinical features

- **Chest pain** Typically central and 'crushing' in nature and often radiates to arms, shoulders, neck or jaw
- **Shortness of breath**
- **Nausea**
- **Palpitations**
- **Sweating**

Note: Some patient groups, e.g. elderly, diabetics, females and those with CKD, may have little or no chest pain, and may present with atypical features such as abdominal pain, altered mental state or jaw pain, so-called 'silent MI'

Epidemiology

- Coronary heart disease is the most common cause of death in the UK
- Incidence increases with age, and elderly people also tend to have higher rates of morbidity and mortality from their infarcts

Investigations

ECG

- **Unstable angina and NSTEMI** May be normal, show ST-segment depression or non-specific abnormalities e.g. T-wave inversion
- **STEMI** Acute ST-segment elevation or new left bundle branch block (LBBB) (see *Figs. 1–3*)

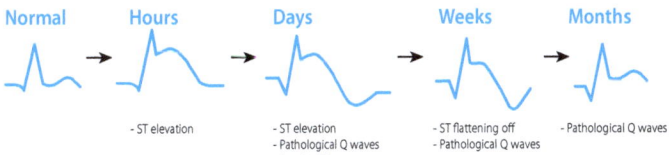

Normal	Hours	Days	Weeks	Months
	- ST elevation	- ST elevation - Pathological Q waves - Inverted T waves	- ST flattening off - Pathological Q waves	- Pathological Q waves

Fig. 1 ECG changes in MI

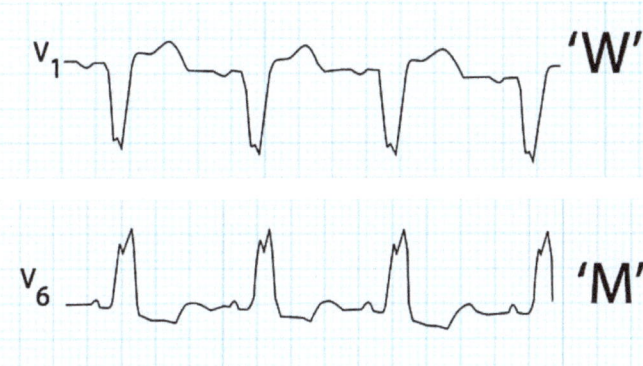

Fig. 2 LBBB on ECG

Bloods

- **Routine** FBC (to exclude anaemia), U&Es (to assess renal function), fasting lipids (risk stratification), LFTs (baseline before starting statins), TFTs
- **Troponin and other cardiac enzymes** Cardiac troponins T and I are highly sensitive and specific for MI (normal in unstable angina); other cardiac enzymes such as creatinine kinase will also be raised but this is less specific

CXR

- To assess for presence or absence of heart failure/pulmonary oedema and exclude other diagnoses

ECHO

- Can assess for regional wall abnormalities and define the extent of the infarction and assess overall ventricular function and can identify complications

Coronary angiography

- Cardiac angiography defines the patient's coronary anatomy and the extent of the disease

Acute coronary syndrome notes

NICE guideline (NG185) on the acute management of ACS

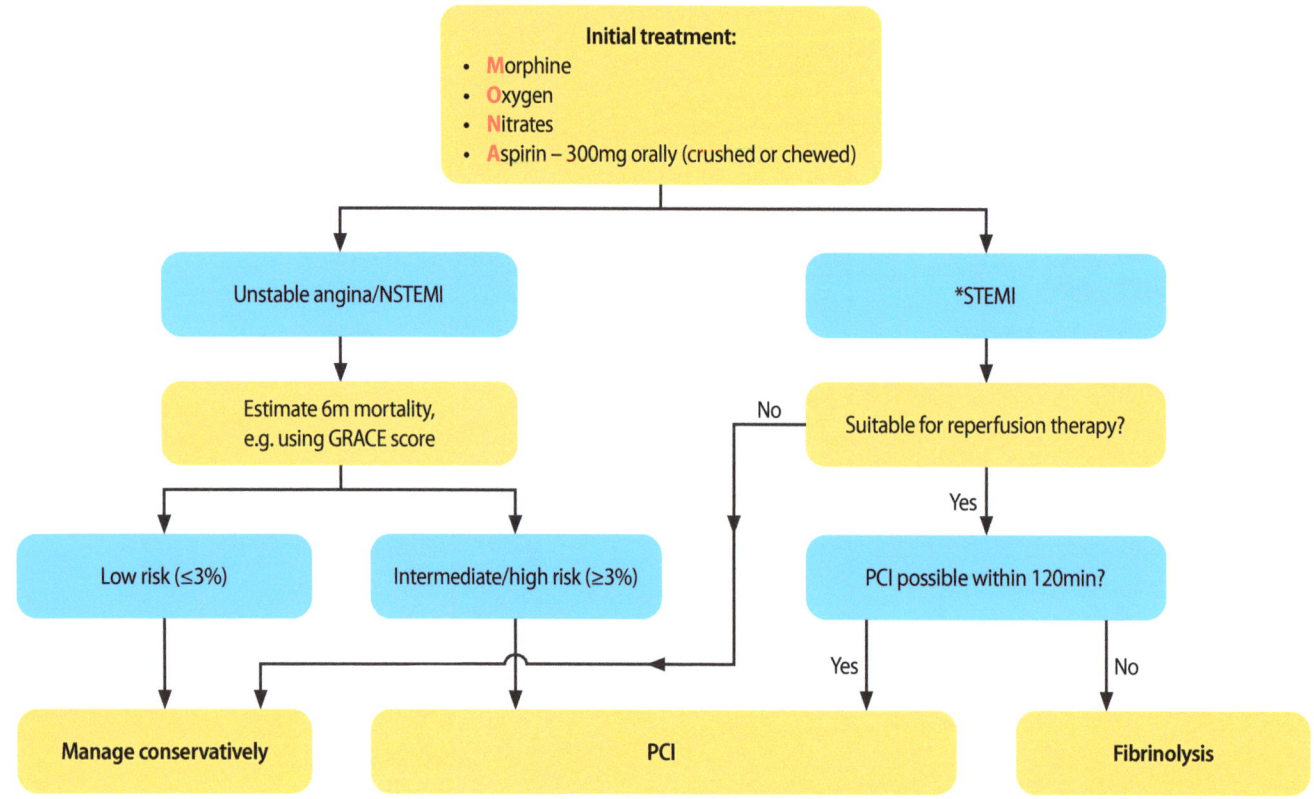

Initial treatment:
- **M**orphine
- **O**xygen
- **N**itrates
- **A**spirin – 300mg orally (crushed or chewed)

Unstable angina/NSTEMI

*STEMI

Estimate 6m mortality, e.g. using GRACE score

Suitable for reperfusion therapy?   No   Yes

Low risk (≤3%)   Intermediate/high risk (≥3%)

PCI possible within 120min?   Yes   No

Manage conservatively   **PCI**   **Fibrinolysis**

Manage conservatively
- Give ticagrelor – initially 180mg for 1 dose, then 90mg twice daily
- Consider clopidogrel 300mg loading dose – with aspirin, or aspirin alone, for high bleeding risk

PCI

For unstable angina/NSTEMI:
- Immediate angiography if unstable, otherwise within 72h if no contraindications
- Give another antiplatelet prior to PCI – prasugrel or ticagrelor (if not taking an oral anticoagulant) or clopidogrel (if taking an oral anticoagulant)
- Offer systemic unfractionated heparin

For STEMI:
- Preferred strategy if <12h of onset of symptoms
- Give another antiplatelet – prasugrel prior to PCI (if not already taking oral anticoagulant) or clopidogrel (if taking an oral anticoagulant)
- Radial access is preferred and offer unfractionated heparin with bailout glycoprotein 2b/3a inhibitor
- Drug-eluting stent should be used in preference

Fibrinolysis

Indicated if <12h of onset of symptoms if primary PCI cannot be delivered within 120min of the time when fibrinolysis could have been given
- Options for fibrinolysis include alteplase, reteplase, streptokinase or tenecteplase
- Give an antithrombin at the same time
- Following procedure, give ticagrelor
- See *Table 2* for typical contraindications to fibrinolysis

*Clinical symptoms consistent with ACS with persistent ECG features in ≥2 contiguous leads of:
- 2.5mm ST elevation in leads V2–3 in men <40y, or ≥2.0mm ST elevation in leads V2–3 in men ≥40y
- 1.5mm ST elevation in V2–3 in women
- 1mm ST elevation in other leads
- new LBBB (LBBB should be considered new unless there is evidence otherwise)

ECG localisation of myocardial infarction

It is possible to localise the ischaemic area of the heart by assessing the leads that show ST segment elevation (see *Table 1*).

Table 1 ECG localisation of myocardial infarction

Leads	Affected myocardial area	Occluded coronary artery
V1-V2	Septal	Proximal LAD
V3-V4	Anterior	LAD
V5-V6	Apical	Distal LAD, LCx or RCA
1, AVL	Lateral	LCx
2, AVF, 3	Inferior	90% RCA, 10% LCx

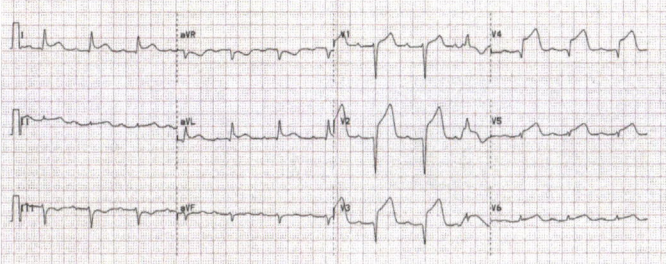

Fig. 3 ECG showing anteroseptal MI

Risk assessment tools for ACS

1. GRACE
- The Global registry of acute coronary events (GRACE) Score is a scoring system to risk stratify patients with diagnosed ACS to estimate their in-hospital and 6-month to 3-year mortality.
- It is based on 8 variables: Age, signs of heart failure, heart rate and BP at presentation, serum creatinine level, ECG changes, troponin concentration and cardiac arrest at presentation

2. TIMI
- The TIMI Risk Score for UA/NSTEMI estimates mortality for patients with unstable angina and NSTEMI.

3. HEART score:
- HEART Score for Major Cardiac Events. Predicts 6-week risk of major adverse cardiac event. It is used in patients ≥21 years old presenting with symptoms suggestive of ACS. **HEART** is an acronym and stands for 5 variables: **H**istory, **E**CG, **A**ge, **R**isk factors, and **T**roponin.

Long-term treatment

Non-pharmacological
- **Smoking cessation**
- **Weight control**
- **Diet** Mediterranean-style diet is advised
- **Exercise** Advise 20–30min/day until patients are 'slightly breathless'; refer to cardiac rehabilitation
- **Driving** If treated successfully by coronary angioplasty, group 1 driving may recommence after 1 week; if not successfully treated, driving may recommence after 4 weeks
- **Sexual activity** May resume 4 weeks after uncomplicated MI; PDE5 inhibitors (e.g. sildenafil) cannot be used until 6 months after MI and should be avoided if patient is on nitrates or nicorandil

Pharmacological (DABS)
- **D**ual antiplatelet therapy (DAPT) Aspirin 75mg OD lifelong and one other antiplatelet (ticagrelor, prasugrel or clopidogrel) for at least 1 year; consider co-prescribing a PPI (e.g. omeprazole) for gastric protection
- **A**ce inhibitor or **A**RB (If intolerant to ACE inhibitor)
- **B**eta blocker e.g. Bisoprolol, carvedilol and metoprolol; start low and increase gradually as blood pressure and pulse allow; if contraindicated consider calcium channel blocker e.g. verapamil or diltiazem
- **S**tatin High dose e.g. atorvastatin 80mg ON
- An **aldosterone antagonist** e.g. Eplerenone for patients who have had an acute MI and evidence of heart failure and left ventricular systolic dysfunction

Typical contraindications to fibrinolytic therapy

Table 2 Typical contraindications to fibrinolytic therapy

Absolute	Relative
• Previous haemorrhagic stroke • Ischaemic stroke in the previous 6 months • Central nervous system trauma or neoplasm • Recent (<3 months) major surgery, head injury or major trauma • Active internal bleeding or GI bleeding within last month • Known or suspected aortic dissection • Known bleeding disorder	• Refractory hypertension (systolic BP >180mmHg) • TIA in preceding 6 months • Oral anticoagulant treatment • Pregnant or <1 week postpartum • Traumatic cardiopulmonary resuscitation (CPR) • Active peptic ulcer disease • Advanced liver disease • Infective endocarditis • Previous allergy to fibrinolytic drugs

Definition

Acute pericarditis is inflammation of the pericardium.

Causes

- Viral infection (e.g. coxsackievirus, mumps, EBV, CMV, varicella, HIV)
- Tuberculosis
- Uraemia (e.g. in severe renal failure)
- Trauma
- Post myocardial infarction, including Dressler syndrome
- Connective tissue disease e.g. SLE, RA, polyarteritis nodosa
- Rheumatic fever
- Hypothyroidism
- Malignancy
- Iatrogenic: radiotherapy, post cardiac surgery, drugs (e.g. procainamide, hydralazine)

Clinical features

Symptoms

- **Chest pain:** may be pleuritic and often relieved by sitting forwards
- Non-specific symptoms: non-productive cough, dyspnoea and flu-like symptoms

Signs

- Pericardial friction rub
- Tachypnoea
- Tachycardia

Acute pericarditis

Complications

- Pericardial effusion and cardiac tamponade
- Chronic pericarditis
- Constrictive pericarditis

Investigations

ECG

- Widespread 'saddle-shaped' ST elevation (see *Fig. 1*)
- Sinus tachycardia is common
- T waves may initially be prominent, upright and peaked
- AF, atrial flutter or atrial topics may occur
- PR depression: most specific ECG marker for pericarditis

Bloods

- FBC, U&Es, CRP/ESR, troponin (may be raised), viral serology, autoantibodies (e.g. ANA, RF, anti-CCP if indicated) and TFTs to assess for underlying causes if indicated

CXR

- May show globular enlargement of the heart if there is presence of pericardial effusion

ECHO

- Confirms the presence of a pericardial effusion

Management

- Treat the underlying cause
- A combination of NSAIDs and colchicine is 1st line for patients with acute idiopathic or suspected viral pericarditis

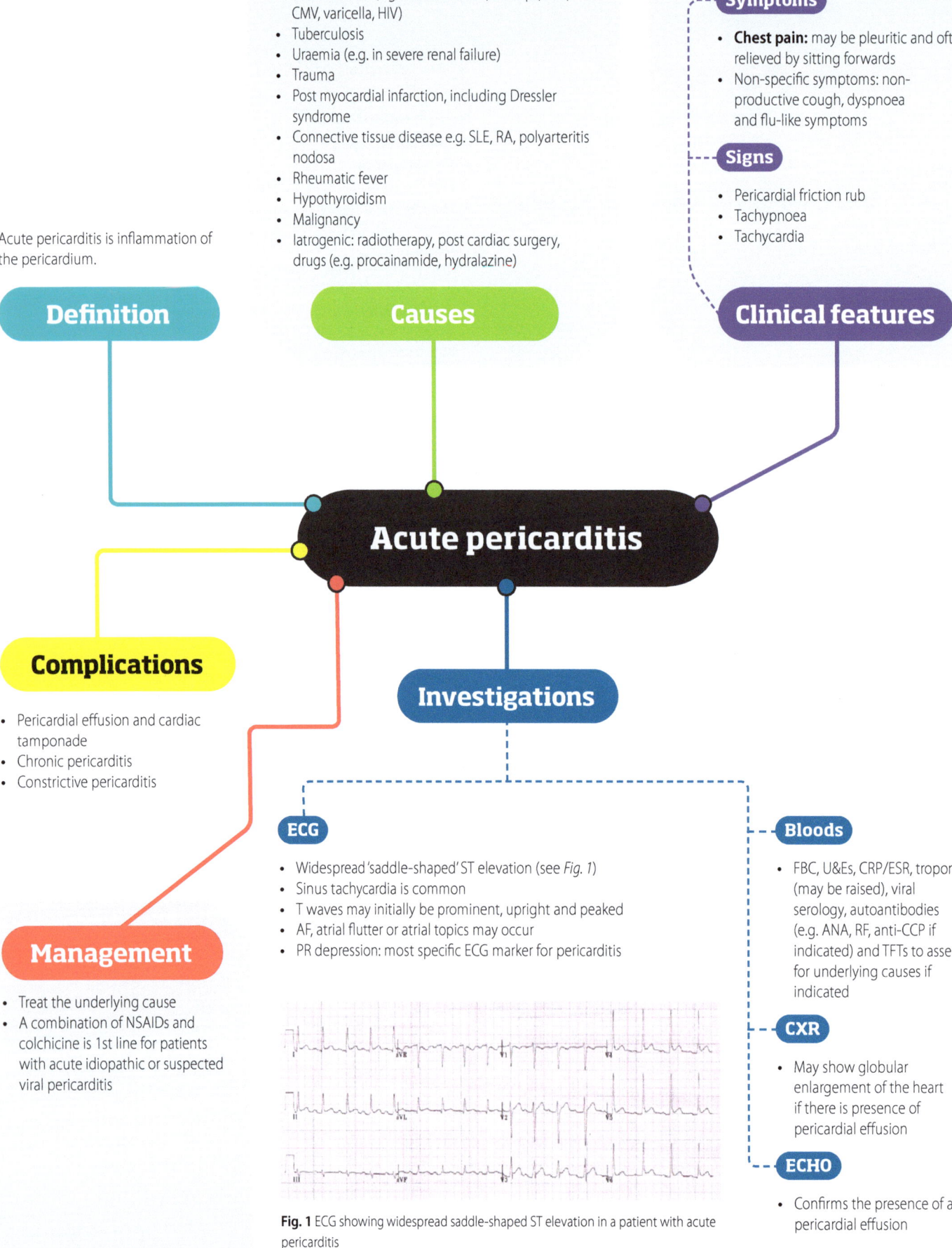

Fig. 1 ECG showing widespread saddle-shaped ST elevation in a patient with acute pericarditis

Pericardial effusion and cardiac tamponade

Definition

Pericardial effusion describes a collection of fluid in the pericardial space which may result from any of the causes of pericarditis. It can lead to cardiac tamponade which is a form of cardiogenic shock from restricted diastolic ventricular filling caused by a large amount of fluid accumulation in the pericardial space. It is a medical emergency.

Clinical features

- Fatigue
- Breathlessness characteristically, occurs on exertion
- Ascites
- Peripheral oedema
- Pulse: pulsus paradoxus, AF, tachycardia
- Kussmaul's sign (a raised JVP with inspiration) – rare
- Cardiac impulses: barely palpable; characteristic is systolic retraction at the apex
- Pericardial knock (loud-high pitched S3) following S2
- Beck's triad is the hallmark of cardiac tamponade (see *Fig. 2*)
- JVP – an absent Y descent

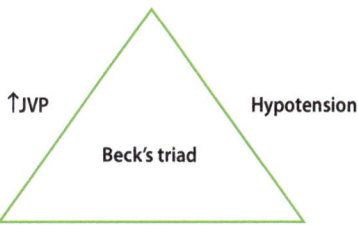

Fig. 2 Beck's triad

Investigations

- CXR: large globular heart
- ECG: may show ST elevation with MI or pericarditis, or loss of voltages; alternating QRS morphologies
- ECHO: diagnostic (echo-free zone surrounds the heart)
- Cardiac MRI or CT: may be superior to ECHO in detecting loculated pericardial effusions and pericardial thickening
- Diagnostic pericardiocentesis: pericardial fluid sent for microbiological and cytological testing

Management

- Urgent therapeutic pericardiocentesis is required

Constrictive pericarditis

Definition

Constrictive pericarditis is caused by a rigid pericardial sac that limits ventricular filling.

Causes

- Tuberculosis
- Viral infection
- Malignancy: carcinomatous invasion of the pericardium
- Radiotherapy of the chest
- Renal failure
- Post cardiac surgery

Clinical features

- Fatigue
- Breathlessness characteristically, occurs on exertion
- Ascites
- Peripheral oedema
- Pulse: AF, tachycardia
- Kussmaul's sign (a raised JVP with inspiration)
- Cardiac impulses: barely palpable; characteristic is systolic retraction at the apex
- Pericardial knock (loud-high pitched S3) following S2

Investigations

- ECG: may show low-voltage QRS complexes and generalised T-wave inversion
- CXR: small cardiac shadow; there may be peripheral calcification
- ECHO: thickened pericardium; a normally contracting ventricle (unlike the ventricle seen in a restrictive cardiomyopathy)

Management

- Pericardiectomy (surgical excision of the pericardium)

Atrial fibrillation (AF) is the most common tachyarrhythmia. It is characterised by an irregular, disorganised electrical activity in the atria. AF can be grouped into:
- **Paroxysmal AF** Episodes lasting >30sec but <7 days that are self-terminating and recurrent
- **Persistent AF** Episodes lasting >7 days
- **Permanent AF** AF that fails to terminate using cardioversion, AF that is terminated but relapses within 24h, or long-standing AF (usually longer than 1 year)

- Results from irregular, disorganised electrical activity in the atria from rapidly firing cells at the junction of the pulmonary veins in the left atrial musculature
- The rapidly firing impulses cause disorganised atrial depolarisation and ineffective atrial contractions
- The atrioventricular (AV) node receives more electrical impulses than it can conduct, resulting in an irregular ventricular rhythm
- This may result in stagnant blood accumulating within the atrial appendage, ↑risk of clot formation and hence embolic stroke

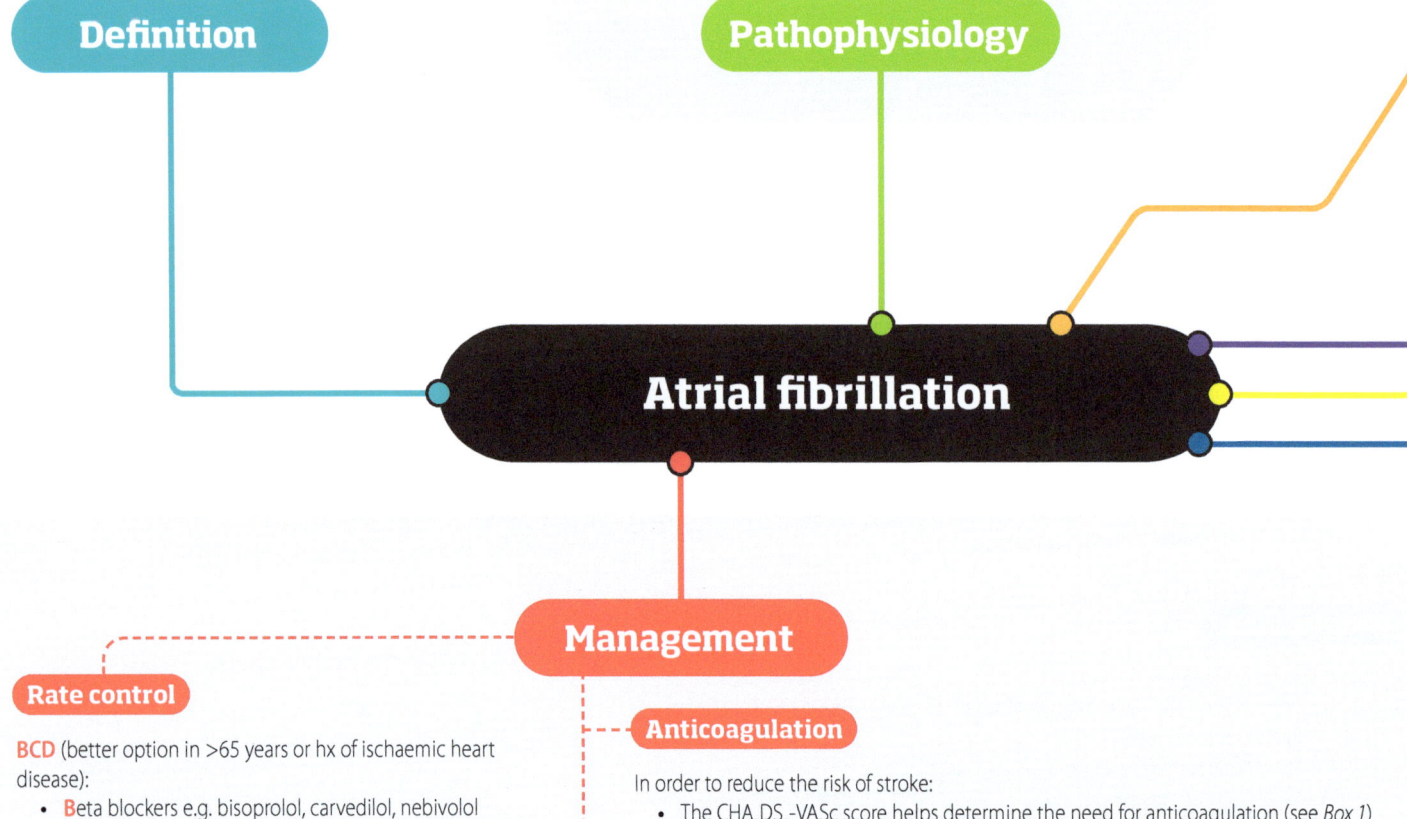

Definition

Pathophysiology

Atrial fibrillation

Management

Rate control

BCD (better option in >65 years or hx of ischaemic heart disease):
- **B**eta blockers e.g. bisoprolol, carvedilol, nebivolol
- **C**alcium channel blockers (rate limiting) e.g. diltiazem, verapamil
- **D**igoxin is preferred if there is co-existing heart failure or hypotension

Rhythm control

This is better option for <65 years, symptomatic, 1st presentation, lone AF or AF 2° to a precipitant or CCF:
- **Chemical:**
  - Sotalol
  - Amiodarone (in the presence or absence of structural heart disease)
  - Flecainide (in the absence of structural heart disease)
- **Electrical:**
  - Can be used in the acute scenario if the patient is haemodynamically unstable
  - Also can be done as an elective procedure where a rhythm control strategy is preferred

Anticoagulation

In order to reduce the risk of stroke:
- The CHA_2DS_2-VASc score helps determine the need for anticoagulation (see *Box 1*)
- The risk of using anticoagulants can be calculated using the HASBLED score (see *Box 2*)
- Patients should be offered a choice of anticoagulation from warfarin and the novel oral anticoagulants (NOACs) e.g. rivaroxaban, apixaban or dabigatran

Box 1 CHA_2DS_2-VASc score

Congestive cardiac failure = 1
HTN (or treated) = 1
Age ≥75 = 2, age 65–74 = 1
Diabetes = 1
S$_2$ Prior stroke or TIA = 2
Vascular disease (including IHD or PVD) = 1
Sex (female) = 1
(≥2 offer anticoagulation)

Box 2 HASBLED score

HTN (systolic BP >160mmHg = 1
Abnormal renal function (=1) or liver function (=1)
Stroke, history of = 1
Bleeding, hx of bleeding or high risk = 1
Labile INRs (<60% in therapeutic range) = 1
Elderly (>65 years) = 1
Drugs predisposing to bleeding (=1) or alcohol use (=1)
(≥3 indicates a 'high risk' of bleeding)

Causes

Cardiac

- Ischaemic heart disease
- Heart failure
- Hypertension
- Valvular heart disease
- Sick sinus syndrome
- Pericarditis
- Infiltrative heart disease
- Cardiomyopathy
- Myocarditis
- Congenital heart disease

Non-cardiac

- Sepsis
- PE
- Thyrotoxicosis
- Lung or pleural disease
- Chest trauma
- Hypokalaemia
- Hypovolaemia
- Hypothermia
- Alcohol abuse
- Drug abuse e.g. cocaine

Clinical features

Symptoms

- Palpitations
- Dyspnoea
- Chest pain
- Dizziness
- Syncope
- Fatigue

Signs

- Irregularly irregular pulse
- Signs of heart failure

Complications

- Stroke (5-fold risk)
- Heart failure
- Tachycardia-induced cardiomyopathy and critical cardiac ischaemia

Investigations

ECG

- Lack of P waves, irregularly irregular rhythm (see *Fig. 1*)

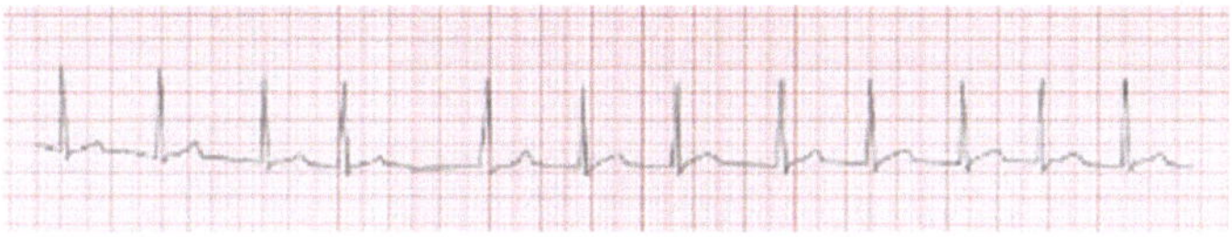

Fig. 1 ECG showing AF (note lack of P waves and irregularly irregular rhythm)

Holter monitoring

- 24–72h ECG for people with suspected paroxysmal AF undetected by standard ECG recordings

Bloods

- FBC, U&Es, TFTs, magnesium, LFTs and coagulation screen

CXR

- May indicate cardiac structural causes of AF, such as mitral valve disease, or heart failure

ECHO

- For whom a rhythm-control strategy that includes cardioversion is being considered, in whom there is a high risk or a suspicion of underlying structural/functional heart disease

CT or MRI brain

- Should be performed if there is any suggestion of stroke or TIA

Valvular heart disease

Aortic stenosis

Causes

- Degenerative calcification (most common cause in patients >65 years)
- Congenital bicuspid valve (most common cause in patients <65 years)
- Post-rheumatic disease
- Williams syndrome (supravalvular aortic stenosis)
- Hypertrophic obstructive cardiomyopathy (HOCM): subvalvular

Clinical features

Symptoms

- Syncope
- Dyspnoea
- Angina

Signs

- Narrow pulse pressure
- Slow rising pulse
- Thrill
- Ejection systolic murmur radiating to carotids
- Soft/absent S2
- S4

Investigations

- **ECG** May show evidence of left ventricular hypertrophy (see *Fig. 1*) or left ventricular strain
- **CXR** May show post-stenotic dilatation of ascending aorta (see *Fig. 2*) and calcification of valve
- **ECHO** Gold standard for diagnosis
- **Multi-slice CT (MSCT)** and **cardiac MRI** May be useful in providing additional information to above prior to surgery
- **Cardiac catheterisation** To measure pressures across the valve to assess the severity of disease and the need for intervention
- **Coronary angiography** May be indicated as part of the assessment of coronary artery disease

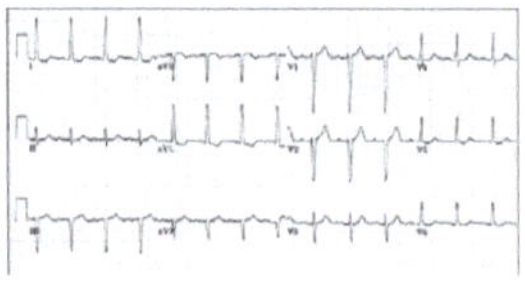

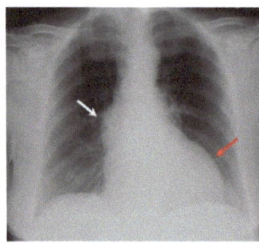

Fig. 1 Left ventricular hypertrophy on ECG

Fig. 2 Post-stenotic dilatation of ascending aorta

Management

- If asymptomatic and the patient has mild to moderate aortic stenosis then the patient should be observed as a general rule
- If symptomatic then patients should have valve replacement; if asymptomatic but severe with valvular gradient >40mmHg and with features such as left ventricular systolic dysfunction then surgery should be considered
- Balloon valvuloplasty is limited to patients with critical aortic stenosis who are not fit for valve replacement
- TAVI (transcatheter aortic valve implantation) is a relatively new procedure which is less invasive, making it a consideration in patients who are unsuitable for surgical aortic valve replacement

Complications

- Heart failure
- Infective endocarditis
- Systemic emboli
- Sudden death

Aortic regurgitation (AR)

Causes

Due to aortic root disease

- Aortic dissection
- Hypertension
- Spondyloarthropathies e.g. ankylosing spondylitis
- Syphilis
- Marfan syndrome, Ehlers–Danlos syndrome

Due to valve disease

- Rheumatic fever
- Infective endocarditis
- Connective tissue diseases e.g. RA/SLE
- Bicuspid aortic valve

Clinical features

Symptoms:

- Dyspnoea
- Angina
- Heart failure

Signs:

- Waterhammer/collapsing pulse
- Wide pulse pressure
- Early diastolic murmur
- Mid-diastolic Austin Flint murmur (in severe AR)
- Traube's sign: 'pistol shot' heard over the femoral artery
- De Musset's sign: head nodding in time with each heart beat
- Quincke's sign: nail bed pulsation

Investigations

- **CXR** May show cardiomegaly, pulmonary oedema and dilatation of the ascending aorta
- **ECG** May show evidence of left ventricular hypertrophy
- **ECHO** Confirms diagnosis and assesses severity
- **MSCT and cardiac MRI** May be required for further evaluation
- **Cardiac catheterisation** May be used to assess coronary anatomy before surgery

Management

- Patients with mild-to-moderate AR can be reviewed on a yearly basis and echocardiography performed every 2 years
- Treat heart failure with diuretics, ACE inhibitors/ARBs and beta blockers
- Surgery is usually indicated in symptomatic patients or asymptomatic patients when left ventricular function begins to deteriorate
- Valve replacement remains the most widely used technique
- Valve-sparing aortic root replacement is increasingly employed in expert centres, particularly in young patients

Complications

- Heart failure
- Arrhythmia
- Infective endocarditis

Mitral stenosis

Causes

- Rheumatic heart disease
- Calcification of valve
- Rheumatoid arthritis
- Ankylosing spondylitis
- SLE
- Malignant carcinoid

Clinical features

Symptoms

- Dyspnoea
- Palpitations (if in AF)
- Heart failure
- Haemoptysis

Signs

- Malar flush
- Tapping apex beat
- Hoarse voice (Ortner syndrome)
- Irregularly irregular pulse
- Loud S1, opening snap
- Mid–late diastolic murmur (best heard in expiration)

Investigations

- **ECG** May show AF or P mitrale (bifid P waves) (see *Fig. 3*)
- **CXR** May show pulmonary oedema and enlarged left atrium
- **ECHO** Confirms diagnosis and assesses severity

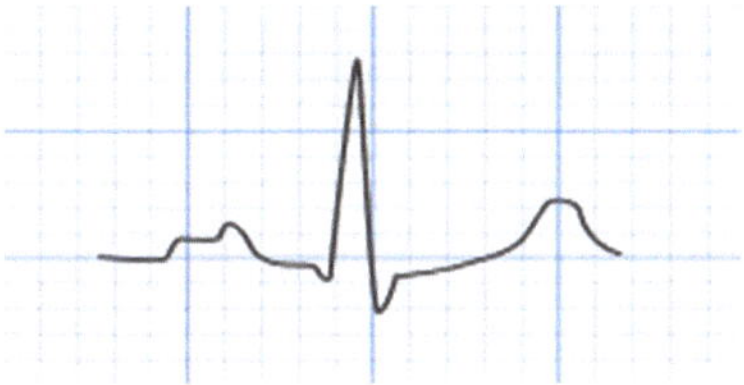

Fig. 3 ECG showing P mitrale

Treatment

- Asymptomatic patients can be managed conservatively by following the patient clinically and with serial ECHO
- Diuretics or long-acting nitrates can be used to alleviate dyspnoea; beta blockers or heart rate regulating calcium-channel blockers, e.g. verapamil, can improve exercise tolerance
- Anticoagulant therapy is indicated in patients with either permanent or paroxysmal AF
- Percutaneous mitral commissurotomy (PMC) should be considered for symptomatic patients with severe mitral stenosis or those with pulmonary hypertension
- Surgical valve replacement should be considered for patients who are not candidates for percutaneous intervention

Complications

- AF
- Heart failure
- Infective endocarditis

Mitral regurgitation (MR)

Causes

- Rheumatic heart disease
- Papillary muscle rupture or rupture of chordae tendineae
- Infective endocarditis
- Mitral valve prolapse (common condition occurring mainly in young women)
- Hypertrophic cardiomyopathy
- Ehlers–Danlos syndrome

Clinical features

Symptoms

- Dyspnoea
- Palpitations (if AF present)
- Heart failure symptoms

Signs

- Irregularly irregular pulse (if AF present)
- Displaced apex beat
- Harsh pansystolic murmur radiating to the axilla
- Soft S1, split S2

Investigations

- **ECG** AF, P mitrale (bifid P waves)
- **CXR** May see cardiomegaly, and pulmonary oedema (if HF present)
- **ECHO** Confirms diagnosis and assesses severity

Management

- In acute cases, medical management with nitrates, diuretics, positive inotropes and an intra-aortic balloon pump can be used to increase cardiac output
- If patients are in heart failure ACE inhibitors, beta blockers and spironolactone should be considered
- The evidence for repair over replacement is strong in degenerative regurgitation due to lower mortality and higher survival rates
- When this is not possible, valve replacement with either an artificial valve or a pig valve is considered
- In acute severe regurgitation, emergency valve replacement is necessary

Complications

- AF
- Heart failure
- Infective endocarditis
- Pulmonary hypertension

Heart failure (HF) is the inability of the heart to provide adequate circulation at normal filling pressures to meet the body's metabolic demands. It is caused by structural or functional abnormalities of the heart.

Definition

Classification

Systolic vs diastolic HF

- **Systolic HF or 'HF with impaired ejection fraction'** Inability of the ventricles to contract properly resulting in ↓cardiac output; ejection fraction <40%; causes include ischaemic heart disease and cardiomyopathy
- **Diastolic HF or 'HF with preserved ejection fraction'** Inability of the ventricles to relax therefore fill adequately; ejection fraction >40%; causes include cardiac tamponade, constrictive pericarditis and restrictive cardiomyopathy

Left HF vs right HF

- Left ventricular failure or right ventricular failure may occur independently or together as congestive cardiac failure (CCF)

Acute HF vs chronic HF

- **Acute HF** Results from sudden failure to maintain cardiac output; there is insufficient time for compensatory mechanisms to develop
- **Chronic HF** Cardiac output declines gradually; symptoms related to compensatory mechanisms predominating

Low-output HF vs high-output HF

- **Low-output HF** Cardiac output is decreased and unable to meet the demands of the body
- **High-output HF** Rare; output is normal or increased in the face of increased needs e.g. Paget's disease, hyperthyroidism, anaemia

Prognosis

- Prognosis is poor on the whole, with approximately 50% of people with HF dying within 4 years of diagnosis
- The mortality rate in the UK appears to be improving and this is mainly down to pharmacological agents and designated HF multidisciplinary teams

Heart failure

Management

Acute heart failure

1. Sit patient up
2. High-flow oxygen
3. IV furosemide e.g. 40mg IV (further boluses or IV infusion may be given)
4. Diamorphine e.g. 2.5–5mg IV (if patient has chest pain or is distressed and is not confused or drowsy) with an anti-emetic
5. If BP stable (i.e. >100 systolic) consider GTN spray e.g. 2 puffs sublingual or an infusion
6. Consider catheterisation to monitor urine output carefully
7. Treat underlying causes e.g. MI or arrhythmias
8. Consider CPAP
9. If BP low (i.e. <100 systolic) consider ITU admission and inotropes, e.g. IV dobutamine for treatment of cardiogenic shock

Chronic heart failure

Conservative:

- **Stop any offending drugs** if possible, such as NSAIDs, some calcium channel blockers, e.g. verapamil
- **Smoking cessation**

- **Diet and fluid intake** Cachectic patients should be assessed by a dietitian; restrict dietary salt; patients with severe CCF should restrict their fluid intake; encourage weight monitoring
- **Alcohol** Restrict alcohol intake or advise abstention
- **Exercise** Aerobic exercise, preferably a supervised cardiac rehabilitation programme
- **Travel** NYHA class I and II are not restricted in plane travel; O_2 may be required for class III and is recommended (with in-flight medical assistance) for class IV
- **Sexual health** No specific restrictions for sexual activity but slight risk of decompensation with NYHA class III–IV patients; sexual dysfunction is common in HF patients due to the condition itself or from the side effects of treatment
- **Mental health and wellbeing** Depression is very common in HF; screen and manage accordingly
- **Immunisation** Annual influenza vaccination and single pneumococcal vaccination should be given

Pharmacological:

See notes on the next page Pharmacological agents for heart failure.

Drugs that reduce mortality:

- ACE inhibitors/angiotensin receptor blockers (ARBs)
- Beta blockers
- Spironolactone
- Hydralazine with nitrates

Drugs for symptomatic relief only:

- Loop or thiazide diuretics
- Digoxin
- Ivabradine

Surgical:

- **Revascularisation** Coronary artery disease is the most common cause of HF and if this is the cause, revascularisation with angioplasty and stenting or coronary artery bypass surgery (CABG) can result in improvement
- **Cardiac resynchronisation therapy** Also known as biventricular pacing; it aims to improve the coordination of the atria and ventricles; it is indicated for patients with systolic HF who have moderate–severe symptoms and a widened QRS complex on ECG
- **Implantable cardioverter-defibrillator (ICD)** For patients at high risk of lethal arrhythmias such as ventricular tachycardia
- **Cardiac transplantation** The treatment of choice for younger patients with intractable HF
- **Left ventricular assist device and artificial heart** For severe HF not controlled with above measures; it is occasionally given to people on the waiting list for a heart transplant

Causes

- **Myocardial disease:** coronary artery disease (most common), hypertension, cardiomyopathies
- **Valvular heart disease:** e.g. aortic stenosis
- **Arrhythmias:** e.g. AF and other arrhythmias
- **Pericardial disease:** pericardial effusion, constrictive pericarditis and cardiac tamponade
- **Congenital heart disease:** e.g. atrial septal defect (ASD) and ventricular septal defect (VSD)
- **High-output states:** anaemia, thyrotoxicosis, liver failure, Paget's disease, beriberi
- **Drugs:** alcohol, steroids, chemotherapy, NSAIDs
- **Severe lung disease:** e.g. COPD, obstructive sleep apnoea, pulmonary embolism

Pathophysiology

- HF results from injury to the myocardium from a variety of causes (see *Causes*)
- As the heart fails, there are several compensatory mechanisms that occur as the failing heart attempts to maintain adequate function
- These include increasing cardiac output via the Frank–Starling mechanism, increasing ventricular volume and eventually increased wall thickness through ventricular remodelling, and maintaining tissue perfusion with increased mean arterial pressure through activation of sympathetic nervous system (SNS) and the renin–angiotensin–aldosterone system (RAAS)
- Although initially beneficial in the early stages of HF, all of these compensatory mechanisms eventually lead to a vicious cycle of worsening HF (see *Fig. 1*).

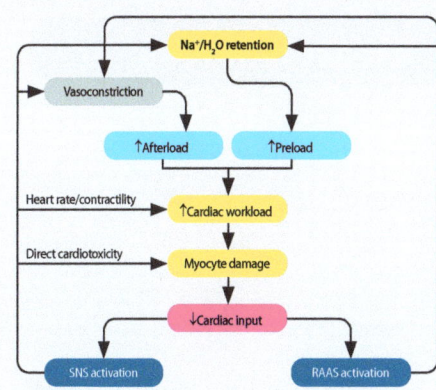

Fig. 1 Pathophysiology of heart failure outlined

Clinical features

Symptoms

- Dyspnoea
- Fatigue
- Oedema
- Nocturnal cough ± pink frothy sputum or wheeze
- Orthopnoea
- Paroxysmal nocturnal dyspnoea (PND)
- Nocturia, cold peripheries, weight loss and muscle wasting

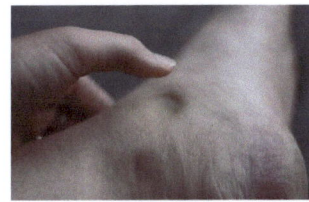

Fig. 2 Pitting oedema of the lower limbs

Signs

Left heart failure

- Displaced apex beat
- Gallop rhythm (3rd heart sound)
- Inspiratory crackles/wheeze
- Pitting oedema (see *Fig. 2*)

Right heart failure

- Raised jugular venous pressure (JVP) (see *Fig. 3*)
- Hepatic enlargement
- Ascites
- Pitting oedema

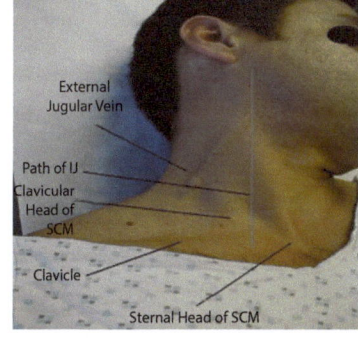

Fig. 3 Jugular venous distension; SCM, sternocleidomastoid muscle; IJ, internal jugular

Staging severity

The New York Heart Association (NYHA) Classification of HF is used to stage HF according to symptoms:

- **Class I** No limitations; ordinary physical activity does not cause symptoms
- **Class II** Symptomatically 'mild'; slight limitation of physical activity but comfortable at rest
- **Class III** Symptomatically 'moderate'; marked limitation of physical activity
- **Class IV** Symptomatically 'severe'; symptoms of HF are present even at rest

Investigations

- **Bloods** FBC, U&Es, LFTs, TFTs, lipid profile, BNP (B-type natriuretic peptide) or N-terminal pro-BNP (NT-proBNP)
- **Urinalysis** Nephrotic syndrome may present with fluid overload
- **CXR** (**ABCD**) **A**lveolar oedema, Kerley **B** lines, **C**ardiomegaly, **D**ilated upper lobe vessels, pleural **E**ffusion (see *Fig. 4*)
- **ECG** May indicate cause e.g. MI, AF or show LVH
- **ECHO** May indicate the cause (MI, valvular heart disease) and confirm the presence or absence of systolic or diastolic function and assess severity
- **Lung function tests** To rule out respiratory disease
- **Cardiac MRI** The gold standard for assessing ventricular volumes, mass and wall motion; can also be used to identify inflammation, infiltration and scarring of the myocardium

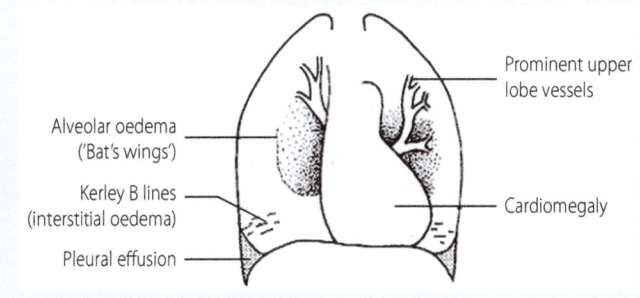

Fig. 4 Signs of heart failure seen on CXR

Heart failure notes

Natriuretic peptides

- B-type natriuretic peptide (BNP) is released into the blood when the ventricular myocardium is stressed
- The physiological action of BNP is to reduce systemic vascular resistance and central venous pressure as well as an increase in natriuresis
- The net effect is a decrease in blood pressure and a decrease in preload and afterload of the heart
- The N-terminal prohormone of brain natriuretic peptide (NT-proBNP) is a prohormone with an N-terminal inactive protein that is cleaved from the molecule to release BNP
- Raised levels of BNP and NT-proBNP are suggestive of heart failure (see *Table 1*) and very high levels are associated with a poor prognosis
- BNP may also be lowered and raised by other factors and it is important to take these into account when interpreting the result (see *Table 2*)

Table 1 Cut off-values for BNP and NT-proBNP

	BNP	NT-proBNP
High level	>400pg/ml	>2000pg/ml
Raised level	100–400pg/ml	400–2000pg/ml
Normal level	<100pg/ml	<400pg/ml

Table 2 Factors that increase and decrease BNP/NT-proBNP

Increase BNP levels	Decrease BNP levels
Left ventricular hypertrophy	Obesity
Ischaemia	Diuretics
Tachycardia	ACE inhibitors
Right ventricular overload	Beta blockers
Hypoxaemia (including PE)	Angiotensin 2 receptor blockers
GFR <60ml/min	Aldosterone antagonists
Sepsis	
COPD	
Diabetes	
Age >70 years	
Liver cirrhosis	

Management of chronic heart failure: a stepwise approach

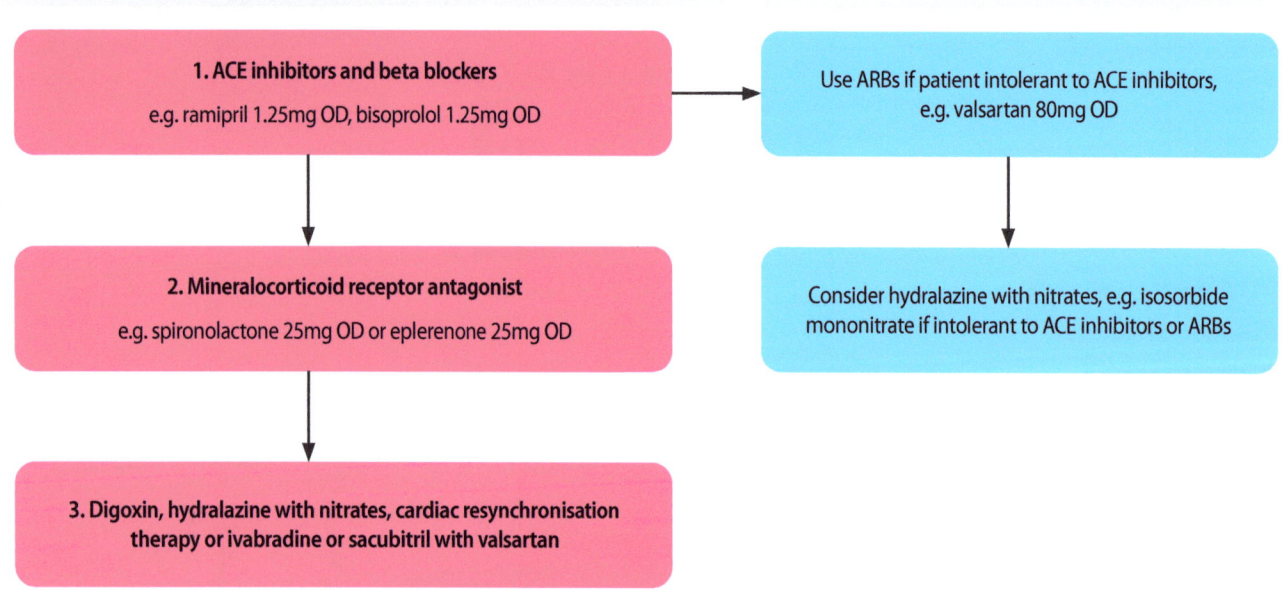

1. ACE inhibitors and beta blockers
e.g. ramipril 1.25mg OD, bisoprolol 1.25mg OD

Use ARBs if patient intolerant to ACE inhibitors, e.g. valsartan 80mg OD

2. Mineralocorticoid receptor antagonist
e.g. spironolactone 25mg OD or eplerenone 25mg OD

Consider hydralazine with nitrates, e.g. isosorbide mononitrate if intolerant to ACE inhibitors or ARBs

3. Digoxin, hydralazine with nitrates, cardiac resynchronisation therapy or ivabradine or sacubitril with valsartan

ACE inhibitors
- Examples include ramipril, lisinopril and enalapril
- All patients with left ventricular ejection fraction (LVEF) ≤40%, regardless of symptom severity, should receive an ACE inhibitor unless contraindicated or not tolerated
- ACE inhibitors improve ventricular function and patient wellbeing and reduce mortality
- Start at low dose and titrate upwards at short intervals (e.g. every 2 weeks) until target or maximum tolerated dose is reached
- Common side effects include a dry cough (around 15% of patients and may occur up to a year after starting treatment), angioedema, hyperkalaemia and hypotension

Angiotensin receptor blockers (ARBs)
- Candesartan and valsartan are examples of ARBs that are licensed for HF
- Indicated for patients who cannot tolerate an ACE inhibitor because of side effects; they do not cause the chronic cough side effect associated with ACE inhibitors

Beta blockers
- Examples of beta blockers licensed for heart failure include bisoprolol, nebivolol and carvedilol
- Beta blockers should be used in all patients with symptomatic HF and LVEF ≤40%, where tolerated and not contraindicated
- Common side effects include: bronchospasm, fatigue, cold peripheries and sleep disturbances
- Asthma, 2nd- or 3rd-degree heart block, sick sinus syndrome (without a pacemaker) and sinus bradycardia (<50bpm) are contraindications to beta-blocker use

Mineralocorticoid (aldosterone) receptor antagonists
- Include spironolactone and eplerenone
- Relatively weak diuretics with a K^+-sparing action
- Spironolactone e.g. 25mg reduces mortality in patients with HF with impaired ejection fraction
- Epleronone reduces mortality in patients with acute MI and HF
- Gynaecomastia is a common side effect
- Main contraindication is hyperkalaemia

Vasodilators
- Nitrates e.g. isosorbide mononitrate (reduces preload) in combination with hydralazine (reduces afterload) improve symptoms and survival in patients with systolic HF
- Should be considered in patients who are intolerant to ACE inhibitors or ARBs

Digoxin
- Considered as an add-on treatment in patients who remain symptomatic despite above treatments
- Useful in patients who have a combination of AF and HF

Ivabradine
- Should be considered in patients that remain symptomatic despite already on suitable therapy (ACE inhibitor, beta blocker + aldosterone antagonist), and have a heart rate >75/min and a left ventricular fraction <35%

Sacubitril / valsartan (*Entresto*®)
- Contains sacubitril and valsartan (ARB)
- Sacubitril (a prodrug) inhibits the breakdown of natriuretic peptides resulting in varied effects including increased diuresis, natriuresis and vasodilatation
- Indications include symptomatic chronic HF with ejection fraction <35% and patients not currently taking an ACE inhibitor or ARB, or stabilised on low doses of either of these agents

Diuretics
- Includes loop diuretics e.g. furosemide 40mg (oral, IV bolus or infusion) and bumetanide 1mg (oral)
- Thiazide diuretics e.g. bendroflumethiazide or indapamide are mild diuretics; the exception is metolazone which causes profound diuresis and is only used for severe and resistant cases by specialists
- Spironolactone and eplerenone are relatively weak diuretics with K^+-sparing action

Hypertrophic obstructive cardiomyopathy (HOCM) is an **autosomal dominant** disorder of muscle tissue leading to left ventricular hypertrophy. It is the most common genetic heart disease and the main cause of sudden cardiac death in the young.

- The most common defects involve a mutation in the gene encoding beta-myosin heavy chain protein or myosin-binding protein C
- It is characterised by myofibrillar hypertrophy with chaotic and disorganised myocytes ('disarray') and fibrosis on biopsy
- This results in:
  - Left ventricular hypertrophy (LVH) → decreased compliance → impairs diastolic filling → decreased cardiac output
- Sudden death is most commonly due to ventricular arrhythmias

- Often asymptomatic (and detected through family screening)
- Exertional dyspnoea
- Angina
- Syncope (typically following exercise)
- Sudden death, arrhythmias, heart failure
- Jerky pulse, large 'a' waves, double apex beat
- Ejection systolic murmur: increases with Valsalva manoeuvre and decreases on squatting
- Pansystolic murmur if mitral regurgitation is present (hypertrophic cardiomyopathy may impair mitral valve closure)

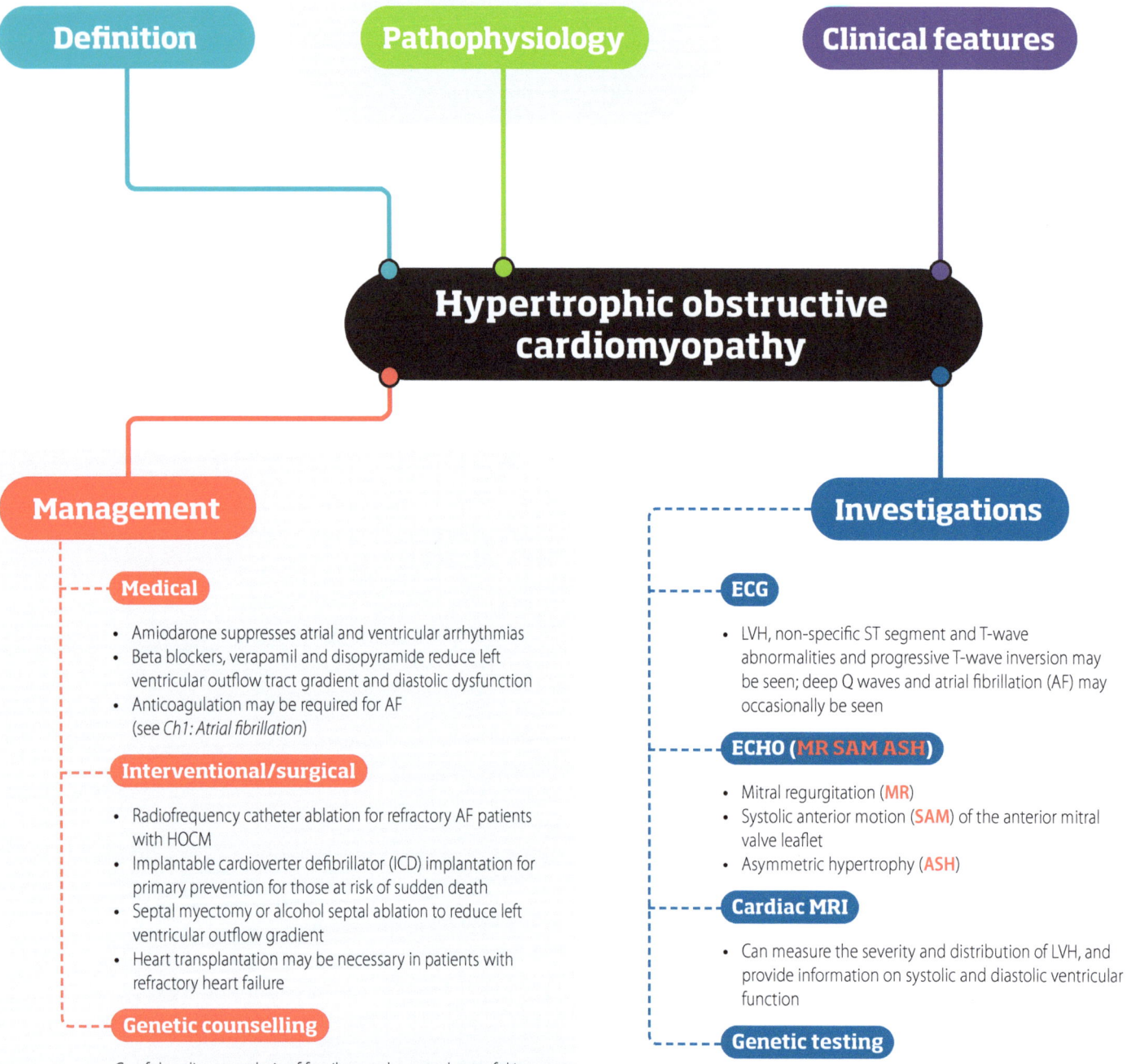

Definition

Pathophysiology

Clinical features

Hypertrophic obstructive cardiomyopathy

Management

Medical

- Amiodarone suppresses atrial and ventricular arrhythmias
- Beta blockers, verapamil and disopyramide reduce left ventricular outflow tract gradient and diastolic dysfunction
- Anticoagulation may be required for AF (see *Ch1: Atrial fibrillation*)

Interventional/surgical

- Radiofrequency catheter ablation for refractory AF patients with HOCM
- Implantable cardioverter defibrillator (ICD) implantation for primary prevention for those at risk of sudden death
- Septal myectomy or alcohol septal ablation to reduce left ventricular outflow gradient
- Heart transplantation may be necessary in patients with refractory heart failure

Genetic counselling

Careful pedigree analysis of family members can be useful in identifying those at risk of inheriting the disease; 1st-degree relatives of patients with HOCM should be regularly screened with ECG and echocardiography

Investigations

ECG

- LVH, non-specific ST segment and T-wave abnormalities and progressive T-wave inversion may be seen; deep Q waves and atrial fibrillation (AF) may occasionally be seen

ECHO (MR SAM ASH)

- Mitral regurgitation (MR)
- Systolic anterior motion (SAM) of the anterior mitral valve leaflet
- Asymmetric hypertrophy (ASH)

Cardiac MRI

- Can measure the severity and distribution of LVH, and provide information on systolic and diastolic ventricular function

Genetic testing

- Genetic mutations can be identified in approximately 60% of patients.

Dilated cardiomyopathy

Dilated cardiomyopathy (DCM) is the most common form of cardiomyopathy (accounting for 90% of cases). It is characterised by a dilated left ventricle which contracts poorly.

Causes

- Idiopathic: the most common cause
- Myocarditis: e.g. Coxsackie B, HIV, diphtheria, Chagas' disease
- Ischaemic heart disease
- Peripartum
- Hypertension
- Drugs: iatrogenic (e.g. doxorubicin), substance misuse (e.g. alcohol and cocaine)
- Inherited: the majority of defects are inherited in an autosomal dominant fashion although other patterns of inheritance are seen
- Infiltrative: e.g. haemochromatosis, sarcoidosis
- Nutritional: e.g. wet beriberi (thiamine deficiency)

Clinical features

- Classic findings of heart failure
- Systolic murmur: from mitral and tricuspid regurgitation
- S3

Investigations

- CXR: cardiomegaly, pulmonary oedema
- BNP: may be raised (especially in heart failure) and useful for prognosis
- ECG: may show sinus tachycardia, an intraventricular conduction delay, LBBB or non-specific changes in ST and T waves
- ECHO: marked dilatation of the left ventricular cavity and reduced systolic and diastolic function; may also show mitral regurgitation, tricuspid regurgitation and mural thrombus
- Cardiac MRI: dilated ventricles with global hypokinesis
- Endomyocardial biopsies may diagnose infiltrative disease

Management

- Heart failure and AF treated in conventional way (see *Ch1: Atrial fibrillation* and *Heart failure*)
- Biventricular pacing (using a cardiac resynchronisation device) can improve symptoms in patients with class III and IV heart failure with marked QRS prolongation, improve survival and increase exercise tolerance
- ICD reduces risk of sudden death in high-risk patients
- Mitral annuloplasty or valve replacement can improve symptoms in patients with severe mitral regurgitation
- Heart transplantation or left ventricular assist devices may be required in severe cases

Restrictive cardiomyopathy

Definition

Restrictive cardiomyopathy is a condition characterised by normal left ventricular cavity size and systolic function but with increased myocardial stiffness.

Causes

- Idiopathic (most common)
- Endomyocardial fibrosis (associated with Löffler syndrome)
- Infiltrative myocardial disease e.g. iron in haemochromatosis, glycogen in Pompe and Cori disease, or glycolipids in Fabry disease
- Amyloid heart disease is the most common cause of restrictive cardiomyopathy in the West
- Sarcoidosis

Clinical features

- Features of right ventricular failure predominate
- Clinical features resemble those of constrictive pericarditis (see *Ch1: Acute pericarditis: constrictive pericarditis*)
- AF is common (see *Ch1: Atrial fibrillation*)

Investigations

- Initial investigations as for heart failure: ECG, CXR, blood tests (see *Ch1: Heart failure*)
- Echocardiography usually shows thickened ventricular walls, valves and atrial septum with small cavities
- Cardiac MRI is useful at distinguishing restrictive cardiomyopathy from constrictive pericarditis

Management

- Prognosis is poor and there is no specific treatment
- Heart failure and AF are treated in the usual way
- Amiodarone can reduce ventricular arrhythmias in high-risk patients
- ICD to prevent sudden death in high-risk patients
- Transplantation may be indicated for some patients

Arrhythmogenic right ventricular cardiomyopathy

Definition

Arrhythmogenic right ventricular cardiomyopathy (ARVC) is caused by fibro-fatty replacement of right ventricular (RV) myocytes due to apoptosis, inflammation (due to unknown cause) or a genetic cause.

Clinical presentation and diagnosis

- It usually presents with symptomatic arrhythmias e.g. ventricular tachycardia or sudden death
- Diagnosing ARVC is challenging due to non-specific disease features and phenotypic manifestations
- ECHO features include increased RV dimensions, RV regional wall motion abnormalities and dysfunction
- RV angiography has often been considered the gold standard for diagnosis, but cardiac MRI has better sensitivity and specificity
- ECG-V1–3 abnormalities (typically T wave inversion), epsilon wave may be present (described as terminal notch buried in the QRS complex)

Management

- In ARVC, severe RV dysfunction is treated with standard heart failure medications
- Cardiac transplantation is considered if treatment is refractory
- Beta blockers are used in asymptomatic patients and an ICD is recommended in high-risk patients

Hypertension (HTN) is persistently raised arterial blood pressure (BP). It is one of the most common conditions and one of several risk factors for diseases such as heart failure, myocardial infarction, stroke and chronic kidney disease.

- **Stage 1 HTN** Clinic BP ≥140/90mmHg, or ambulatory BP monitoring (ABPM) daytime average/home BP monitoring (HBPM) average ≥135/85mmHg
- **Stage 2 HTN** Clinic BP ≥160/100mmHg, or ABPM daytime average/HBPM average BP ≥150/95mmHg
- **Severe 3 HTN** Clinic systolic BP ≥180mmHg, or clinic diastolic BP ≥120mmHg

- **Hypertensive urgency** A clinical situation in which BP is very high (e.g. ≥180/≥120mmHg) with no signs or symptoms indicating acute organ damage
- **Hypertensive emergency** (or malignant HTN) Severe HTN with potentially life-threatening symptoms and signs indicative of acute impairment of one or more organ systems

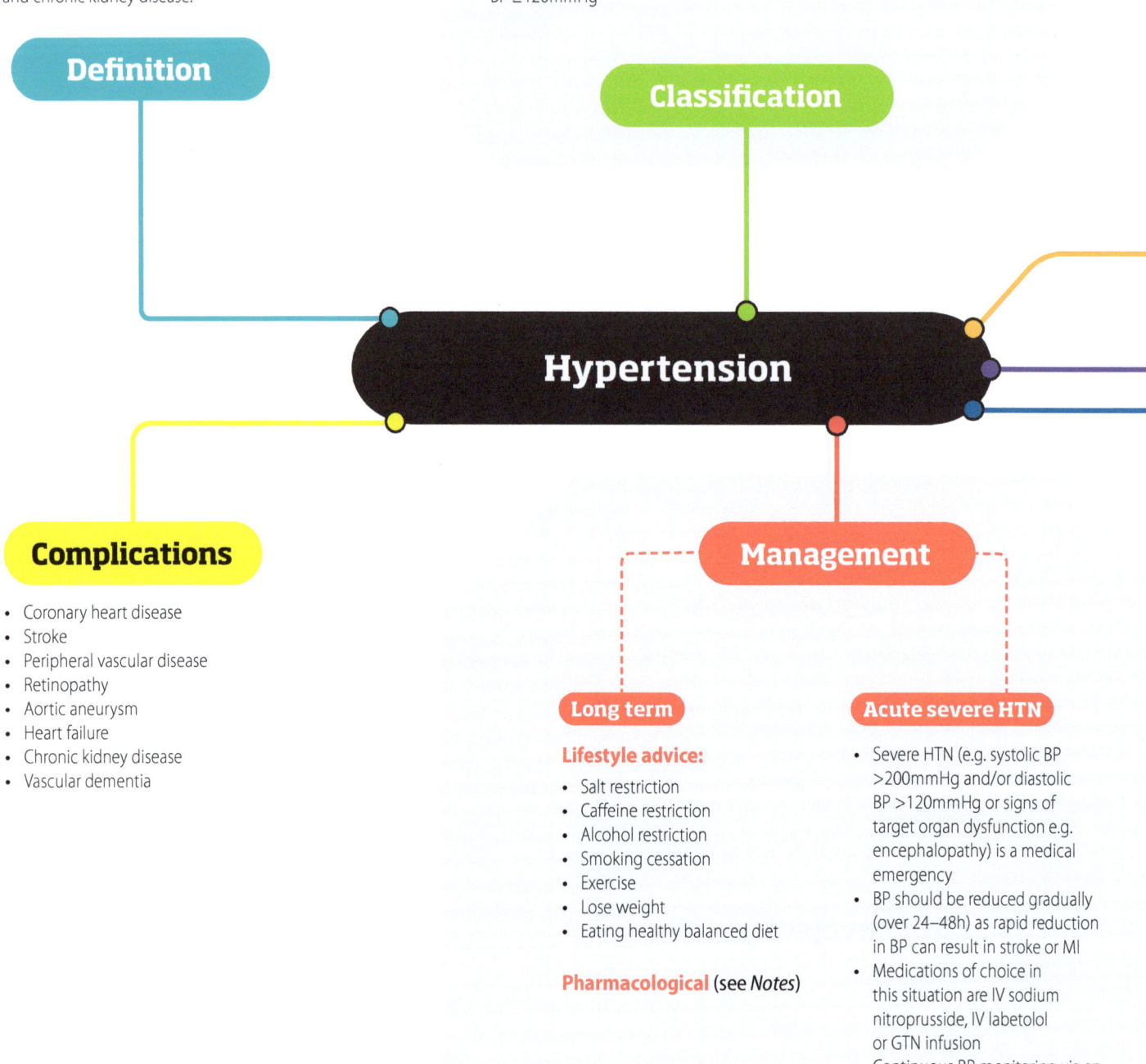

Definition

Classification

Hypertension

Complications

- Coronary heart disease
- Stroke
- Peripheral vascular disease
- Retinopathy
- Aortic aneurysm
- Heart failure
- Chronic kidney disease
- Vascular dementia

Management

Long term

Lifestyle advice:

- Salt restriction
- Caffeine restriction
- Alcohol restriction
- Smoking cessation
- Exercise
- Lose weight
- Eating healthy balanced diet

Pharmacological (see *Notes*)

Acute severe HTN

- Severe HTN (e.g. systolic BP >200mmHg and/or diastolic BP >120mmHg or signs of target organ dysfunction e.g. encephalopathy) is a medical emergency
- BP should be reduced gradually (over 24–48h) as rapid reduction in BP can result in stroke or MI
- Medications of choice in this situation are IV sodium nitroprusside, IV labetolol or GTN infusion
- Continuous BP monitoring via an arterial line and admission to high dependency unit (HDU) or ITU may be required

Aetiology

Primary (essential) HTN

- No direct underlying cause (accounts for about 95% of cases)
- Linked to genetics, low birthweight, obesity, excessive alcohol, excessive salt and metabolic syndrome

Secondary HTN

This is secondary to a specific underlying cause:
- **Vascular** Coarctation of the aorta, renal artery stenosis
- **Renal** Chronic pyelonephritis, diabetic nephropathy, glomerulonephritis, polycystic kidney disease, renal cell carcinoma
- **Endocrine** Primary hyperaldosteronism, phaeochromocytoma, Cushing syndrome, Liddle syndrome, congenital adrenal hyperplasia, acromegaly, thyroid disease
- **Drugs** COCP, NSAIDs, corticosteroids
- **Pregnancy** Either as gestational HTN or pre-eclampsia

Clinical features

Symptoms

- Usually asymptomatic
- Headaches
- Visual disturbance
- Dizziness
- Seizures

Signs

Signs of underlying disease:

- Risk factors e.g. obesity
- Signs of Cushing syndrome
- Radiofemoral delay or weak femoral pulses (coarctation of aorta)
- Renal bruits (renovascular disease)
- Palpable kidney

Signs of end-organ damage:

- Signs of retinopathy: grade 1 (silver or copper wiring), grade 2 (A-V nipping), grade 3 (flame haemorrhages and cotton wool spots), grade 4 (papilloedema)
- Signs of heart failure
- Signs of renal failure e.g. proteinuria

Investigations

Confirming hypertension

To avoid 'white coat' hypertension, patients with stage 1 HTN should have one of the following to confirm hypertension:
- **24-h ambulatory BP** At least two measurements per hour during the person's usual waking hours (for example, between 08:00 and 22:00); the average value of at least 14 measurements should be used
- **Home readings** For each BP recording, two consecutive measurements need to be taken, at least 1 min apart (with person seated); BP should be recorded twice daily, ideally in the morning and evening; BP should be recorded for at least 4 days (ideally 7 days); the first day recording should be discarded and the average should be taken of all the other values

Checking for end-organ damage

- Examination of the fundi for the presence of hypertensive retinopathy
- Urine dipstick/microscopy to detect proteinuria and haematuria
- Urine albumin: creatinine ratio (ACR) to detect microalbuminuria
- Serum U&Es to check for renal disease
- 12-lead ECG to look for left ventricular hypertrophy or signs of ischaemic heart disease
- ECHO to look for left ventricular hypertrophy/signs of heart failure

Looking for secondary causes

For young patients (<40) with HTN or secondary causes suspected:

- Thyroid function tests (exclude thyroid disease)
- 24-h urinary metanephrines (exclude phaeochromocytoma)
- Urinary free cortisol (exclude Cushing syndrome)
- Renin/aldosterone level (exclude primary hyperaldosteronism)
- U&Es ($\downarrow K^+$ in primary hyperaldosteronism; impaired creatinine/eGFR in renal disease)
- Plasma calcium (exclude hyperparathyroidism)
- Renal ultrasound (exclude renal disease e.g. polycystic kidneys)
- MRI renal arteries (exclude renal artery stenosis)

Assess cardiac risk profile

- Fasting blood glucose/HbA1c
- Fasting lipid profile

Hypertension notes

Diagnosis of hypertension

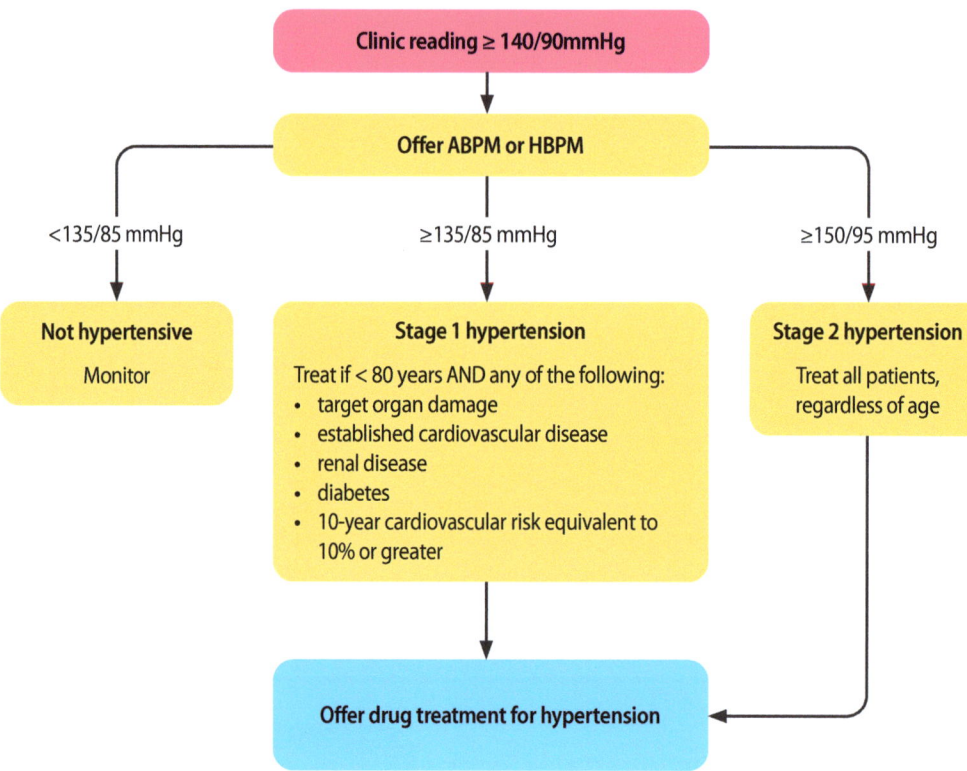

Clinic reading ≥ 140/90mmHg

Offer ABPM or HBPM

<135/85 mmHg → Not hypertensive — Monitor

≥135/85 mmHg → **Stage 1 hypertension**
Treat if < 80 years AND any of the following:
- target organ damage
- established cardiovascular disease
- renal disease
- diabetes
- 10-year cardiovascular risk equivalent to 10% or greater

≥150/95 mmHg → **Stage 2 hypertension**
Treat all patients, regardless of age

Offer drug treatment for hypertension

Pharmacological step-wise approach

- **BP targets**
Reduce and maintain BP to the following targets:
- **Age <80y:**
  - Clinic BP <140/90mmHg
  - ABPM/HBPM <135/85mmHg
- **Age ≥80y:**
  - Clinic BP <150/90mmHg
  - ABPM/HBPM <145/85mmHg
- **Postural hypertension:**
  - Base target on standing BP
- **Frailty or multimorbidity:**
  - Use clinical judgement

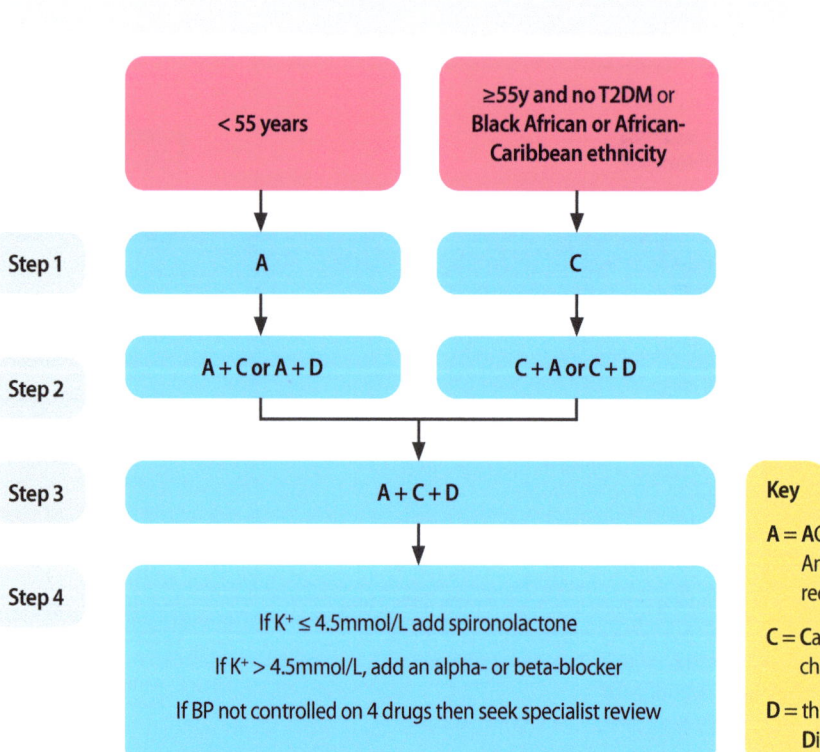

	< 55 years	≥55y and no T2DM or Black African or African-Caribbean ethnicity
Step 1	A	C
Step 2	A + C or A + D	C + A or C + D
Step 3	A + C + D	
Step 4	If K⁺ ≤ 4.5mmol/L add spironolactone If K⁺ > 4.5mmol/L, add an alpha- or beta-blocker If BP not controlled on 4 drugs then seek specialist review	

Key

A = **A**CE inhibitor or Angiotensin 2 receptor blocker

C = **C**alcium channel blocker

D = thiazide-like **D**iuretic

ACE inhibitors

- Include ramipril, lisinopril, perindopril
- Inhibit the conversion angiotensin I to angiotensin II and therefore the activation of the RAAS system
- 1st-line treatment in younger patients (<55 years) and diabetic patients with hypertension
- Side effects include dry cough, angioedema and hyperkalaemia
- Renal function must be checked 2–3 weeks after starting due to the risk of worsening renal function in patients with renovascular disease (acceptable changes are an increase in serum creatinine up to 30% from baseline and an increase in K^+ up to 5.5mmol/L)

Angiotensin receptor blockers (ARBs)

- Include losartan, candesartan, valsartan
- Block effects of angiotensin II at the AT1 receptor and therefore the activation of the RAAS system
- Angiotensin II receptor blockers are generally used in situations where patients have not tolerated an ACE inhibitor, usually due to the development of a cough
- Side effects similar to ACE inhibitors (minus cough)
- Like ACE inhibitors, renal function must be checked 2–3 weeks after starting due to the risk of worsening renal function in patients with renovascular disease

Calcium channel blockers

- Include amlodipine (most commonly used), nifedipine
- Block voltage-gated Ca^{2+} channels relaxing vascular smooth muscle and the force of myocardial contraction
- 1st-line treatment in older patients (≥55 years)
- Common side effects include headache, flushing and ankle swelling

Thiazide diuretics

- Include indapamide (thiazide of choice), chlorthalidone, bendroflumethiazide (no longer favoured by NICE)
- Thiazides inhibit reabsorption of Na^+ and Cl^- from the distal convoluted tubules in the kidneys, by blocking the NaCl symporter
- A step 3 treatment for patients who are already on ACE inhibitors/ARBs and Ca^{2+} channel blockers
- Common side effects include hyponatraemia, hypokalaemia and dehydration

Spironolactone

- An aldosterone antagonist, relatively weak diuretic with K^+-sparing action
- Used as step 4 treatment in patients with K^+ <4.5mmol/L
- Main side effects are hyperkalaemia and gynaecomastia

Beta blockers

- Include bisoprolol, carvedilol, atenolol, propranolol
- Competitive antagonists that block the receptor sites for adrenaline and noradrenaline on adrenergic beta receptors
- Used as step 4 treatment where patients are intolerant or contraindicated to using diuretics

Alpha blockers

- Include doxazosin (alpha-1 selective alpha blocker), methyldopa (alpha-2 adrenergic receptor agonist), moxonidine (alpha-2/imidazoline receptor agonist)
- Alpha-1 adrenergic receptor blockers inhibit the binding of noradrenaline to the alpha-1 receptors on vascular smooth muscle cells, resulting in vasodilatation, which decreases peripheral vascular resistance, leading to decreased BP
- Used as add-on therapy if above measures have failed to control BP or are not tolerated/contraindicated

Direct renin inhibitors

- Include aliskiren
- Relatively newer drug which works by inhibiting renin and thus blocks the conversion of angiotensinogen to angiotensin I
- Can be used alone or in combination with other antihypertensives
- Initial trials suggest aliskiren reduces BP to a similar extent as ACE inhibitors or ARBs
- Main side effect is diarrhoea

Infective endocarditis (IE) is an infection of the endocardium of the heart usually involving the heart valves. It may occur as a fulminating or acute infection but more commonly runs an insidious course which is known as subacute endocarditis.

- IE typically develops on the valvular surfaces of the heart that have sustained endothelial damage secondary to turbulent blood flow
- A mass of fibrin, platelets and infectious organisms form vegetations along the edges of the valve (see *Fig. 1*)
- The valves most commonly affected by IE are (in decreasing order of frequency): 1 mitral valve, 2 aortic valve, 3 combined mitral and aortic valve, 4 tricuspid valve (more common in IV drug users), pulmonary valve (rare)

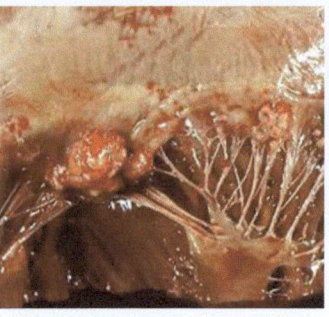

Fig. 1 Acute infective endocarditis causing vegetations along the mitral valve

Definition

Pathophysiology

Infective endocarditis

Complications

- MI, pericarditis, cardiac arrhythmias
- Heart valve insufficiency
- Congestive cardiac failure
- Sinus of Valsalva aneurysm
- Aortic root or myocardial abscess
- Arterial emboli, infarctions, mycotic aneurysms
- Arthritis, myositis
- Glomerulonephritis, acute kidney injury
- Stroke
- Mesenteric or splenic abscess or infarction

Management

- **Antibiotics** Give IV for first 2 weeks and orally for further 2–4 weeks; empirical antibiotic therapy should be given while awaiting blood cultures, usually a combination of IV benzylpenicillin and gentamicin (local hospital protocol should be followed and advice sought from a microbiologist); subsequent treatment depends on cultures and sensitivity
- **Surgery** Valve repair or valve replacement

Investigations

- **Bloods** FBC (↓Hb, ↑WCC), CRP/ESR (↑), U&Es (possible AKI), serum immunoglobulins (↑), complement levels (↓)
- **Blood cultures** 3 sets taken at different sites and different times
- **Urinalysis** Microscopic haematuria
- **ECG** 10% of patients will develop conduction defects
- **CXR** Possible heart failure or evidence of septic emboli in right-sided endocarditis
- **ECHO** Transthoracic ECHO should be performed within 24h; identifies vegetations and underlying valvular abnormalities
- **Serology** Useful if unusual organisms are suspected e.g. *Coxiella* spp., *Bartonella* spp. or *Legionella* spp.
- MRI, nuclear imaging and multi-slice CT coronary angiography are other imaging modalities which may be used

- *Staphylococcus aureus* (most common cause overall)
- Streptococci: most commonly viridans streptococci
- Coagulase-negative staphylococci (account for 30% of cases of IE in prosthetic valves)
- *Pseudomonas aeruginosa*
- HACEK organisms: *Haemophilus* spp., *Aggregatibacter* spp., *Cardiobacterium* spp., *Eikenella corrodens* and *Kingella* spp.
- Enterococci
- Fungi

Causative organisms

Symptoms

- Fever
- Rigors
- Night sweats
- Malaise
- Weight loss
- Loss of appetite
- Fatigue
- Flu-like illness
- Joint pain

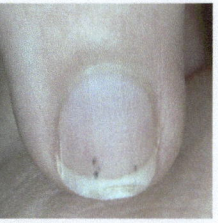

Fig. 2 Splinter haemorrhage

Signs

- Fever
- Heart murmurs
- Petechiae
- Splinter haemorrhages (see *Fig. 2*)
- Osler nodes
- Janeway lesions
- Clubbing (see *Fig. 3*)
- Arthritis
- Splenomegaly
- Meningism
- Roth spots (see *Fig. 4*)

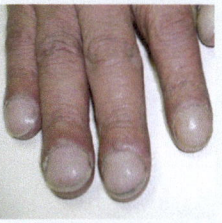

Fig. 3 Clubbing

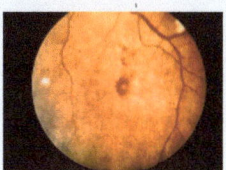

Fig. 4 Roth spot

Clinical features

Diagnostic criteria

Duke's criteria of IE (must meet 2 major criteria, or 1 major and 3 minor criteria, or 5 minor criteria):

Major criteria

- **Positive blood culture:**
  - Typical micro-organism for IE from 2 separate blood cultures *or*
  - Persistently positive blood cultures
- **Evidence of endocardial involvement:**
  - Oscillating intracardiac mass on valve/supporting structures *or*
  - Abscess *or*
  - New partial dehiscence of prosthetic valve or new valvular regurgitation

Minor criteria

- **Predisposing heart condition/IV drug use**
- **Fever** (>38℃)
- **Vascular phenomenon** Major arterial emboli, septic pulmonary infarcts, mycotic aneurysm, intracranial haemorrhage, conjunctival haemorrhage, Janeway lesions
- **Immunological phenomenon** Glomerulonephritis, Osler nodes, Roth spots, rheumatoid factor
- **Positive blood cultures** Not meeting major criteria
- **ECHO** Consistent with IE but not meeting major criterion

Risk factors

- Valvular heart disease with stenosis or regurgitation
- Valve replacement
- Structural congenital heart disease
- Previous IE
- Hypertrophic cardiomyopathy
- Recreational drug abuse
- Invasive vascular procedures

Chapter 2

Respiratory

Acute respiratory distress syndrome (ARDS) is an acute life-threatening, diffuse, inflammatory form of lung injury that is associated with a variety of causes (but often caused by infection). It is characterised by increased lung microvascular permeability, resulting in hypoxaemic respiratory failure.

- Acute inflammation or injury at the lung's alveolar-capillary membrane increases the permeability of the pulmonary microvasculature causing leakage of fluid across the membrane
- The resulting acute inflammatory exudate inactivates surfactant leading to collapse and consolidation of distal lung parenchyma with progressive loss of lung gas exchange surface area

- This loss also impairs compensatory pulmonary vasoconstriction in response to hypoxia
- The combination of these two processes causes profound hypoxaemia in association with high permeability pulmonary oedema
- The predominant cause of death in ARDS is multiple organ failure

Definition

Pathophysiology

Acute respiratory distress syndrome

Diagnostic criteria

Requires all 3 to exist:

- Acute onset: 20–50% of acute lung injury patients will develop ARDS within 7 days
- CXR shows bilateral infiltrates (*Fig. 1*)
- Refractory hypoxaemia: $P_aO_2{:}F_iO_2 < 200$

Management

Admit to ITU, give supportive therapy (*see below*) and treat the underlying cause

Respiratory support

- Prone positioning can improve oxygenation
- **CPAP** Can be used to treat early ARDS
- **Ventilation** Indications for ventilation include P_aO_2 <8.3 despite 60% F_iO_2 or a P_aCO_2 >6kPa

Circulatory support

- Invasive haemodynamic monitoring with an arterial line and Swan–Ganz catheter to monitor pulmonary capillary wedge pressure and cardiac output
- IV fluids
- Inotropes e.g. dobutamine
- Vasodilators e.g. low-dose nitric oxide

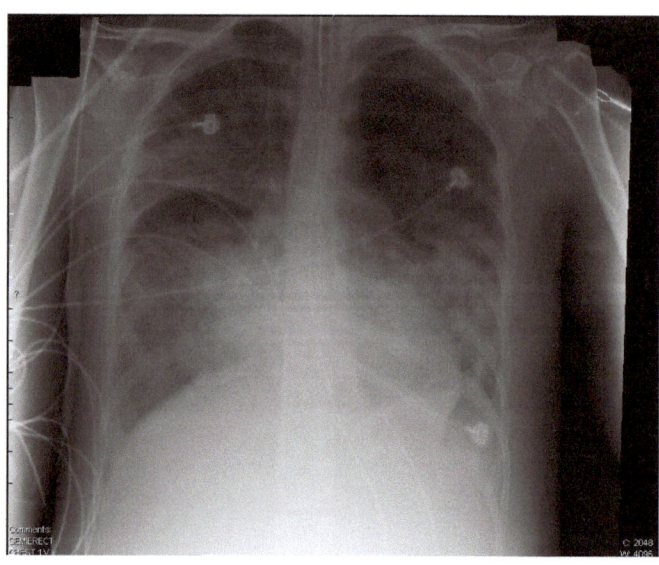

Fig. 1 ARDS on CXR

- Sepsis (most common)
- Trauma
- Hypovolaemic shock
- Pneumonia
- Gastric aspiration
- Fat or amniotic fluid embolism
- Acute pancreatitis
- Burns
- Smoke inhalation
- Cardiopulmonary bypass
- Diabetic ketoacidosis

- Cyanosis
- Tachypnoea
- Tachycardia
- Bilateral fine inspiratory crackles

- **Bloods** FBC, U&Es, LFTs, amylase, clotting, CRP, blood cultures
- **ABG** Type 1 respiratory failure
- **CXR** Bilateral alveolar shadowing, often with air bronchograms (see *Fig. 1*)

Risk factors

Clinical features

Investigations

Notes

Acute respiratory distress syndrome

Asthma is a chronic inflammatory condition of the airways characterised by hyper-responsiveness and constriction in response to a variety of stimuli. Narrowing of the airways is usually reversible (either spontaneously or with medication) leading to intermittent symptoms, but in some people with chronic asthma, the inflammation may lead to irreversible airflow obstruction.

- Atopic asthma is the result of airway inflammation caused by exposure to an environmental allergen
- Patients with asthma have an exuberant Th2-mediated Ig immune response
- IgE binds to bronchial mast cells resulting in degranulation and the release of pro-inflammatory mediators
- There are 2 phases of inflammation:
  - **Acute phase** Characterised by bronchoconstriction and airway oedema; this process begins within minutes of allergen exposure and resolves within hours
  - **Delayed phase** Pro-inflammatory mediators, such as IL-5, released by mast cells recruit eosinophils, basophils and Th2 lymphocytes, resulting in ongoing inflammation, sensitisation of sensory nerve endings, resulting in bronchial hyper-responsiveness

Definition

Pathophysiology

Asthma

Investigations

Acute asthma

- **Bloods** FBC: raised WCC and typically eosinophilia; U&Es: salbutamol can cause hypokalaemia; CRP: to rule out infection
- **ABG** Patients with S_pO_2 <92% or other features of life-threatening asthma require ABG measurement
- **CXR** To rule out pneumonia/ pneumothorax; typically normal or shows hyperinflation and flattened diaphragm (see *Fig. 2*)
- **Peak flow** Peak expiratory flow (PEF) expressed as a % of the patient's previous best value is most useful clinically; in the absence of this, PEF as a % of predicted is also useful
- **ECG** Often sinus tachycardia

Chronic asthma

Spirometry:

The bronchodilator reversibility (BDR) test is preferred over peak flow measurement for initial confirmation of obstruction of airways in the diagnosis of asthma. An FEV_1/FVC ratio <70% is considered obstructive. A positive bronchodilator reversibility test is indicated by an improvement in FEV_1 of 12% or more and increase in volume of 200ml or more.

Peak flow:

Measurement of peak expiratory flow rate (PEFR) via a peak flow meter (see *Fig. 1*) is the simplest and most basic test for diagnosing asthma; diurnal variation typically in the early morning is suggestive of asthma. However, PEFR is more useful in the monitoring of patients with established asthma.

FeNO:

The FeNO (fractional exhaled nitric oxide) test is a relatively new test which measures the level of NO in the exhaled breath and provides an indication of eosinophilic inflammation in the lungs; in adults a level of ≥40 parts per billion (ppb) is considered positive.

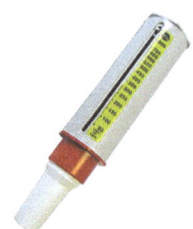

Fig. 1 Peak flow meter

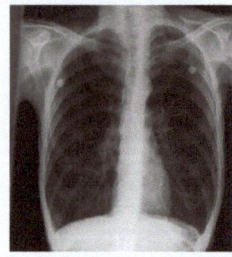

Fig. 2 CXR showing hyperinflation

Risk factors

- Personal history of atopy e.g. eczema and hay fever
- Family history of asthma or atopy
- Inner city environment, socio-economic deprivation
- Obesity
- Prematurity and low birth weight
- Viral infections in early childhood
- Smoking
- Maternal smoking
- Early exposure to broad-spectrum antibiotics

Triggers

- Respiratory infections
- Cold air
- Exercise
- Pollution e.g. cigarette smoke, fumes
- Allergens e.g. pollen, dust mite, animals
- Time of day
- Work-related (occupational)
- Drugs e.g. beta blockers and NSAIDs
- Emotional factors e.g. stress, laughter
- Gastro-oesophageal reflux disease

Clinical features

Symptoms

- Intermittent SOB
- Wheeze: polyphonic
- Cough: often nocturnal ± sputum

Signs

- ↓Chest expansion
- Bilateral polyphonic wheeze
- Tachypnoea
- Tachycardia
- Reduced air entry
- Hyperinflated chest

Complications

- Pneumonia
- Pneumothorax
- Pneumomediastinum
- Respiratory failure and arrest
- Pulmonary collapse

Notes

Asthma

Asthma notes

Grading severity of asthma attack

Moderate	Severe	Life-threatening	Near fatal
• PEFR 50–75% best or predicted • Speech normal • RR <25/min • Pulse <110bpm	• PEFR 33–50% best or predicted • Can't complete sentences • RR >25/min • Pulse >110bpm	• PEF <33% best or predicted • S_pO_2 <92% • P_aO_2 <8kPa • 'Normal' P_aCO_2 (4.6–6.0kPa) • Altered conscious level • Exhaustion • Arrhythmia • Hypotension • Cyanosis • Silent chest • Poor respiratory effort	• Raised P_aCO_2 and/or requiring mechanical ventilation with raised inflation pressures

Management of acute asthma

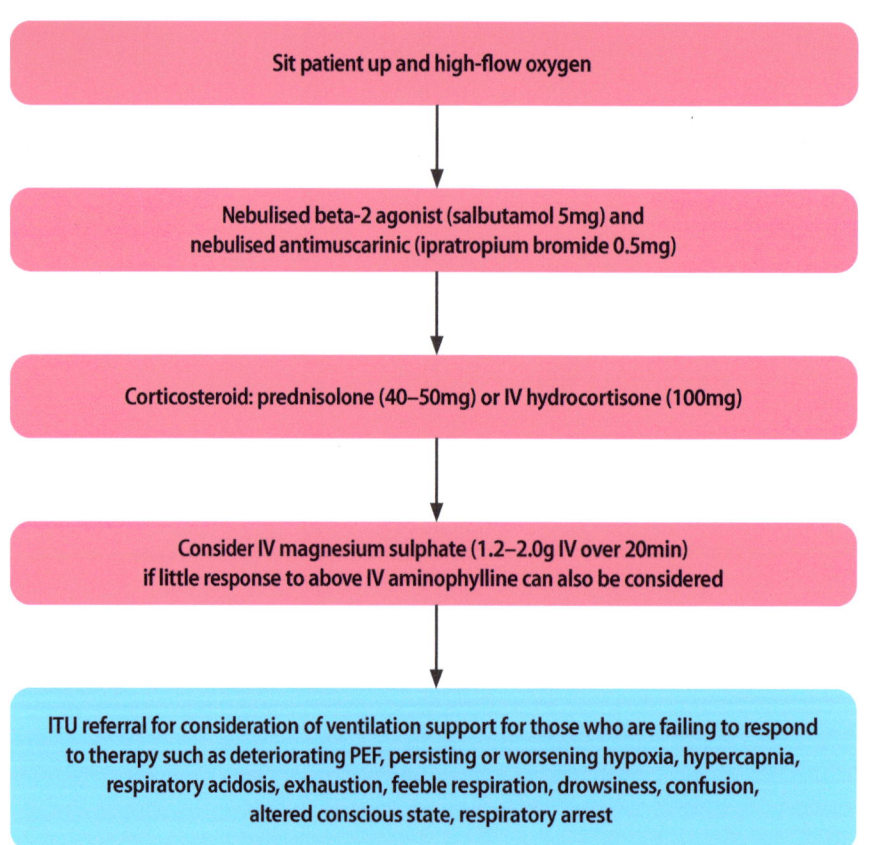

Sit patient up and high-flow oxygen

↓

Nebulised beta-2 agonist (salbutamol 5mg) and nebulised antimuscarinic (ipratropium bromide 0.5mg)

↓

Corticosteroid: prednisolone (40–50mg) or IV hydrocortisone (100mg)

↓

Consider IV magnesium sulphate (1.2–2.0g IV over 20min) if little response to above IV aminophylline can also be considered

↓

ITU referral for consideration of ventilation support for those who are failing to respond to therapy such as deteriorating PEF, persisting or worsening hypoxia, hypercapnia, respiratory acidosis, exhaustion, feeble respiration, drowsiness, confusion, altered conscious state, respiratory arrest

Management of chronic asthma: stepwise approach

Step	Details
1. Newly diagnosed asthma	Short-acting beta agonist (SABA) i.e. salbutamol PRN
2. Not controlled on step 1 OR newly diagnosed asthma with symptoms ≥3/week or night-time waking	SABA + low-dose* inhaled corticosteroid (ICS) e.g. beclomethasone or budesonide
3	SABA + low-dose ICS + leukotriene receptor antagonist (LTRA) e.g. montelukast 10mg OD
4	• SABA + low-dose ICS + long-acting beta agonist (LABA) e.g. formoterol • Continue LTRA depending on patient's response to LTRA
5	• SABA ± LTRA • Switch ICS/LABA for a maintenance and reliever therapy (MART) that includes a low-dose ICS e.g. symbicort (budesonide with formoterol)
6	• SABA ± LTRA + moderate-dose** ICS MART *or* • Consider changing back to a fixed dose of a moderate-dose ICS and a separate LABA
7	SABA ± LTRA + one of the following options: • Increase ICS to high-dose*** (only as a fixed-dose regime, not as part of MART) • Trial an additional drug such as a long-acting muscarinic receptor antagonist e.g. tiotropium or theophylline • Seek advice from a healthcare professional with expertise in asthma

*Low dose ≤400µg budesonide or equivalent
**Moderate dose 400–800µg budesonide or equivalent
***High dose >800µg budesonide or equivalent

Definition

Bronchiectasis is a permanent dilatation and thickening of the airways characterised by chronic cough, excessive sputum production, bacterial colonisation and recurrent acute infections. It is caused by chronic inflammation of the airways and is associated with, or caused by, a large number of diseases. It may be widespread throughout the lungs (diffuse) or more localised (focal).

Pathophysiology

- This is dependent on the cause; the most common cause is infection
- Infection of the small distal airways results in inflammation and release of inflammatory mediators
- This impairs ciliary action resulting in bacterial proliferation and tissue damage which cause bronchial dilatation
- The most common organisms isolated from patients with bronchiectasis include: *Haemophilus influenzae* (most common), *Pseudomonas aeruginosa*, *Klebsiella pneumoniae* and *Streptococcus pneumoniae*

Bronchiectasis

Management

Conservative

- Physical training (e.g. inspiratory muscle training) and chest physiotherapy
- Postural drainage should be performed regularly

Medical

- **Antibiotics** For exacerbations (empirical while awaiting sensitivities) + long-term rotating antibiotics in severe cases
- **Bronchodilators** For patients who have a degree of reversibility
- **Immunisation** Against influenza and pneumococcus

Surgical

- **Lung resection surgery** Considered for localised disease when symptoms are not controlled by medical treatment
- **Bronchial artery embolisation/ surgery** 1st line for management of massive haemoptysis
- **Lung transplantation** Considered for end-stage disease if pulmonary function is very poor (FEV$_1$ <30% of predicted)

Congenital

- **Kartagener's syndrome (primary ciliary dyskinesia)** Impaired ciliary mobility resulting in ↑susceptibility to infection; results in situs inversus
- **Alpha-1 antitrypsin (A1AT) deficiency**
- **Yellow nail syndrome** Associated with azoospermia
- **Cystic fibrosis** (see *Ch2: Cystic fibrosis*)

Acquired

- **Post infection** Childhood respiratory infections e.g. measles, pertussis, TB, bacterial pneumonia
- **Immunodeficiency** Including HIV
- **Connective tissue disorders** e.g. RA, SLE, Sjögren syndrome
- **Asthma**
- **Allergic bronchopulmonary aspergillosis**
- **Gastric aspiration**
- **Bronchial obstruction** Tumour, lymphadenopathy, foreign body
- **Inflammatory bowel disease**

Causes

Symptoms

- Persistent cough
- Copious purulent sputum
- Intermittent haemoptysis
- Fever
- Malaise

Signs

- Finger clubbing (see *Fig. 1*)
- Coarse inspiratory crackles
- Wheeze

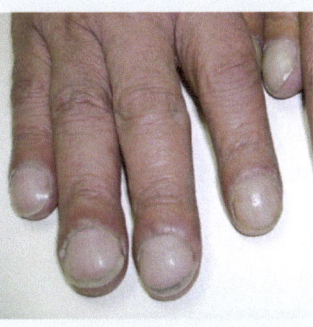

Fig. 1 Finger clubbing

Clinical features

Investigations

- **Imaging**:
  - **CXR** May be normal or show ring or tubular opacities, tramlines and fluid levels
  - **High-resolution CT** The diagnostic gold standard (see *Fig. 2*)
- **Sputum microbiology** To identify causative organisms
- **Routine bloods** FBC (↑WCC in presence of infection), polycythaemia (in advanced cases), CRP (↑ in presence of infection)
- **Immunological tests** Serum immunoglobulins (IgG, IgA, IgM) and serum electrophoresis; serum IgE, skin prick testing/serum IgE testing to *Aspergillus fumigatus* and aspergillosis precipitins
- **Lung function tests** Often show an obstructive pattern; reversibility should be assessed
- **Bronchoscopy** To locate the site of haemoptysis or exclude obstruction
- **Testing for cystic fibrosis** (see *Ch2: Cystic fibrosis*)

Complications

- Repeated infections
- Empyema
- Lung abscess
- Pneumothorax
- Life-threatening haemoptysis
- Respiratory failure
- Right heart failure
- Cerebral abscess
- Amyloidosis (rare)
- Reduced quality of life

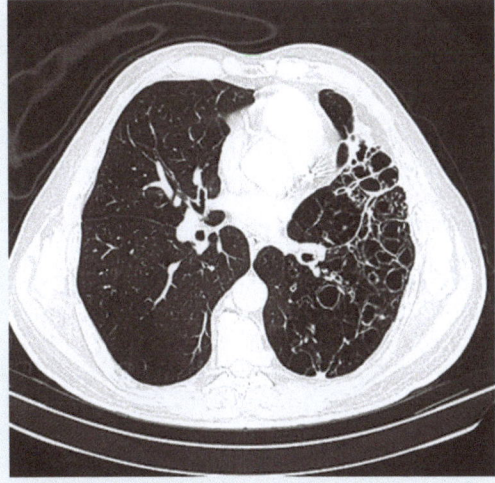

Fig. 2 Distortion of lung parenchyma caused by cystic bronchiectasis with predominant involvement of the lower lobes

Chronic obstructive pulmonary disease (COPD) is characterised by airflow obstruction that is not fully reversible. The airflow obstruction does not change markedly over several months and is usually progressive in the long term. COPD is predominantly caused by smoking. COPD consists of two subtypes which may occur independently or together:

- **Chronic bronchitis** Defined clinically as cough productive of sputum for at least 3 months in each year for 2 consecutive years
- **Emphysema** Enlargement of the air spaces distal to the terminal bronchioles in the lungs, either from dilatation, destruction or distension of their walls

- **Tobacco smoking** About 90% of cases are caused by cigarette smoking
- **Occupational exposure** Dust, chemicals, noxious gases and particles (such as coal, grains, silica, welding fume, isocyanates and polycyclic aromatic hydrocarbons) have been associated with the development of COPD
- **Air pollution** Indoor and outdoor air pollution may contribute to the development of COPD
- **Genetics** Homozygous alpha-1antitrypsin (A1AT) deficiency accounts for less than 1% of COPD cases

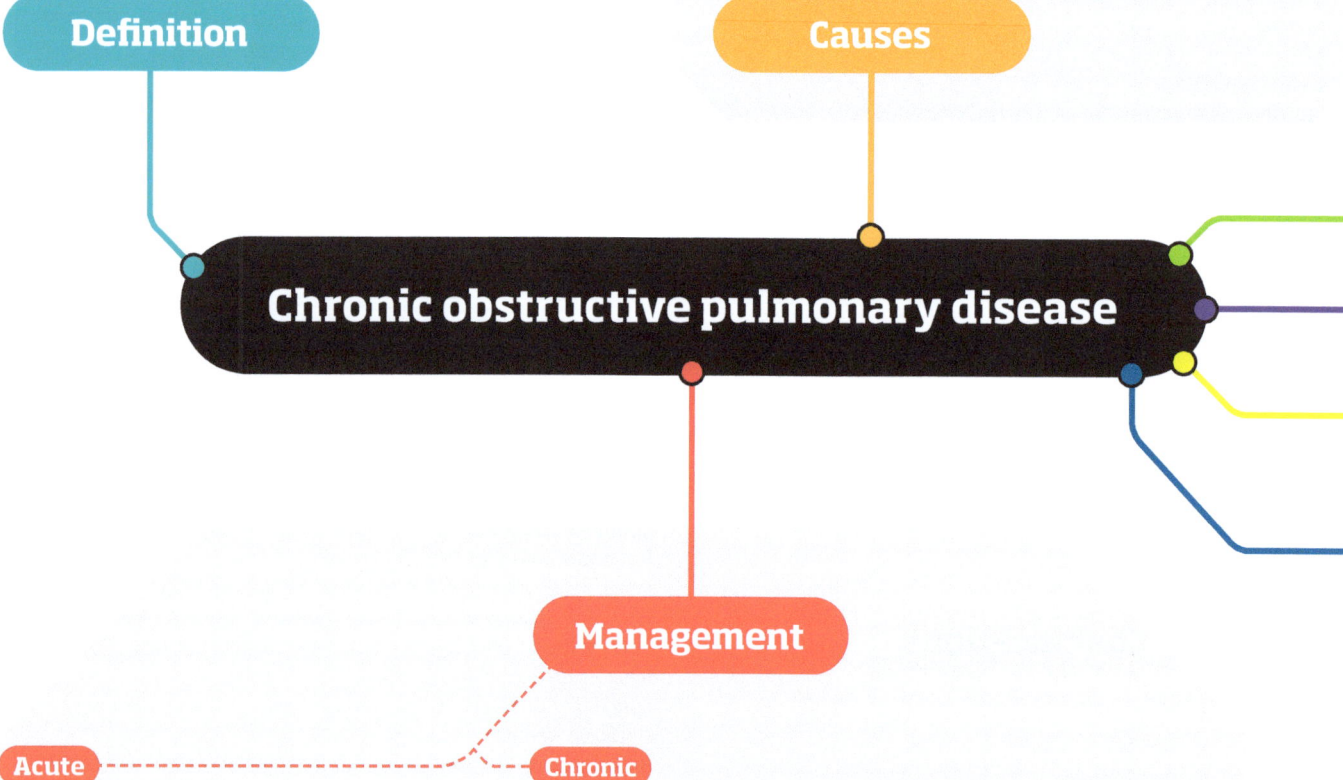

Definition

Causes

Chronic obstructive pulmonary disease

Management

Acute

- **Controlled O_2 therapy** Start at 24–28% via venturi mask and increase accordingly (aim for O_2 saturations of 88–92%)
- **Nebulised bronchodilators** Salbutamol 5mg and ipratropium bromide 500µg; repeat as required
- **Steroids** Oral prednisolone 40mg, or 200mg IV hydrocortisone
- **Antibiotics** If evidence of infection
- Consider **IV aminophylline or salbutamol** if there is inadequate response to nebulisers
- **Non-invasive positive pressure ventilation (NIPPV)** If no response to above and if respiratory rate >30 or pH <7.35; settings are guided by arterial blood gases
- Consider ITU, intubation and ventilation if inadequate response to above

Chronic

- **General management** Smoking cessation advice; annual influenza vaccination + one-off pneumococcal vaccination
- **Inhaler therapy** Short-acting beta-2 agonist (SABA), short-acting muscarinic antagonist (SAMA), long-acting beta-2 agonist (LABA) and inhaled corticosteroids (see *Notes*)
- **Oral theophylline** NICE recommends theophylline only after trials of short- and long-acting bronchodilators or those who cannot use inhaled therapy
- **Mucolytics** Should be 'considered' in patients with a chronic productive cough
- **Long-term O_2 therapy (LTOT)** Offer to patients with a PO_2 of <7.3kPa or to those with a PO_2 of 7.3–8kPa and one of the following: secondary polycythaemia, nocturnal hypoxaemia, peripheral oedema, pulmonary hypertension
- **Prophylactic antibiotic** e.g. Azithromycin prophylaxis recommended in select patients
- **Pulmonary rehabilitation**
- **Surgery** Resection of large bullae or lung volume reduction surgery

Pathophysiology

Chronic bronchitis

- Airflow limitations are seen mainly in the small airways caused by inflammation, narrowing and inflammatory exudates
- There is an increased number of goblet cells and size of bronchial submucosal glands resulting in mucous hypersecretion; this causes bronchial wall narrowing
- This is compounded by ciliary dysfunction caused by squamous metaplasia of the epithelium; this overall causes bronchial wall narrowing

Emphysema

- Alveolar walls are destroyed resulting in bullae formation and fusion of adjacent alveoli
- This results in reduced exchange, decreased elastic recoil, progressive air trapping and hyperinflation
- May be caused by A1AT deficiency

Clinical features

Symptoms

- Breathlessness
- Cough: usually worse in the mornings and productive of small amount of colourless sputum
- Wheeze: may occur typically on exertion or in exacerbations

Signs

- Tachypnoea
- Breathlessness on exertion
- Increased use of accessory muscles of respiration
- Pursed lip breathing
- Cyanosis
- Wheeze
- Hyperinflation (barrel chest)
- Abnormal posture: patients may lean forward and rest their arms on the table to ease breathing
- Drowsiness, flapping tremor and mental confusion ($\uparrow CO_2$)
- Signs of cor pulmonale: peripheral oedema, raised JVP

Complications

- Acute exacerbations ± infections
- Polycythaemia
- Respiratory failure (type 2)
- Cor pulmonale: right-sided heart failure 2° to chronic pulmonary hypertension
- Pneumothorax
- Lung cancer

Investigations

- **CXR** To explore other diagnoses – may be normal or show hyperinflation, flattened diaphragms, bullae (see *Fig. 1*)
- **Bloods** FBC (in the chronic setting) to exclude anaemia and polycythaemia; eosinophils may be raised if asthmatic component present; in the acute setting, WCC may be raised if underlying infection, CRP is useful acutely to identify infection; U&Es, A1AT in younger patients, or in those who are not exposed to cigarette smoke
- **Sputum** Microscopy, culture and sensitivity if suspected infection
- **ABG** Typically shows type 2 respiratory failure; very important to guide O_2 therapy and need for non-invasive ventilation
- **ECG** May show signs of cor pulmonale (P pulmonale, right ventricular hypertrophy, right bundle branch block)
- **Spirometry** Aids diagnosis to demonstrate airflow obstruction: FEV_1/FVC ratio less than 70%; also used to determine severity (see *Notes*)
- **CT** To investigate abnormalities seen on CXR, may confirm emphysematous bullae
- **ECHO** To assess cardiac status if features of cor pulmonale

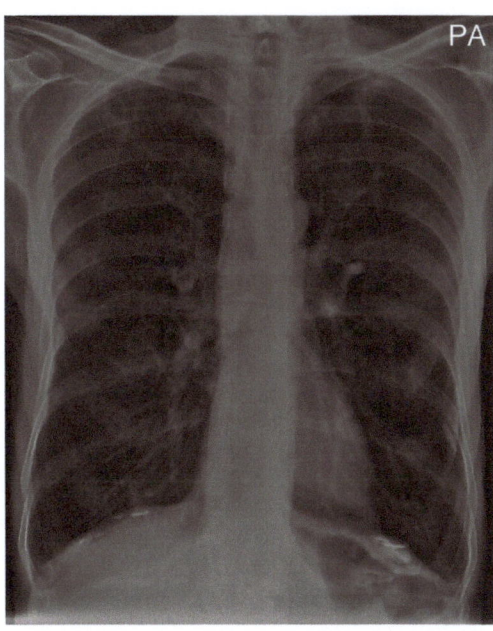

Fig. 1 COPD with marked hyperinflation and flattened diaphragms

Chronic obstructive pulmonary disease notes

Severity of COPD by spirometry

The severity of COPD is categorised using FEV_1:

Post-bronchodilator FEV_1/FVC	FEV_1 (of predicted)	Severity
<0.7	≥80%	Stage 1: Mild*
<0.7	50–79%	Stage 2: Moderate
<0.7	30–49%	Stage 3: Severe
<0.7	<30%	Stage 4: Very severe

*Symptoms should be present to diagnose COPD in these patients

Severity of COPD by clinical features

For this the Medical Research Council (MRC) dyspnoea scale is used:

MRC dyspnoea scale	
Grade 1	Not troubled by breathlessness except on strenuous exertion
Grade 2	Short of breath when hurrying on level ground or walking up a slight incline
Grade 3	Walks slower than contemporaries because of breathlessness, or has to stop for breath when walking at own pace
Grade 4	Stops for breath after walking about 100m or stops after a few minutes of walking on level ground
Grade 5	Too breathless to leave the house or breathless on dressing or undressing

Stepwise inhaler therapy

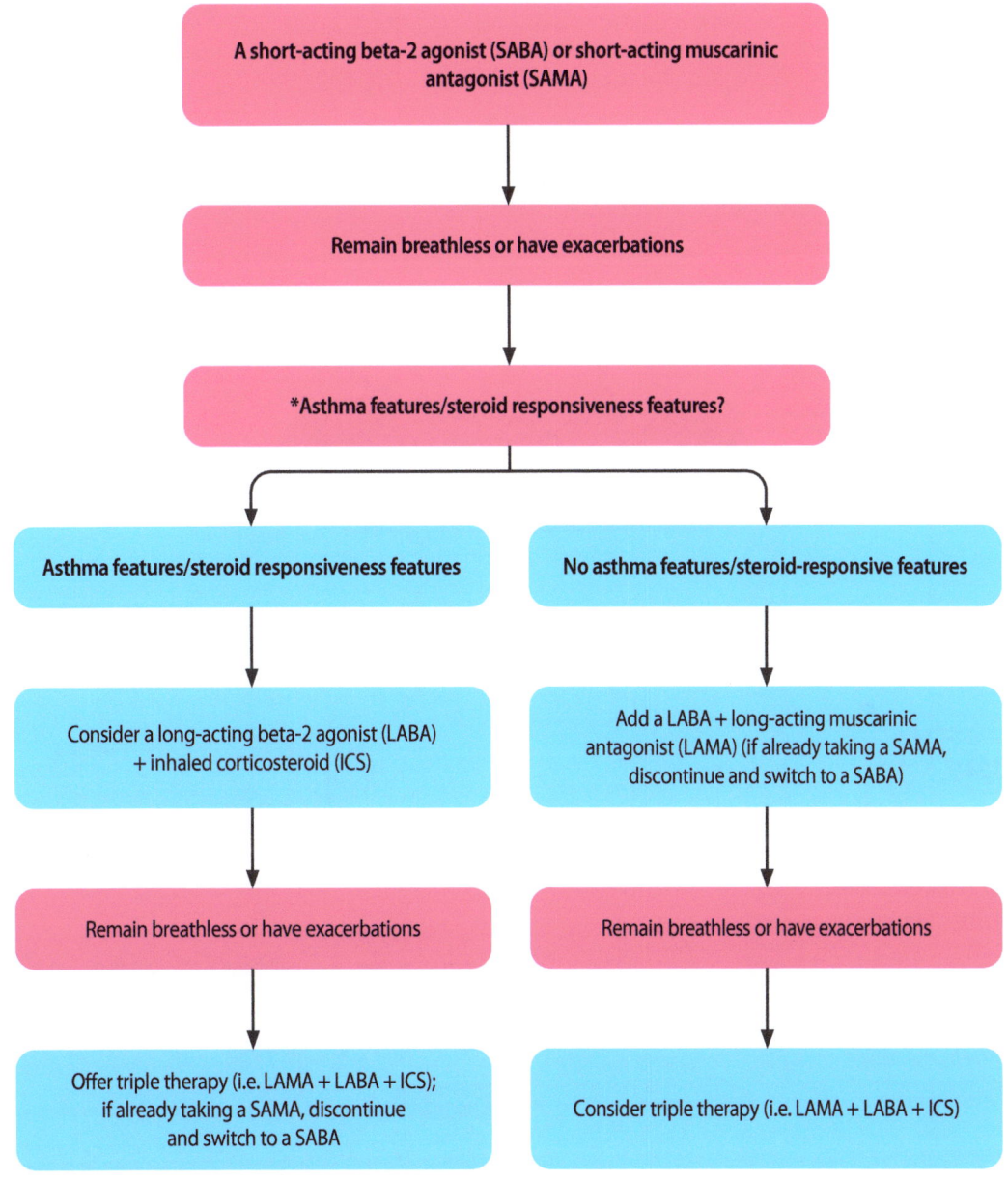

A short-acting beta-2 agonist (SABA) or short-acting muscarinic antagonist (SAMA)

↓

Remain breathless or have exacerbations

↓

*Asthma features/steroid responsiveness features?

Asthma features/steroid responsiveness features

↓

Consider a long-acting beta-2 agonist (LABA) + inhaled corticosteroid (ICS)

↓

Remain breathless or have exacerbations

↓

Offer triple therapy (i.e. LAMA + LABA + ICS); if already taking a SAMA, discontinue and switch to a SABA

No asthma features/steroid-responsive features

↓

Add a LABA + long-acting muscarinic antagonist (LAMA) (if already taking a SAMA, discontinue and switch to a SABA)

↓

Remain breathless or have exacerbations

↓

Consider triple therapy (i.e. LAMA + LABA + ICS)

*Determining whether a patient has asthmatic/steroid-responsive features:
- Any previous secure diagnosis of asthma or atopy
- A higher blood eosinophil count
- Substantial variation in FEV_1 over time (at least 400ml)
- Substantial diurnal variation in peak expiratory flow (at least 20%)

Cystic fibrosis (CF) is an **autosomal recessive disorder** and the most common inherited condition in Caucasian individuals. It is due to a defect in **cystic fibrosis transmembrane conductance regulator (CFTR)**, a chloride channel found in cells lining the lungs, intestines, pancreatic ducts, sweat glands and reproductive organs.

- The defective protein is a cAMP-regulated Cl⁻ channel, CFTR, whose gene is on the long arm (q) of chromosome 7
- There are many types of defect in the *CFTR* gene, of which the most common, a deletion of phenylalanine at position 508, accounts for about 70% of the total
- The abnormal CFTR channel in the cell membrane leads to the production of excessively viscid secretions in the body with a high concentration of Na^+ and a low concentration of Cl^- in exocrine secretions
- As the Cl⁻ channel is found in cells lining the lungs, intestines, pancreatic ducts, sweat glands and reproductive organs, it has various complications affecting these organs

- CF is the most common inherited disease in Caucasians
- Prevalence is 1 in 2500 newborn infants
- Carrier frequency is 1 in 25

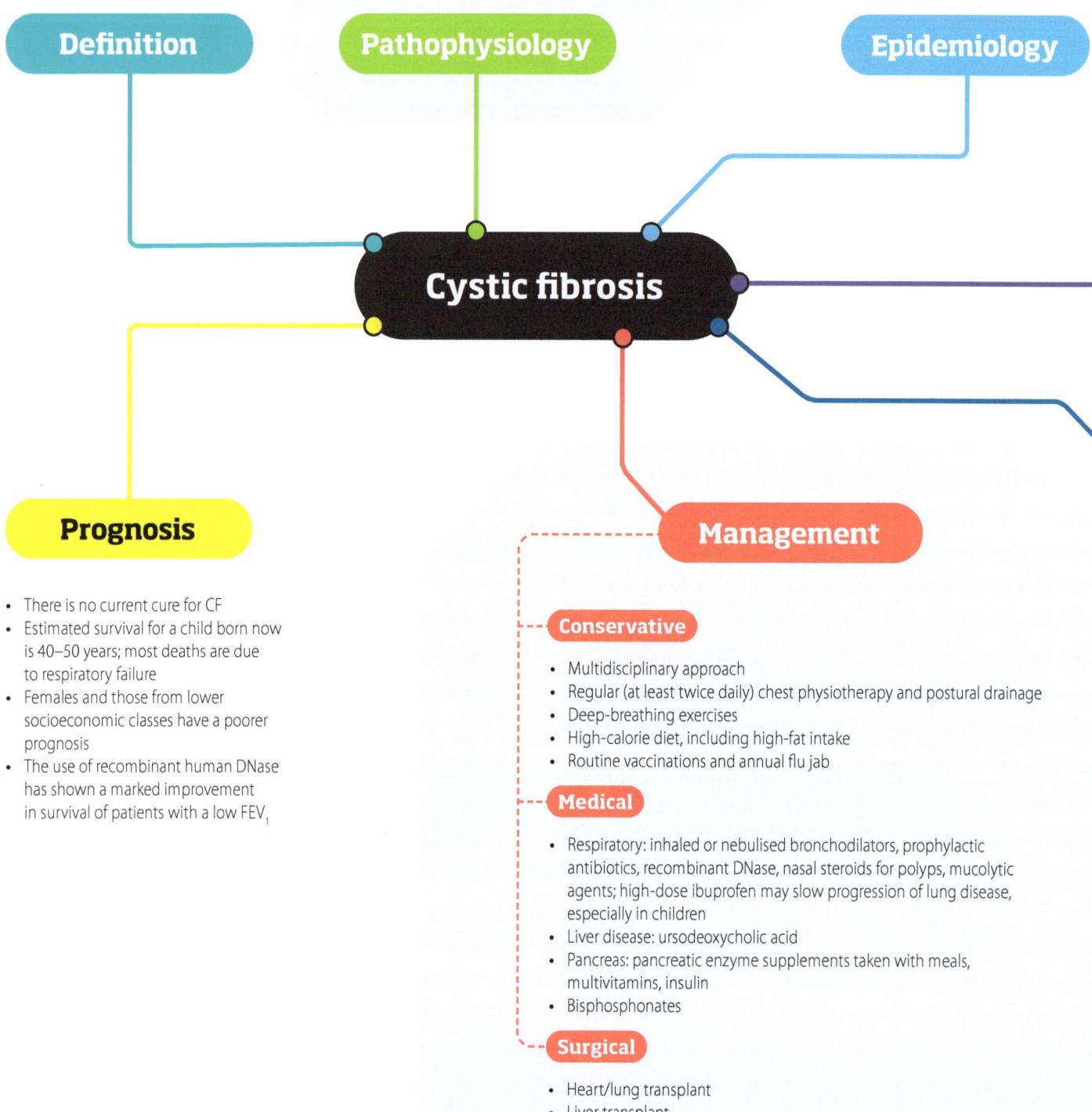

Definition

Pathophysiology

Epidemiology

Cystic fibrosis

Prognosis

- There is no current cure for CF
- Estimated survival for a child born now is 40–50 years; most deaths are due to respiratory failure
- Females and those from lower socioeconomic classes have a poorer prognosis
- The use of recombinant human DNase has shown a marked improvement in survival of patients with a low FEV_1

Management

Conservative

- Multidisciplinary approach
- Regular (at least twice daily) chest physiotherapy and postural drainage
- Deep-breathing exercises
- High-calorie diet, including high-fat intake
- Routine vaccinations and annual flu jab

Medical

- Respiratory: inhaled or nebulised bronchodilators, prophylactic antibiotics, recombinant DNase, nasal steroids for polyps, mucolytic agents; high-dose ibuprofen may slow progression of lung disease, especially in children
- Liver disease: ursodeoxycholic acid
- Pancreas: pancreatic enzyme supplements taken with meals, multivitamins, insulin
- Bisphosphonates

Surgical

- Heart/lung transplant
- Liver transplant

Respiratory/ENT

- Cough with purulent sputum
- Wheeze
- Recurrent chest infections (organisms which may colonise CF patients: *Staphylococcus aureus*, *Pseudomonas aeruginosa*, *Burkholderia cepacia*, *Aspergillus* spp.)
- Reduced exercise tolerance
- Nasal polyps
- Sinusitis
- Bronchiectasis
- Pneumothorax
- Respiratory failure
- Cor pulmonale

Gastrointestinal

- Pancreatic insufficiency (diabetes mellitus, steatorrhoea)
- Meconium ileus (in neonates)
- Rectal prolapse (infants)
- Distal intestinal obstruction syndrome
- Gallstones
- Cirrhosis

Miscellaneous

- Male infertility (congenital absence of vas deferens)
- Osteoporosis
- Arthritis
- Vasculitis
- Failure to thrive (neonates/children)
- Hypertrophic pulmonary osteoarthropathy (HPOA)
- Finger clubbing

Clinical features

Investigations

- **Antenatal screening or newborn screening test** May pick up CF
- **Sweat testing** Confirms the diagnosis and is 98% sensitive; Cl^- >60mmol/L with Na^+ < Cl^- on two separate occasions
- **Molecular genetic testing** *CFTR* gene
- **Sinus X-ray or CT** Opacification of the sinuses is present in almost all patients with CF
- **CXR** Hyperinflation and bronchiectasis changes
- **CT thorax** To help diagnose bronchiectasis
- **Bloods** FBC, U&Es, fasting glucose, LFTs and vitamins A, D and E
- **Lung function testing** Spirometry is unreliable in children <6 years
- **Sputum microbiology** To isolate common pathogens that cause chest infections
- **Semen analysis** (if appropriate)

Notes

Cystic fibrosis

Definition

Interstitial lung disease refers to a group of chronic conditions which produce interstitial lung damage and fibrosis resulting in loss of the elasticity of the lungs. It may be secondary to a wide range of diseases or may be idiopathic with no known underlying cause. Pulmonary fibrosis can be localised, segmental, lobar, or affect the entirety of the lung(s).

Interstitial lung disease

Classification by cause

Known causes

- **Industrial dust diseases** Including coal worker's pneumoconiosis, silicosis, asbestosis and berylliosis
- **Drugs** Including nitrofurantoin, bleomycin, amiodarone and sulfasalazine
- **Hypersensitivity pneumonitis**
- **Infections** Fungal e.g. histoplasmosis; bacterial e.g. TB; or viral e.g. COVID-19
- **Radiation**
- **Malignancy** e.g. Metastases or lymphangitis carcinomatosis
- **Paraquat poisoning**

Associated with systemic inflammatory disorders

- Sarcoidosis
- RA
- SLE
- Systemic sclerosis and mixed connective tissue disease
- Ankylosing spondylitis

Idiopathic

- Idiopathic pulmonary fibrosis (IPF)
- Cryptogenic organising pneumonia
- Acute interstitial pneumonia, desquamative interstitial pneumonia and respiratory bronchiolitis

Management

- Treat underlying cause if possible e.g. antibiotics for infection, treat malignancy, stop offending drugs, steroids or immunosuppressant for autoimmune disorders
- Avoid exposure to irritants e.g. asbestosis, coal etc.
- Supportive treatment, including oxygen therapy and pulmonary rehabilitation
- Claim compensation for occupational-related illness
- Lung transplantation

- **CXR and high-resolution CT** (see *Fig. 1, Table 1*) Features include honeycombing, traction bronchiectasis, lung architectural distortion, reticulation and interlobular septal thickening
- **Lung function tests** Spirometry shows a restrictive pattern with reduced transfer factor for carbon monoxide
- **ABG** May show type 1 respiratory failure
- **Lung biopsy** May confirm diagnosis

Table 1 Causes of fibrotic shadowing on CXR depending on predominant location

Upper-zone predominant	Mid-zone predominant	Lower-zone predominant
• TB • Hypersensitivity pneumonitis • Ankylosing spondylitis • Sarcoidosis • Histoplasmosis • Silicosis	• Progressive massive pulmonary fibrosis	• IPF • Asbestosis • Scleroderma • RA-associated interstitial disease

- Dyspnoea on exertion
- Cough (non-productive)
- Crepitations on auscultation (specific sounds depend on underlying cause)

Clinical features

Investigations

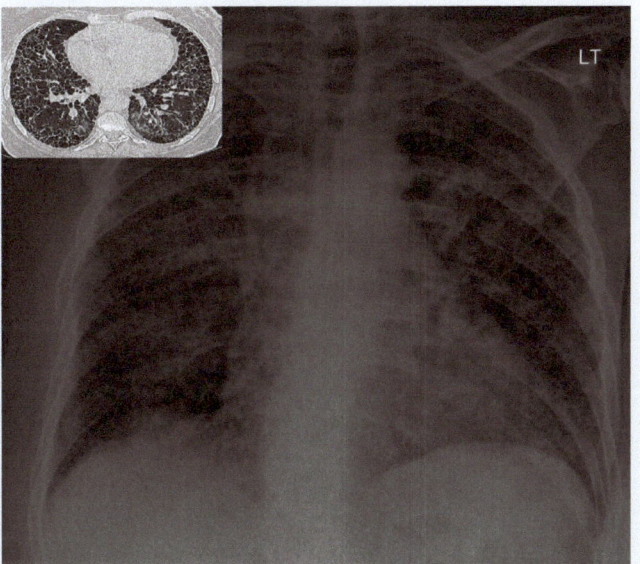

Fig. 1 Pulmonary fibrosis on CXR, with CT inset

Hypersensitivity pneumonitis

Definition

Hypersensitivity pneumonitis, also known as extrinsic allergic alveolitis, is a condition caused by hypersensitivity-induced lung damage due to a variety of inhaled organic particles.

Pathophysiology

It is thought to be largely caused by immune-complex-mediated tissue damage (type III hypersensitivity) though a delayed hypersensitivity (type IV) is also thought to play a role, particularly in the chronic phase.

Types

- **Farmer's lung** One of the most common forms; due to exposure to mouldy hay; the major antigen is *Saccharopolyspora rectivirgula*
- **Bird-fancier's lung** Caused by exposure to avian proteins e.g. pigeons and parakeets
- **Cheese-worker's lung** Caused by exposure to cheese mould, *Penicillium casei*
- **Malt worker's lung** Caused by exposure to *Aspergillus clavatus* in mouldy malt
- **Hot tub lung** Caused by exposure to *Mycobacterium avium* in poorly maintained hot tubs
- **Chemical worker's lung** Due to exposure to trimellitic anhydride, diisocyanate and methylene diisocyanate during the manufacture of plastics, polyurethane foam and rubber
- **Mushroom worker's lung** Due to exposure to thermophilic actinomycetes in mushroom compost

Clinical features/diagnosis

- **Acute presentation** (several hours after exposure to antigen) Fever, malaise, cough, shortness of breath and coarse end-inspiratory crackles
- **Chronic presentation** Progressive exertional dyspnoea, weight loss and cough
- Bloods may show raised WCC in acute phase and CXR typically shows upper/middle zone fibrosis
- Bronchoalveolar lavage may show lymphocytosis

Management

- Allergy avoidance and may require change of job
- Prednisolone may be used for treatment in severe cases

Idiopathic pulmonary fibrosis (IPF)

Industrial dust diseases

Definition

IPF (previously termed cryptogenic fibrosing alveolitis) is a chronic lung condition characterised by progressive fibrosis of the interstitium of the lungs. The term IPF is reserved for when no underlying cause exists.

Clinical features/diagnosis

- Highest incidence in late-middle age
- Progressive exertional dyspnoea
- Dry cough
- Bibasal fine end-inspiratory crepitations on auscultation
- Clubbing
- **CXR and CT** Shows bilateral interstitial shadowing – typically small, irregular, peripheral opacities ('ground-glass') later progressing to 'honeycombing'
- ANA positive in approx. 30% and RF positive in approx. 10%

Management

- Pulmonary rehabilitation
- Treatment is limited: pirfenidone (an antifibrotic agent) may be useful in selected patients
- Many patients will require oxygen therapy and eventually lung transplant if suitable

Coal worker's pneumoconiosis (CWP)

Definition

A common dust disease in countries that have or have had underground coal mines. It results from inhalation of coal dust over years (approx. 15–20 years).

Pathophysiology

- Tiny particles of coal dust (2–5μm diam.) are retained in the alveoli
- They are engulfed by macrophages but, eventually, the system is overwhelmed and an immune response follows; this produces pulmonary fibrosis
- **Caplan syndrome** When CWP is associated with RA, and pulmonary rheumatoid nodules

Clinical features/diagnosis

- Patients with simple CWP are often asymptomatic and incidentally found on CXR although co-existing chronic bronchitis is common
- CXR in CWP shows many small round opacities (1–10mm) in the upper zones
- CWP may progress to **progressive massive pulmonary fibrosis** caused by continuous exposure; it is characterised by large fibrotic masses (1–10cm) predominantly in the upper lobes
- Symptoms of progressive massive pulmonary fibrosis include breathlessness, cough productive of black sputum and cor pulmonale

Management

- There is no specific treatment; patients should avoid exposure to coal dust and co-existing chronic bronchitis should be treated
- Patients may be eligible for compensation in the UK via the Industrial Injuries Act

Notes

Silicosis

Silicosis is a fibrotic lung disease caused by the inhalation of fine particles of crystalline silicon dioxide (silica).

Pathophysiology

- Dust containing crystalline silica is highly fibrogenic
- When silica dust is inhaled, the particles deposit within the distal airways
- Macrophages ingest these particles and initiate an inflammatory response by releasing pro-inflammatory molecules leading to the formation of nodular lesions and tissue fibrosis
- Occupations at risk of silicosis include those who worked in mining, slate works, foundries and potteries

Clinical features/diagnosis

- **Simple nodular silicosis** Usually asymptomatic and may be incidentally found on CXR
- **Advanced nodular silicosis** Cough and exertional dyspnoea are common
- There is increased risk of TB and COPD
- **CXR** Miliary or nodular pattern in upper and mid zones and thin streaks of calcification are seen around the hilar lymph nodes ('eggshell' calcification)

Management

- There is no specific cure
- Management involves avoiding further exposure, smoking cessation, treating co-existing TB or bacterial infections, bronchodilators, oxygen therapy, and in some cases lung transplant
- Patients are usually eligible for compensation as in CWP

Asbestosis

Definition

Asbestosis is a typical pneumoconiosis caused by inhalation of asbestos fibres. Asbestos can cause a variety of other lung diseases including **benign pleural plaques**, **pleural thickening**, **asbestosis**, **mesothelioma** and **bronchial adenocarcinoma**.

Pathophysiology

- The result of exposure to asbestos with **blue asbestos (crocidolite)** being the most fibrogenic, **white (chrystotile)** being least and **brown (amosite)** being intermediate
- The development of pulmonary fibrosis appears to be related to the severity and duration of exposure; the latent period is typically 15–30 years

Clinical features/diagnosis

- Most people have occupational exposure such as fitting or working with asbestos insulation e.g. builders, plumbers and electricians
- It usually presents with progressive dyspnoea, dry cough, repetitive inspiratory basal crackles and clubbing of the fingers (advanced feature)
- CXR shows diffuse bilateral shadowing and honeycomb lung; pleural plaques may be present which are an indicator of previous exposure to asbestos

Management

- There is no specific treatment; management is largely supportive including avoidance of asbestos, pulmonary rehabilitation and oxygen therapy; smoking cessation is important and patients may benefit from influenza and pneumococcal vaccinations
- Monitoring to assess for risk of mesothelioma or lung cancer
- Compensation can be claimed as with CWP

Interstitial lung disease

SCLC (15%)

- Arise from Kulchitsky cells
- Rapidly growing and highly malignant (almost always inoperable at presentation but chemoresponsive)
- SCLCs tend to contain membrane-bound neurosecretory granules that can release calcitonin, ADH, ACTH and PTH-related peptide (PTHrP)

NSCLC (85%)

Squamous cell carcinoma (42%):

- Typically arise in proximal segmental bronchi; most present at obstructive lesions of the bronchus
- Local spread is common, distant metastases occur late
- They can also release PTHrP

Adenocarcinoma (39%):

- Arise from mucous cells of bronchial epithelium
- The most common bronchial carcinoma associated with asbestos and more common in non-smokers
- Even small resectable lesions carry a risk of early occult metastases (most commonly spread to the brain and bones)

Large cell carcinoma (8%):

- These consist of sheets of large, round to polygonal cells with large nuclei and prominent nucleoli
- They frequently arise centrally and are poorly differentiated

Classification/pathophysiology

Most cases of lung cancer are bronchial carcinomas which are malignant tumours originating from the epithelial cell lining of the lower respiratory tract. They are divided primarily into **small cell lung carcinoma (SCLC)** and **non-small cell lung carcinoma (NSCLC)** depending on histology.

Definition

Lung cancer

Management

Management options are described in full on the following *Notes* pages

Investigations

Bloods

FBC May show anaemia, raised platelets
U&Es May show hyponatraemia in ADH-producing tumours
Calcium May be ↑ in PTHrP-secreting tumour, or if there is bone metastasis
Albumin May be low

Imaging

- **CXR** Often 1st investigation done in patients with suspected lung cancer (see *Fig. 1*)
- **CT chest** The investigation of choice to investigate suspected lung cancer
- **PET scan** Typically done in NSCLC to establish eligibility for curative treatment

Histology

- **Bronchoscopy** Used to obtain biopsies and washings for cytology
- **Pleural effusion analysis** (see *Ch2: Pleural effusion*)
- **Sputum** Used for people with suspected lung cancer who have centrally placed nodules or masses and who decline/cannot tolerate bronchoscopy/other invasive tests
- **Transthoracic fine needle aspiration biopsy** (under imaging) To obtain histology for peripheral lesions

Epidemiology

- Lung cancer is the 3rd most common cancer in the UK, accounting for 13% of all new cancer cases
- Lung cancer is the most common cause of cancer death in the UK

Risk factors

- Cigarette smoking (approx. 90% of lung cancers are caused by smoking)
- COPD
- Previous malignancy, particularly head and neck
- Industrial dust diseases: asbestos, chromium, arsenic, radon gas
- Family history
- Increasing age

Clinical features

Symptoms

- Cough (80%)
- Haemoptysis (70%)
- Dyspnoea (60%)
- Chest pain (40%)
- Recurrent or slow-resolving pneumonia
- Anorexia
- Weight loss

Signs

Locoregional spread:

- Shoulder/inner arm pain/weakness (brachial plexus compression)
- Horner syndrome (sympathetic ganglion compression)
- Hoarseness (recurrent laryngeal nerve compression)
- Upper limb oedema, facial congestion and distended neck veins (superior vena cava obstruction)

Distant metastases:

- Personality change, seizures, headaches, focal neurological signs (brain metastases)
- Bone pain, back pain, leg weakness (bone metastases and spinal cord compression)

Paraneoplastic syndrome:

- Finger clubbing
- Signs of hypercalcaemia (see *Ch5: Hypercalcaemia and hyperparathyroidism*): due to bone metastases or PTHrP release (in small cell carcinoma or squamous cell carcinoma)
- Hypertrophic osteoarthropathy

Staging and prognosis

- The TNM (tumour, node, metastasis) staging system is used for staging lung cancer
- Lung cancer should be staged by a contrast-enhanced CT scan of the patient's chest, liver and adrenal glands and by selected imaging of any symptomatic area
- Prognosis depends on cancer type and the stage of cancer
- Overall, the 10-year survival rate for lung cancer in the UK is around 5.5%
- SCLC has a much poorer prognosis than NSCLC with 65–70% of patients having disseminated or extensive disease at presentation

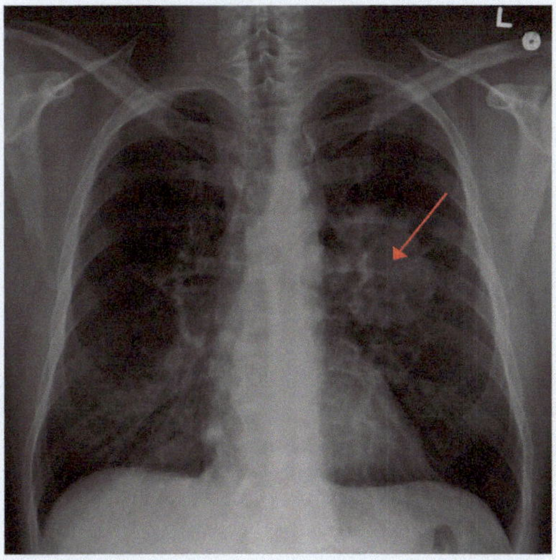

Fig. 1 Bronchial carcinoma of the left lung

Management of lung cancer

General management

- Smoking cessation
- Access to multidisciplinary team
- There is currently no national screening but NHS England is looking at using low-dose CT scans as a possible screening test for lung cancer for those of a certain age and who smoke or used to smoke

NSCLC

- **Surgery** The treatment of choice for patients with stage I or II disease; lobar resection is the procedure of choice
- All patients undergoing surgical resection should have hilar and mediastinal lymph node sampling to provide accurate pathological staging
- **Radiotherapy** Should be offered to all patients with stage I–III NSCLC who are not suitable for surgery
- **Chemotherapy** Should be offered to patients with stage III or IV NSCLC and good performance status, to improve survival, disease control and quality of life
- **Tyrosine kinase inhibitors** e.g. Afatinib, erlotinib and gefitinib are indicated for metastatic NSCLC in individuals with an epidermal growth factor receptor mutation

SCLC

- Surgery is often not possible (as SCLC metastasises early)
- **Chemotherapy** Usually 1st line; SCLC is much more chemotherapy sensitive than NSCLC
- Multi-drug treatments are often used
- **Radiotherapy** is an option if there is good response to initial chemotherapy

Supportive palliative treatment

- **Palliative care team** For patients with advanced disease
- **Radiotherapy** Used for bronchial obstruction, cough, chest pain, haemoptysis, superior vena cava (SVC) obstruction, bone and brain metastases, and spinal cord compression
- **Debulking surgery** Considered in bronchial obstruction or for haemoptysis
- **Stent insertion** An option for bronchial obstruction and in SVC obstruction
- **Opiates** e.g. Morphine can be used for breathlessness and cough in addition to pain
- **Aspiration or drainage ± pleurodesis** Can provide symptomatic relief from pleural effusions
- **Bisphosphonates** should be considered for bone metastases

Mesothelioma

Definition

Mesothelioma is malignancy of mesothelial cells which usually occurs in the pleura. It can also occur in other sites, including the peritoneum, pericardium and testes.

Epidemiology and Risk factors

- Malignant mesothelioma is three times more common in men than in women
- More than 2600 people are diagnosed with the condition each year in the UK
- Almost half of cases of mesothelioma are diagnosed in people aged ≥75
- Occupational exposure to asbestos accounts for more than 80% of cases; there may be a time lag of 20–40 years between exposure and development of tumour
- Crocidolite (blue) asbestos is the most dangerous form

Clinical features

- Shortness of breath (progressive)
- Chest pain
- Fatigue, fever and sweats may occur
- Finger clubbing
- Signs of pleural effusion (see *Ch 2: Pleural effusion*)
- Palpable chest wall mass
- Signs of metastases: lymphadenopathy, hepatomegaly, bone pain, bone tenderness, abdominal pain and gastrointestinal obstruction

Investigations

- **CXR** and **CT scan** may show pleural effusion, lobulated or nodular pleural thickening, a pleural mass and rib destruction
- **MRI/PET scan** may provide further detail
- **Pleural fluid:** straw coloured or bloodstained; cytological analysis may be useful for diagnosis
- **Pleural biopsy:** ultrasound or CT-guided percutaneous biopsy to confirm diagnosis
- **Mediastinoscopy** and **video-assisted thoracoscopy** may be useful in determining the stage

Management

Management options are limited:
- **Surgery** Curative surgery may be possible only in stage I; extrapleural pneumonectomy may lengthen time to recurrence
- **Chemotherapy** Palliative chemotherapy has been shown to improve survival of patients with unresectable mesothelioma
- **Radiotherapy** May be given in an adjuvant setting after surgery or chemosurgery although there is little good evidence to support this practice
- Patients are often eligible for compensation in the UK under the **UK Industrial Injuries Act**

Staging and prognosis

- The **TNM staging** is used for staging mesothelioma
- The prognosis remains poor and is typically around 1 year

- Obstructive sleep apnoea (OSA) syndrome is a clinical condition in which there is intermittent and repeated upper airway collapse during sleep; this results in irregular breathing at night and excessive sleepiness during the day
- **Complete apnoea** is defined as a 10-sec pause in breathing activity
- **Partial apnoea**, also known as **hypopnoea**, is characterised by a 10-sec period in which ventilation is reduced by at least 50%

- Irregular breathing results from the upper airway collapsing during sleep
- This occurs during sleep as the muscles that hold the airway open are hypotonic
- Collapse of the airways can be **partial (hypopnoea)** or **complete (apnoea)**, leading to a temporary arousal from sleep which allows restoration of normal airway muscular tone
- These cycles can occur hundreds of times throughout the night but they can be so brief that the patient is unaware of them
- This disturbance to normal sleep pattern leads to reduced sleep quality, excessive daytime sleepiness and reduced concentration and alertness as a result
- There are several contributing factors to this (see *Risk factors*)

Definition

Pathophysiology

Obstructive sleep apnoea

Complications

- Pulmonary hypertension
- Type 2 respiratory failure
- Hypertension
- Myocardial infarction
- Stroke
- Road traffic accidents

Management

- **Behavioural interventions** Weight loss, smoking cessation, avoid alcohol during evenings, sleep on side
- **CPAP** Still recognised as the gold standard treatment; nasal CPAP (nCPAP) is highly effective in controlling symptoms, improving quality of life and reducing the clinical sequelae of sleep apnoea
- **Bilevel positive airway pressure (BIPAP)** Provides two different levels of pressure and is an alternative in patients intolerant to CPAP and also in patients with associated hypoventilation or COPD
- **Mandibular advancement devices** – increase airway diameter with soft tissue displacement by mandibular protrusion
- **Pharmacological** Role is limited; modafinil may afford some benefit in some patients
- **Surgery** Removal of markedly enlarged tonsils and correction of facial abnormalities

Diagnosis

- Simple studies, e.g. pulse oximetry, video recordings, may be all that are required
- The **Epworth Sleepiness Scale** is a simple tool to help discriminate between OSA and simple snoring
- **Polysomnography (PSG)** is the traditional gold standard investigation; it usually involves an electroencephalogram (EEG), two electro-oculograms (EOGs) to measure horizontal and vertical eye movements and an electromyogram to monitor muscle movement (during sleep): at the end of the investigation, the number of apnoea/hypopnoea episodes is quoted as the apnoea/hypopnoea index (AHI)
- **Arterial blood gases** may show type 2 respiratory failure

- Male sex (male to female ratio is 2–3:1)
- Obesity
- Large neck circumference
- Family history of OSA
- Smoking
- Alcohol intake before bed
- Sleeping supine
- Hypothyroidism
- Acromegaly
- In children: obesity, adenotonsillar hypertrophy and congenital conditions e.g. Down syndrome, craniofacial abnormalities, and Prader–Willi syndrome

Risk factors

Clinical features

Symptoms

- Loud snoring
- Daytime somnolence
- Poor sleeping quality
- Morning headache
- Decreased libido
- Decreased cognitive performance
- Irritability/personality change

Signs

- Obesity
- Fat deposition anterolateral to the upper airway may signify obstruction
- Large neck circumference
- Certain craniofacial or pharyngeal abnormalities e.g. retrognathia, micrognathia, enlarged tonsils, macroglossia, thickening or lengthening of the soft palate or uvula
- Nasal polyps, rhinitis or any deformity of the nose

Pleural effusion is the presence of excessive fluid between the visceral and parietal pleura (pleural space). It can comprise a variety of liquids including blood (**haemothorax**), pus (**empyema**) and chyle (**chylothorax**) in the pleural space. Both blood and air in the pleural space is called **haemopneumothorax**.

Normally, the pleural space contains a small physiological amount of pleural fluid. Pleural effusion occurs when there is discrepancy between the formation and resorption of pleural fluid. The fluid may be either transudative or exudative:

- **Transudate** Results from abnormal accumulation of pleural fluid due to high capillary and interstitial hydrostatic pressures (e.g. in heart failure) or abnormally decreased capillary oncotic pressure (e.g. in nephrotic syndrome)
- **Exudate** Results from inflammatory and malignant processes which adjust the permeability of the local capillary and pleural membrane or by lymphatic blockage

Transudates

- Heart failure
- Hypoalbuminaemia: cirrhosis, nephrotic syndrome, malabsorption
- Constrictive pericarditis
- Ascites
- Hypothyroidism
- End-stage kidney disease
- Meigs syndrome (ovarian fibroma producing right-sided pleural effusion)
- Peritoneal dialysis
- Superior vena cava obstruction

Definition

Pathophysiology

Causes

Pleural effusion

Management

Acute

- Treat underlying cause: e.g. infection with antibiotics, and diuretics for heart failure
- Therapeutic pleural aspiration or intercostal drainage: if effusion is symptomatic or large; it is best removed slowly

Long-term

- **Pleurodesis:** chemical pleurodesis with tetracycline, bleomycin or talc for recurrent effusions
- **Pleurectomy:** for exceptional cases e.g. in mesothelioma and in patients in good general condition where pleurodesis has failed

Bloods

- **FBC** WCC raised in infection/inflammation
- **U&Es** Impaired in renal disease
- **CRP** Raised in infection, inflammation and malignancy
- **LFTs** To rule out liver disease
- **BNP/NT-pro BNP** To help rule out heart failure
- **Serum protein***
- **Serum LDH***

Urine

- **Dipstick** Protein-positive in nephrotic syndrome
- **Urine protein: creatinine ratio** Raised in nephrotic syndrome

Exudates

- **Infection** Empyema, pneumonia, paraneoplastic effusion, TB
- **Malignancy** Lung carcinoma, lymphoma, leukaemia, mesothelioma, lung metastases
- **Inflammatory** ARDS, pancreatitis, sarcoidosis, radiation
- **Connective tissue disease** Churg–Strauss disease, SLE, rheumatoid arthritis, granulomatosis with polyangiitis
- **Pulmonary embolus** With infarction
- **Drugs** Methotrexate, amiodarone, nitrofurantoin, beta blockers

Clinical features

Symptoms

- May be asymptomatic
- Shortness of breath
- Pleuritic chest pain
- Cough (non-productive)

Signs

- ↓Chest expansion on affected side(s)
- Stony dull on percussion
- ↓Breath sounds on affected side(s)
- Reduced vocal and tactile fremitus on affected side(s)
- Mediastinal shift to opposite side of effusion (large effusions)
- Signs of underlying cause e.g. malignancy, hypothyroidism, cardiac failure etc.

Investigations

Imaging

- **CXR** Loss of costophrenic angle, homogenous white shadow with a concave-upwards upper border (meniscal sign), tracheal deviation away from affected side (may occur in massive pleural effusions) (see *Fig. 1*)
- **US** Used for determining pleural effusion and guiding diagnostic or therapeutic aspiration
- **CT chest** To provide more detailed images and help to identify underlying causes e.g. malignancy
- **Transthoracic ECHO** To determine if there is heart failure
- **Pleural biopsy** Obtained by CT-guided, blind or video-assisted thoracoscopic approach; provides tissue diagnosis (TB smear, culture and histology)

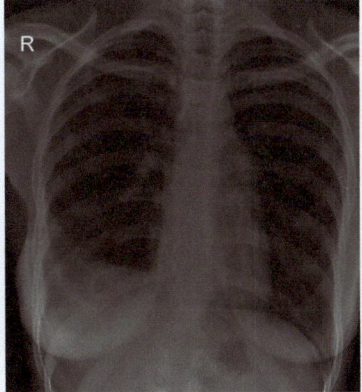

Fig. 1 Chest X-ray showing a moderate right pleural effusion

*Light's criteria: helps to determine exudate vs transudate

Light's criteria are used when it is unclear whether the pleural effusion is a transudate or an exudate. It uses protein and LDH in the serum and in the pleural fluid. A pleural effusion is likely exudative if at least one of the following exists:

Pleural fluid protein divided by serum protein >0.5 *or*
Pleural fluid LDH divided by serum LDH >0.6 *or*
Pleural fluid LDH more than two-thirds the upper limits of normal serum LDH

Pleural aspiration and analysis

- **Gross appearance** Turbid/yellow (empyema, parapneumonic effusion), haemorrhagic (trauma, malignancy, pulmonary infarction)
- **Microbiology:**
  - **White cells** Raised in empyema and exudates; neutrophils raised in parapneumonic effusion, pulmonary embolism (PE) and abdominal diseases; lymphocytes raised in malignancy, TB, PE
  - **Red cells** Raised in malignancy, trauma, parapneumonic effusion, PE
  - **Culture** To identify causative organism in infection
- **Biochemistry:**
  - **Protein** <25g/L = transudate, >35g/L = exudate
  - **Glucose** <3.3mmol/L: empyema, malignancy, TB, RA
  - **pH** <7.2: empyema, malignancy, TB
  - **↑LDH*** Any exudative cause
  - **↑Amylase** Pancreatitis, carcinoma, bacterial pneumonia
- **Cytology** To help determine whether there is malignancy
- **Immunology** RA, ANA, complement levels

Definition

An acute lower respiratory tract infection of the lung parenchyma associated with radiographic changes.

Classification

Community-acquired pneumonia (CAP)

Typical:

- *Streptococcus pneumoniae* (80%)
- *Haemophilus influenzae*
- *Moraxella catarrhalis*
- *Staphylococcus aureus*
- Viruses e.g. influenza A, coronavirus (COVID-19)

Atypical:

- *Chlamydia pneumoniae*
- *Legionella pneumophila* (typically fresh water and man-made water systems)
- *Mycoplasma pneumoniae*

Hospital-acquired pneumonia (HAP)

- At least 48–72 h after being admitted
- *Staphylococcus aureus*
- Gram-negative enterobacteria
- *Klebsiella pneumoniae*
- *Pseudomonas* spp.

Pneumonia

Management

Acute

- **Oxygen** Keep O$_2$ sats ≥96% (88–92% in those with COPD)
- **IV fluids** As per SEPSIS 6 if septic or if patient is dehydrated
- **Antibiotics** Local microbiology guidelines should be followed but examples include amoxicillin for uncomplicated CAP (doxycycline or clarithromycin if penicillin allergic), clarithromycin for atypical organisms, co-amoxiclav for HAP (<5 days admission); ≥5 days after admission: tazocin *or* a broad-spectrum cephalosporin *or* a quinolone; amoxicillin and metronidazole or co-amoxiclav for aspiration pneumonia
- **Analgesia** and **antipyretics** e.g. NSAIDs, paracetamol
- **Nebulised saline** May aid expectoration
- In severe cases, patients may require **non-invasive ventilation**, or **intubation** and **ventilation** in ITU

Prevention

- Influenza and pneumococcal vaccination
- Smoking cessation

Complications (SLAPPED HER)

- **S**eptic shock
- **L**ung abscess
- **A**cute kidney injury, **A**cute respiratory distress syndrome
- **P**neumothorax
- **P**ost-infective bronchiectasis
- Pleural **E**ffusion
- **D**eep vein thrombosis
- **H**ypotension
- **E**mpyema
- **R**espiratory failure

Pneumonia in the immunocompromised

- For example in AIDS, lymphomas, leukaemias, patients taking immunosuppressive drugs
- *Pneumocystis jirovecii* (common opportunistic infection in AIDS)
- Adenovirus
- CMV
- Herpes simplex virus
- *Mycobacterium tuberculosis*

Aspiration pneumonia

- ↑Risk with impairment of swallowing from neurological abnormalities (e.g. stroke, dementia, Parkinson's disease), ↓consciousness, oesophageal disease or iatrogenic intervention (e.g. NG tube, bronchoscopy)
- Oropharyngeal anaerobes

Symptoms

- Shortness of breath
- Purulent cough (typically green or rust-coloured sputum)
- Haemoptysis
- Fever ± rigors
- Chest pain (pleuritic)
- Systemic: malaise, anorexia, fatigue

Signs

- Look – Cyanosis, ↑RR, confusion
- Feel – Fever, tachycardia, dullness on percussion, ↑tactile fremitus, ↓chest expansion
- Listen – Bronchial breathing, ↓air entry, ↑vocal resonance, pleural rub

Clinical features

Investigations

- **Bloods**:
  - FBC: typically ↑WCC
  - CRP: typically raised
  - LFTs: may be deranged in legionella and sepsis
  - U&Es: assessing severity (urea), ↓Na^+ in legionella pneumonia
  - Serology: for mycoplasma
  - Blood culture
- **Sputum** Gram stain, culture and sensitivity
- **CXR** Lobar/multi-lobar infiltrates, air bronchogram, pleural effusion, consolidation (see *Fig. 1*) – repeat 6 weeks after treatment to ensure resolution
- **Urine** For pneumococcal or legionella antigen
- **ABG** Type 1 respiratory failure (↓PO_2 with ↔ or ↓PCO_2)

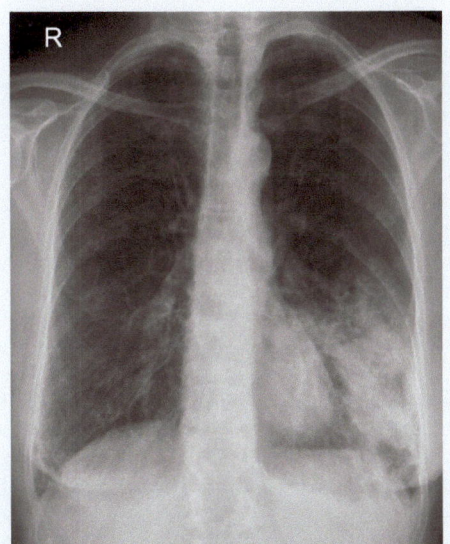

Fig. 1 Chest X-ray of a patient with CAP showing left lower lobe consolidation

Severity (CURB 65)

- **C**onfusion: Abbreviated mental test score (AMTS) ≤8
- **U**rea: >7mmol/L
- **R**espiratory rate: ≥30/min
- **B**lood pressure: systolic <90mmHg or diastolic ≤60mmHg
- **65** years or above

(Each of the above is worth 1 point: 0–1 outpatient care, 1–2 admission, ≥3 consider ITU treatment)

Spontaneous pneumothorax

▶Primary:

Occurs in the absence of known lung disease; risk factors include:
- Tall, thin stature
- Smoking
- Marfan syndrome
- Pregnancy
- Familial pneumothorax

▶Secondary:

- **Airway disease** COPD, asthma, cystic fibrosis
- **Infection** Pneumonia, TB
- **Malignancy** Lung cancer

- **Interstitial lung disease** e.g. Sarcoidosis, idiopathic pulmonary fibrosis
- **Connective tissue disease** e.g. RA, ankylosing spondylitis, Marfan syndrome, Ehlers–Danlos syndrome

Non-spontaneous pneumothorax

- **Traumatic pneumothorax** Follows a penetrating chest trauma such as a stab wound, gunshot injury or a fractured rib
- **Iatrogenic pneumothorax** A complication of medical or surgical procedures e.g. central line placement, lung biopsy and percutaneous liver biopsy
- **Catamenial pneumothorax** Refers to pneumothorax at the time of menstruation; due to thoracic endometriosis leading to necrotic holes in the diaphragm

Causes

A pneumothorax is a life-threatening condition that refers to a collection of air in the pleural cavity (between the lung and the chest wall) resulting in collapse of the lung on the affected side.

Definition

Pneumothorax

Complications

- Further pneumothorax
- Respiratory failure
- Cardiac arrest

Management

Immediate (see *Notes* for algorithm)

- **High-flow oxygen**
- **Tension pneumothorax** requires **immediate aspiration** in the 2nd intercostal space mid-clavicular line on the suspected side of pneumothorax (do not delay by obtaining a CXR)
- Observation for patients with a small PSP without breathlessness
- **Needle aspiration** For PSP (any size) and small SSP in patients <50 years
- **Chest drain** Indications include: in any ventilated patient, tension pneumothorax after initial needle relief, persistent or recurrent pneumothorax after simple aspiration, large SSP in patients >50 years

Long-term

- **Pleurodesis** If there has been recurrence or if high risk; involves prevention of further pneumothorax by obliterating the pleural space; surgical options are more effective but medical pleurodesis using talc and bleomycin may be appropriate for patients who are either unwilling or unable to undergo surgery
- **Surgery** For more difficult cases referral to thoracic surgeons may be considered; open thoracotomy or video-assisted thoracoscopic surgery (VATS) with pleurectomy and pleural abrasion; indications include bilateral pneumothoraces, failure of intercostal drainage, 2 or more previous pneumothoraces on same side or history of pneumothorax on other side
- **Smoking cessation** Reduces risk of a first pneumothorax and that of a recurrence

- The pathophysiology of pneumothorax depends on the underlying cause
- **Primary spontaneous pneumothorax (PSP)** occurs in the absence of known lung disease but in most patients occurs from the rupture of blebs and bullae; it typically occurs in tall, young people without parenchymal lung disease and is thought to be related to increased shear forces in the apex
- **Secondary spontaneous pneumothorax (SSP)** occurs in the presence of lung disease, most commonly COPD
- **Tension pneumothorax** typically occurs in blunt traumatic injuries e.g. a stab wound; air cannot escape on expiration due to a one-way valve mechanism; this results in mediastinal shift and significant lung collapse

Pathophysiology

Symptoms

- Acute SOB
- Acute pleuritic chest pain
- Sudden deterioration in patient with asthma or COPD

Signs

- ↓Expansion on affected side
- Hyper-resonance on affected side
- ↓Breath sounds on affected side
- Tracheal deviation to unaffected side (tension pneumothorax)
- Hypotension (tension pneumothorax)
- Distended neck veins (tension pneumothorax)

Clinical features

Investigations

- **CXR** Pleural line, reduced vascular markings on affected side (see *Fig. 1*) and deviation of trachea away from affected side in tension pneumothorax (see *Fig. 2*)
- **ABG** Type 1 respiratory failure
- **US chest** Main value is in management of supine trauma patients
- **CT chest** Recommended for uncertain or complex cases

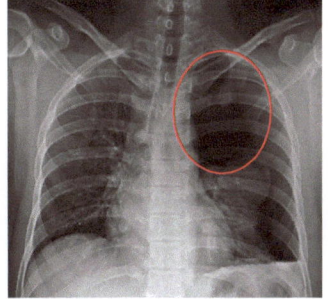

Fig. 1 Left-sided pneumothorax

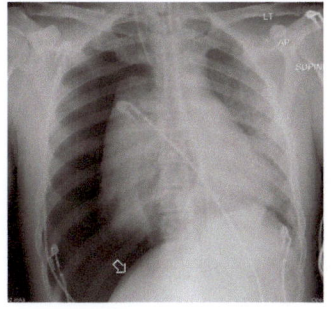

Fig. 2 Right-sided tension pneumothorax

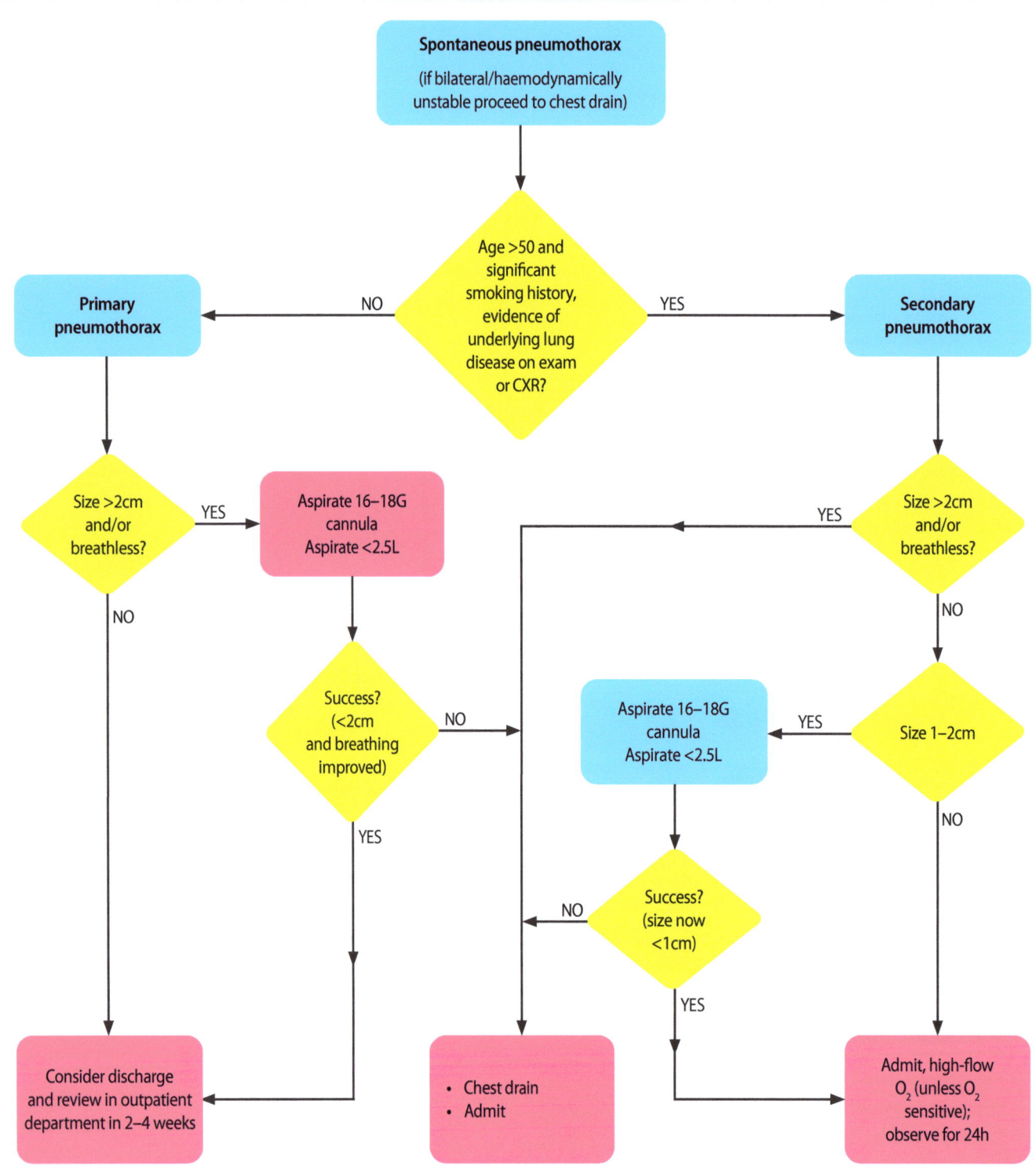

Management of spontaneous pneumothorax: British Thoracic Society pleural disease guideline 2010.

Definition

Pulmonary embolism (PE) is a condition in which one or more emboli, usually arising from a thrombus (blood clot) formed in the veins (or, rarely, in the right heart), are lodged in and obstruct the pulmonary arterial system.

Sources of emboli

- **Deep vein thrombosis (DVT)** The most common source of pulmonary emboli is a DVT in the lower limbs
- **Tumours** Most commonly prostate and breast cancers
- **Fat** From long-bone fractures
- **Amniotic fluid** In pregnant women
- **Sepsis** For example: tricuspid valve endocarditis in people who inject illicit drugs IV
- **Foreign body** e.g. During IV drug use, or from broken catheters, guide wires, vena cava filters etc.
- **Air**

(This mind map focuses on thrombotic PE)

Risk factors

- DVT
- Previous DVT/PE
- Surgery
- Obstetrics: late pregnancy, postpartum, caesarean
- Active cancer
- Immobility
- Increasing age
- Oestrogen: COCP, HRT
- Obesity
- Significant comorbidities: e.g. heart disease; metabolic, endocrine, neurological disability

Pulmonary embolism

Management

Acute

- **Oxygen**
- **Heparin:** anticoagulate with SC low molecular weight heparin (LMWH) (e.g. tinzaparin 175U/kg or enoxaparin 1.5U/kg) or IV heparin infusion
- **Thrombolysis:** e.g. alteplase, consider if critically ill or massive PE; 1st-line treatment for massive PE where there is circulatory failure (e.g. hypotension); may be considered also if there is evidence of right heart strain (on CTPA or ECHO); the Pulmonary Embolism Severity Index (PESI) score can be used to predict the outcome of PE and need for thrombolysis

Long-term

- **Warfarin** or a **direct oral anticoagulant (DOAC)** should ideally be commenced within 24h of diagnosis
- Examples of DOACs include rivaroxaban, apixaban and dabigatran; once started, heparin can be discontinued
- **Heparin** should be continued with warfarin however for 5 days or until the INR is in the therapeutic range (INR 2–3)
- In some cases, e.g. in a patient with active cancer, LMWH should be used long term instead of warfarin or DOACs
- The length of treatment depends on whether the PE is provoked, unprovoked or recurrent:
  - **Provoked PE:** warfarin or DOAC for 3 months; at 3 months clinicians should assess risks and benefits of extending treatment
  - **Unprovoked PEs:** warfarin or DOAC for 6 months and rule out underlying cancer
  - **Recurrent PEs:** lifelong warfarin or DOAC
  - **Patients with active cancer:** LMWH for 6 months

Symptoms

- Dyspnoea
- Chest pain: pleuritic chest pain, retrosternal chest pain
- Cough and haemoptysis
- Dizziness or syncope (right heart failure in severe cases)

Signs

- Tachypnoea, tachycardia
- Hypoxia
- Pyrexia
- Elevated jugular venous pressure
- Gallop heart rhythm, a widely split second heart sound, tricuspid regurgitant murmur
- Pleural rub
- Systemic hypotension and cardiogenic shock (massive PE)

Clinical features

Two-level Wells score (see *Fig. 1*)

- Clinically suspected DVT = 3.0
- Alternative diagnosis less likely than PE = 3.0
- Tachycardia (HR >100) = 1.5
- Immobilisation >3 days or surgery ≤4 weeks = 1.5
- History of DVT or PE = 1.0
- Haemoptysis = 1.0
- Malignancy = 1.0

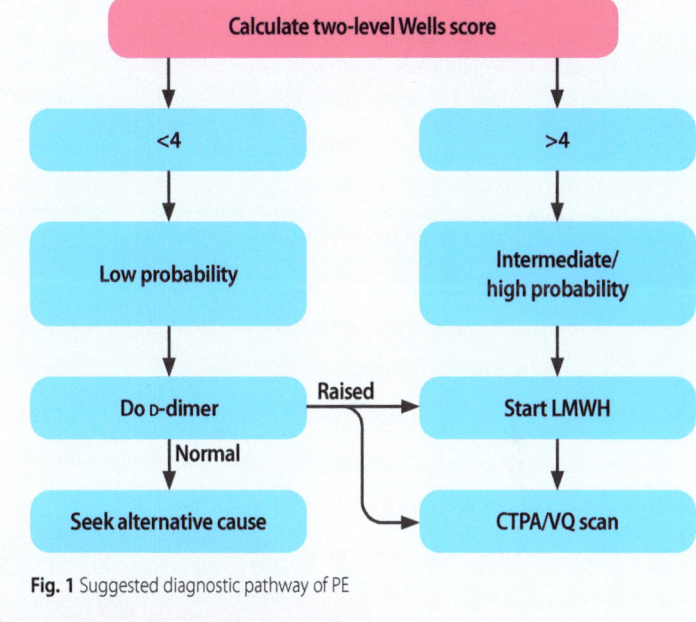

Calculate two-level Wells score

| <4 | >4 |

| Low probability | Intermediate/ high probability |

| Do D-dimer | —Raised→ | Start LMWH |

Normal

| Seek alternative cause | | CTPA/VQ scan |

Fig. 1 Suggested diagnostic pathway of PE

Calculating risk

Investigations

- **Bloods** Routine bloods to exclude other causes; D-dimers ↑sensitivity but ↓specificity; troponin and BNP levels may also be elevated if there is heart strain due to the PE
- **ECG** Any of: normal, sinus tachycardia (most common finding), AF, non-specific ST or T-wave abnormalities, right ventricular strain pattern V1–3, right axis deviation, right bundle branch block (RBBB) or 'S1Q3T3' pattern (see *Fig. 2*)
- **CXR** Usually normal; may show ↓vascular markings, small effusion or wedge-shaped area of infarction; mainly useful to exclude other chest disease
- **ABG** May show hypoxia/type 1 respiratory failure

- **ECHO** May show signs of right ventricular strain or right ventricular hypokinesis
- **CT pulmonary angiogram (CTPA)** Method of choice for imaging the pulmonary vasculature to identify PE (see *Fig. 3*)
- **Ventilation-perfusion (VQ) scan** May be used initially if appropriate facilities exist, the CXR is normal, and there is no significant symptomatic concurrent cardiopulmonary disease
- **Pulmonary angiography** The gold standard for diagnosis but is invasive with significant complication rates compared with above investigations

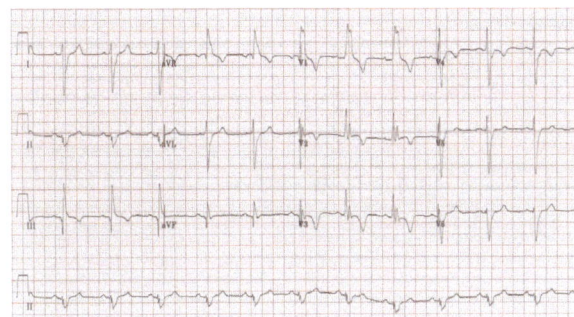

Fig. 2 'S1Q3T3' pattern on ECG

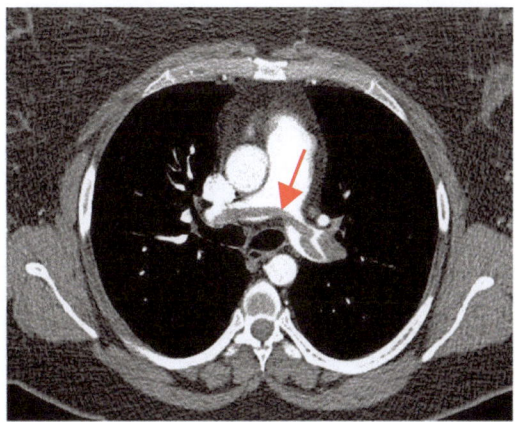

Fig. 3 CTPA showing saddle embolus sitting across main pulmonary arteries

Definition

Respiratory failure occurs when gas exchange is inadequate, resulting in hypoxia. It is defined as a P_aO_2 <8kPa and classified as either **type 1** or **type 2**, based on whether there is a high CO_2 level.

Classification

Type 1 respiratory failure

Defined as hypoxia (P_aO_2 <8kPa) with a **normal or low P_aCO_2**. It is caused primarily by ventilation/perfusion mismatch.

Type 2 respiratory failure

Defined as hypoxia (P_aO_2 <8kPa) with **hypercapnia** (P_aCO_2 >6kPa). This is caused by alveolar hypoventilation with or without ventilation/perfusion mismatch.

Respiratory failure

Management

Type 1 respiratory failure

- Treat the underlying cause
- Give O_2 via facemask to correct hypoxia
- Assisted ventilation if P_aO_2 <8kPa despite 60% O_2

Type 2 respiratory failure

- Treat the underlying cause
- Controlled oxygen therapy via venturi mask; start at 24% O_2; O_2 therapy should be given with care but hypoxia should not be left untreated
- Recheck the arterial blood gas after approx. 20min; if P_aCO_2 is steady or lower, increase O_2 concentration in stages (see *Fig. 1*)
- If P_aCO_2 has risen above 1.5kPa and the patient is still hypoxic, consider a respiratory stimulant or assisted ventilation (e.g. NIPPV, non-invasive positive pressure ventilation)
- If improvement with NIPPV, continue and adjust settings accordingly
- If this fails consider intubation and ventilation if appropriate

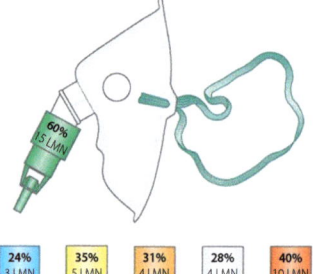

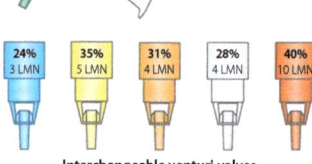

Interchangeable venturi valves

Fig. 1 Venturi masks are used to deliver controlled percentages of O_2 in patients at risk of type 2 respiratory failure

Investigations

- Bloods: FBC, U&Es, CRP
- ABG
- Peak expiratory flow rate
- Chest radiology: CXR, CT
- Microbiology: sputum and blood cultures
- Spirometry
- ECG

Type 1 respiratory failure

- Pneumonia
- Pulmonary oedema
- Pulmonary embolism
- Asthma
- Pulmonary fibrosis
- Pneumothorax
- Bronchiectasis
- Acute respiratory distress syndrome

Type 2 respiratory failure

- **Obstructive pulmonary disease** Asthma (severe), COPD, obstructive sleep apnoea
- **Reduced respiratory drive** Sedative drugs, CNS tumour or trauma
- **Neuromuscular disease** Cervical cord lesion, diaphragmatic paralysis, poliomyelitis, myasthenia gravis, Guillain–Barré syndrome
- **Thoracic wall disease** Flail chest, kyphosis, scoliosis

Causes

Clinical features

Hypoxia

- Dyspnoea
- Restlessness
- Agitation
- Confusion
- Central cyanosis
- Long-standing polycythaemia, pulmonary hypertension, cor pulmonale

Hypercapnia

- Headache
- Peripheral vasodilatation
- Tachycardia
- Bounding pulse
- Tremor/flap
- Papilloedema
- Confusion
- Drowsiness
- Coma

Definition

A **multisystem chronic inflammatory condition** characterised by the formation of **non-caseating epithelioid granulomata** at various sites in the body: most commonly the lungs, lymph nodes, eyes and skin. In approximately 50% of cases the disease is detected incidentally on routine CXR in an asymptomatic individual.

Pathophysiology

- It is thought that one or more unidentified antigen(s) triggers activation of T-helper cells followed by the development of non-caseating granulomata in genetically susceptible individuals
- The granulomas consist of macrophages, epithelioid cells and multinucleated giant cells surrounded by lymphocytes, monocytes, mast cells and fibroblasts
- The accumulation of T lymphocytes, mononuclear phagocytic cells and non-caseating granulomas occurs in involved organs; these granulomas may resolve spontaneously or lead to secondary fibrosis and permanent organ damage
- Sarcoidosis involves the lungs in >90% of cases and commonly the lymphoreticular system, skin, eyes, muscles and joints; less commonly other organs, including the heart, kidneys, brain and the peripheral nervous system

Sarcoidosis

Prognosis

Poor prognostic factors

- Insidious onset, symptoms >6 months
- Absence of erythema nodosum
- Extrapulmonary manifestations e.g. lupus pernio, splenomegaly
- CXR: stage III–IV features
- Black ethnicity

Management

Steroids

- Oral prednisolone or IV hydrocortisone
- Indication for steroids include:
  - CXR stage II or III who have moderate to severe or progressive symptoms
  - Hypercalcaemia
  - Eye, heart or neuro involvement

DMARDs/biological agents

- Antimetabolites, e.g. methotrexate, azathioprine, leflunomide and mycophenolate, are alternatives to steroids
- TNF alpha inhibitors, e.g. infliximab and adalimumab, may be prescribed if patients not responding to antimetabolites

Surgical

- Surgery may be considered with severe progressive lung fibrosis, including lung transplantation (rare)

Investigations

- **Bloods FBC** (WCC usually raised), **CRP/ESR** (usually raised), **calcium** (usually raised), **LFTs** (deranged if liver involvement), **ACE level** raised in approx. 60% of patients with acute disease and decreases in response to treatment/resolution of the disease
- **CXR** (see *Staging*)
- **ECG** To check for early signs of rhythm disturbance due to conducting system disease or effects of hypercalcaemia
- **Tuberculin test** Typically negative in patients with sarcoidosis
- **CT chest** Used to detect and assess the severity of interstitial lung disease
- **Lung function tests** Show restrictive defect in severe, progressive cases
- **Bronchoalveolar lavage** ↑Lymphocytes, ↑CD4:CD8 ratio
- **Biopsy** Transbronchial, lymph node or skin lesion biopsies demonstrate non-caseating granulomas
- **FGD PET scan** Can be used to assess inflammatory activity accurately in patients
- **Gallium scan** May be used to detect extrapulmonary disease and tends to reveal a 'lambda' pattern

- **Constitutional symptoms** Fever, night sweats, malaise, weight loss
- **Lymph nodes** Commonly picked up on CXR but may be symptomatic and affect the axillary, cervical and inguinal nodes
- **Lungs** Cough (usually dry), breathlessness, wheeze, fine crackles
- **Skin** Erythema nodosum (*Fig. 1*), lupus pernio, infiltration of scars by granulomas
- **Eyes** Uveitis (anterior and posterior), dry eyes, glaucoma
- **Heart** Arrhythmia, cardiomyopathy, heart failure, conduction defects
- **Neurological** Meningeal inflammation, seizures, mass lesions, neuropathy, hypothalamic pituitary infiltration
- **Hypercalcaemia** Nephrolithiasis, neuropsychiatric disturbance, abdominal pain, bone pain
- **Liver** Commonly involved but rarely clinically significant, hepatitis, hepatosplenomegaly

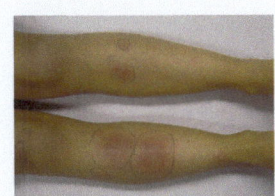

Fig. 1 Erythema nodosum

- **Löfgren syndrome** An acute form of the disease characterised by bilateral hilar lymphadenopathy, erythema nodosum, fever and polyarthralgia; it usually carries an excellent prognosis
- **Mikulicz syndrome** Enlargement of the parotid and lacrimal glands due to sarcoidosis, TB or lymphoma
- **Heerfordt syndrome** Parotid enlargement, fever and uveitis secondary to sarcoidosis

Clinical features

Staging

There are 5 stages of sarcoidosis according to CXR findings (see *Fig. 2*)
- **Stage 0** Normal CXR findings
- **Stage I** Bihilar lymphadenopathy
- **Stage II** Bihilar lymphadenopathy + parenchymal infiltrates
- **Stage III** Parenchymal infiltrates alone
- **Stage IV** Pulmonary fibrosis

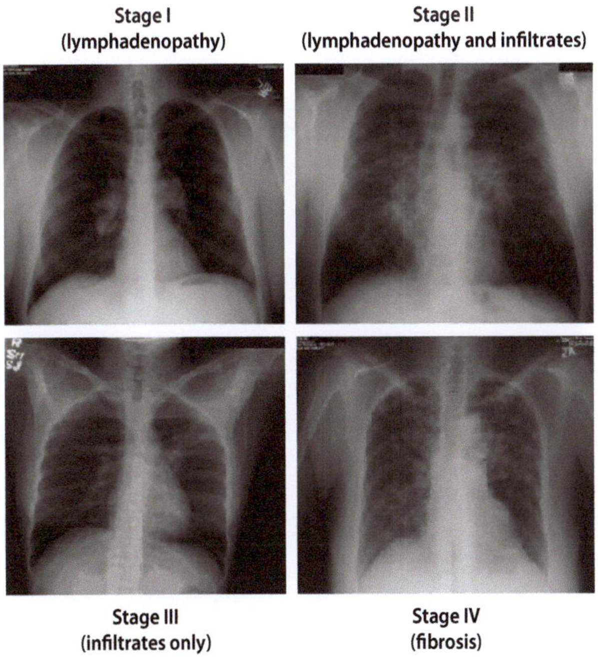

Stage I
(lymphadenopathy)

Stage II
(lymphadenopathy and infiltrates)

Stage III
(infiltrates only)

Stage IV
(fibrosis)

Fig. 2 Stages I–IV of sarcoidosis

Epidemiology and risk factors

- Age: occurs at all ages, although it usually develops before the age of 50 years, with the incidence peaking at 20–39
- Can occur in all ethnic groups but the disease is more severe in African–Caribbeans than Caucasians
- Family history increases risk
- HLA-B8 antigens and HLA-DRB1 and -DQB1 alleles have been shown to confer susceptibility
- Environmental associations: emissions from wood-burning stoves and tree pollen, exposure to inorganic particles, insecticides and mouldy environments have been reported; positive associations have also been made with service in the US Navy, metalworking, firefighting and the handling of building supplies; bacteria such as mycobacteria have also been linked with sarcoidosis

03

Chapter 3

Gastroenterology

Acute liver failure (ALF) is an uncommon but life-threatening illness in which rapid deterioration of the liver function results in coagulopathy and alteration in the mental status of a previously healthy individual.

Definition

Classification

Bernau's classification

- **Fulminant hepatic failure (FHF)** Liver failure takes place within 8 weeks of the onset of the underlying illness
- **Subacute FHF** or **late-onset hepatic failure** Occurs when there has been a gap of 8–26 weeks between the onset of illness and liver failure

O'Grady's classification

- **Hyperacute** Liver failure occurring **<7 days** from disease onset
- **Acute** Liver failure occurring **1–4 weeks** from disease onset
- **Subacute** Liver failure occurring **4–12 weeks** from disease onset

Acute liver failure

Management

Supportive measures and monitoring

- Should be managed in specialised liver unit or ITU setting with regular monitoring
- Patients who have advanced encephalopathy should have airways protected with intubation and NG tube inserted to avoid aspiration and remove any blood from stomach

Treat underlying cause

- e.g. IV NAC for paracetamol overdose, stop offending drugs, steroids for autoimmune hepatitis

Manage complications

- **Treat bleeding/raised INR** Vitamin K e.g. 10mg IV, platelets, fresh frozen and red cells as needed
- **Treat renal failure** Haemofiltration or haemodialysis

- **Manage infections** Broad-spectrum antibiotics e.g. IV ceftriaxone
- **Manage hypoglycaemia** IV dextrose
- **Manage ascites** Restrict fluid, low-salt diet, daily weights, diuretics
- **Manage hypotension** Monitor with arterial line, fluid resuscitation
- **Manage encephalopathy** Avoid sedatives, correct electrolytes, lactulose
- **Treat seizures** Phenytoin
- **Manage cerebral oedema** Patients should be positioned with the head elevated at 30° in ITU; patient should have ICP monitoring; treat with IV mannitol and hyperventilation

Emergency liver transplantation

King's College Criteria for liver transplant
Predicts poor outcome in acute liver failure and should prompt consideration for transplantation

Criteria for paracetamol-induced liver failure

- Arterial pH <7.30 (24h after ingestion)

OR all of the following:
- INR >6.5 (PT >100sec)
- Creatinine >300µmol/L
- Grade III or IV hepatic encephalopathy

Criteria for non-paracetamol-induced liver failure

Prothrombin time >100sec (INR >6.5)
OR any three of the following (**PADDS**):
- **P**rothrombin time >50sec (INR >3.5)
- **A**ge <10 or >40 years
- **D**rug-induced liver failure
- **D**uration of jaundice to hepatic encephalopathy >7 days
- **S**erum bilirubin >300µmol/L

- **Infection** Viral hepatitis (mainly hepatitis A or B, it is extremely uncommon in hepatitis C), leptospirosis, yellow fever, EBV, CMV, herpes simplex virus, dengue virus
- **Drugs** Paracetamol overdose (most common cause in developed countries), halothane, isoniazid, phenytoin, amiodarone, propylthiouracil, Ecstasy, herbal remedies, amoebic infection
- **Toxins** *Amanita phalloides* mushroom toxin, carbon tetrachloride, yellow phosphorus

- **Wilson's disease**
- **Autoimmune hepatitis**
- **Budd–Chiari syndrome**
- **Pregnancy related** Acute fatty liver of pregnancy, HELLP syndrome
- **Reye syndrome** Rare side effect of aspirin
- **Ischaemic hepatitis** e.g. From shock or heart failure
- **Indeterminate**

Causes

- **Jaundice**
- **Encephalopathy** (classification):
  - **Grade 0** No personality or behavioural abnormality detected
  - **Grade 1** Lack of awareness, euphoria or anxiety, shortened attention span, impaired performance of addition
  - **Grade 2** Lethargy or apathy, minimal disorientation for time or place, subtle personality change, inappropriate behaviour, impaired performance of subtraction
  - **Grade 3** Somnolence to semi stupor but responsive to verbal stimuli, confusion, gross disorientation
  - **Grade 4** Coma
- Fetor hepaticus
- Asterixis/hepatic flap
- Constructional apraxia
- Hypoglycaemia
- Bleeding and bruising
- Hepatomegaly
- Ascites

Clinical features

Notes

Acute liver failure

Complications

- Cerebral oedema
- Hypoglycaemia
- Hypotension
- Hepatorenal syndrome
- Sepsis
- Seizures
- Acute respiratory distress syndrome

Investigations

- **Bloods** FBC, ESR, CRP, LFTs, U&Es, glucose, ANA, AMA, SMA, immunoglobulins, prothrombin time/INR, hepatitis screen, EBV and CMV serology, paracetamol and salicylate levels
- **ABG**
- **Ceruloplasmin and 24-h urine copper** If suspected Wilson's disease
- **Blood cultures**
- **Doppler of hepatic veins** If suspected Budd–Chiari syndrome
- **CXR**
- **US abdomen**
- **Ascitic tap** If ascites present

Acute inflammation of the pancreas causing the release of exocrine enzymes that cause autodigestion of the organ. There may be involvement of local tissues and distant organs.

- A trigger, e.g. alcohol or any of the causes listed, is thought to activate a common pathway leading to marked elevation of intracellular calcium leading to activation of intracellular proteases and release of exocrine pancreatic enzymes
- This results in acinar cell injury and necrosis which promote migration of inflammatory cells
- This leads to local inflammatory response and occasionally a systemic inflammatory response, resulting in single or multi-organ failure

- **G**allstones ⎫ By far the most common causes
- **E**thanol ⎬
- **T**rauma
- **S**teroids
- **M**umps (other viruses include Coxsackie B)
- **A**utoimmune (e.g. polyarteritis nodosa), **A**scaris infection
- **S**corpion venom
- **H**ypertriglyceridaemia, **H**yperchylomicronaemia, **H**ypercalcaemia, **H**ypothermia
- **E**RCP
- **D**rugs e.g. azathioprine, bendroflumethiazide, furosemide, mesalazine, steroids, sodium valproate

Definition

Pathophysiology

Causes (GET SMASHED)

Acute pancreatitis

Complications

Local (the Ps)

- **P**seudocyst
- **P**ancreatic abscess
- **P**ancreatic necrosis
- **P**ancreatic fistulae
- Chronic **P**ancreatitis

Systemic (DR SAM)

- **D**isseminated intravascular coagulation
- **R**enal failure (acute)
- **S**epsis
- **A**cute respiratory distress syndrome
- **M**ultiple organ dysfunction

Management

- Initially **nil by mouth** and resuscitation with **IV fluids**
- **Oxygen**
- **Pain relief** e.g. with opioids
- **Antibiotics (broad spectrum)** For treatment of associated cholangitis or other acute infections; if pancreatic necrosis is suspected, IV antibiotics should be given
- Severe cases should be treated in **ITU** or a **HDU**
- **Nutritional support** Oral feeding can commence in people with mild acute pancreatitis (in absence of nausea/ vomiting, or abdominal pain); enteral feeding is otherwise preferable and is possible in the majority of people; parenteral feeding is reserved for people in whom enteral nutrition is not possible

Assessing severity

Glasgow Imrie criteria (PANCREAS) at 48h after admission:
- P_aO_2 (arterial) <8.0kPa
- **A**ge >55 years
- **N**eutrophilia White blood cells >15×10^9/L
- **C**alcium <2.0mmol/L
- **R**enal (serum urea) >16mmol/L
- **E**nzymes LDH >600IU/L
- **A**lbumin <32g/L
- **S**ugar (glucose) >10mmol/L

(≥3 points: high risk for severe pancreatitis)
Other scoring systems for prognosis include: **Ranson's Criteria/Acute Physiology and Chronic Health Evaluation II (APACHE II)** as well as measurement of **CRP**

Symptoms

- Acute upper abdominal pain (may radiate to the back)
- Nausea/vomiting
- Anorexia
- Pyrexia

Signs

- Fever, hypotension, tachycardia, tachypnoea
- Epigastric tenderness, with guarding on abdominal examination
- Decreased bowel sounds
- Jaundice
- Grey Turner's sign (ecchymosis of the flank) and Cullen's sign (ecchymoses in the periumbilical region) (see *Fig. 1*)

Clinical features

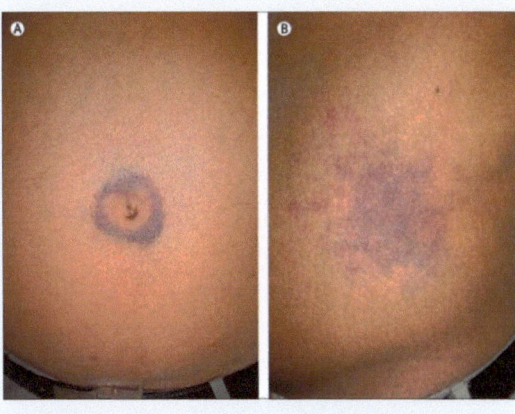

Fig. 1 Cullen's sign (A) and Grey Turner's sign (B): signs of retroperitoneal haemorrhage (a late clinical feature of acute pancreatitis)

Notes

Acute pancreatitis

Investigations

Bloods

- Pancreatic enzymes: **serum amylase** raised (typically ≥3× upper limit of normal); **lipase** levels are more sensitive and more specific
- FBC, U&Es, glucose and CRP indicate prognosis (see *Assessing severity*)
- Raised bilirubin and/or serum aminotransferase (suggest gallstones)
- Calcium (hypocalcaemia is relatively common and may indicate prognosis)

Imaging

- **AXR (erect)** Excludes other differentials, e.g. intestinal obstruction and perforation, and may show pancreatic calcification
- **CXR** May show elevation of one hemidiaphragm, infiltrates ± acute respiratory distress syndrome or pleural effusions (in severe cases)
- **CT pancreas (contrast-enhanced)** Can identify pancreatic swelling, fluid collection and change in density of gland; this has implications for prognosis and predicts the need for surgery
- **US abdomen** Can show a swollen pancreas, dilated common bile duct and free peritoneal fluid; it is also useful for detecting gallstones
- **MRI pancreas** May reveal acute abdominal wall oedema which may be useful in assessing severity

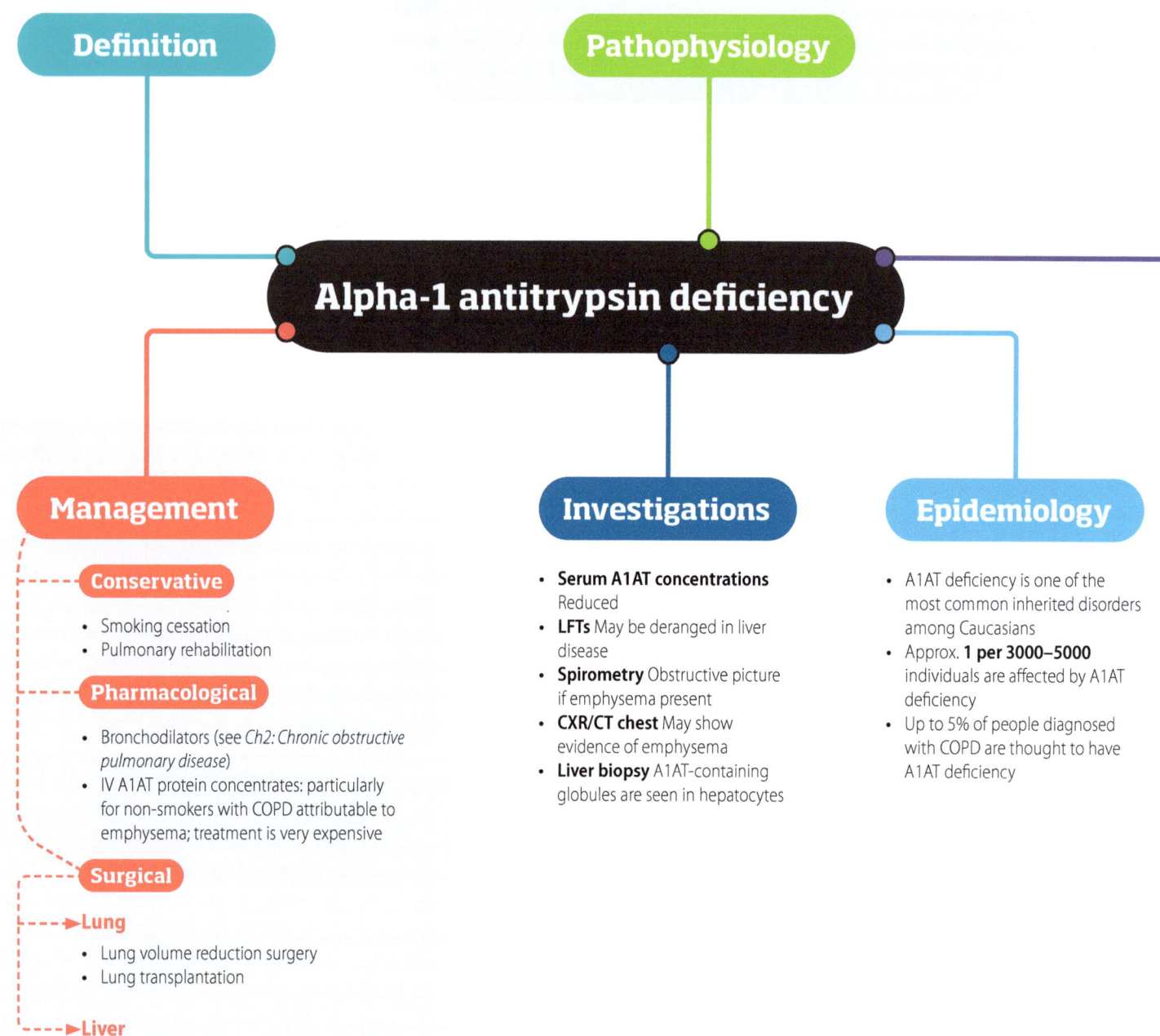

Definition

Alpha-1 antitrypsin (A1AT) deficiency is a common inherited condition caused by lack of the protease inhibitor (Pi) A1AT normally produced by the liver. It classically causes emphysema (i.e. COPD) in patients who are young and non-smokers.

Pathophysiology

- The gene for A1AT is found on chromosome 14 and is inherited in an **autosomal recessive fashion**
- Alleles are classified by their electrophoretic mobility: M, normal; S, slow; and Z, very slow:
  - *Normal* = **PiMM**
  - *Homozygous* **PiSS** (50% normal A1AT levels)
  - *Homozygous* **PiZZ** (10% normal A1AT levels)
- The role of A1AT is to protect cells from enzymes such as neutrophil elastase
- Patients who manifest disease usually have **PiZZ genotype**
- If there is a deficiency of A1AT then elastase can break down elastin unchecked; in the lungs this can cause destruction of alveolar walls resulting in emphysema
- Some people may develop liver disease due to congestion of A1AT in the liver cells causing cell destruction

Alpha-1 antitrypsin deficiency

Management

Conservative

- Smoking cessation
- Pulmonary rehabilitation

Pharmacological

- Bronchodilators (see *Ch2: Chronic obstructive pulmonary disease*)
- IV A1AT protein concentrates: particularly for non-smokers with COPD attributable to emphysema; treatment is very expensive

Surgical

►Lung

- Lung volume reduction surgery
- Lung transplantation

►Liver

- Liver failure may require liver transplantation

Investigations

- **Serum A1AT concentrations** Reduced
- **LFTs** May be deranged in liver disease
- **Spirometry** Obstructive picture if emphysema present
- **CXR/CT chest** May show evidence of emphysema
- **Liver biopsy** A1AT-containing globules are seen in hepatocytes

Epidemiology

- A1AT deficiency is one of the most common inherited disorders among Caucasians
- Approx. **1 per 3000–5000** individuals are affected by A1AT deficiency
- Up to 5% of people diagnosed with COPD are thought to have A1AT deficiency

Lungs

- Lung disease does not usually present until people are in their 30s or 40s, with smokers tending to develop symptoms approx. 10 years earlier than non-smokers
- COPD symptoms: dyspnoea, wheezing and cough most common (see *Ch2: Chronic obstructive pulmonary disease*)
- There is increased risk of lung cancer

Liver

(Not everyone with A1AT deficiency will develop liver disease)

►Neonates/children

- Neonates may present with neonatal jaundice and hepatitis
- Older children may develop hepatitis, cirrhosis and liver failure

►Adults

- May develop hepatitis, fibrosis, cirrhosis and liver failure
- Increased risk of hepatocellular carcinoma (due to above)

Clinical features

Notes

Alpha-1 antitrypsin deficiency

Chronic pancreatitis is a chronic, irreversible inflammation and/or fibrosis of the pancreas, typically characterised by severe abdominal pain and progressive endocrine and exocrine insufficiency.

- The underlying mechanism is unclear
- Abnormalities of bicarbonate excretion caused by functional defects at the level of the cellular wall, e.g. in cystic fibrosis, or mechanical causes e.g. trauma, can result in pancreatic enzyme activation
- Pancreatic enzyme activation leads to pancreatic tissue injury and necrosis
- Pancreatic fibrogenesis is a typical response to injury involving a complex interplay of growth factors, cytokines and chemokines, leading to the deposition of extracellular matrix
- Alcohol causes proteins to precipitate in the ductular structure of the pancreas; this leads to local pancreatic dilatation and fibrosis; there may also be direct toxic effects of alcohol on the pancreas
- Oxidative stress seems to play an important role in the pathogenesis of chronic pancreatitis

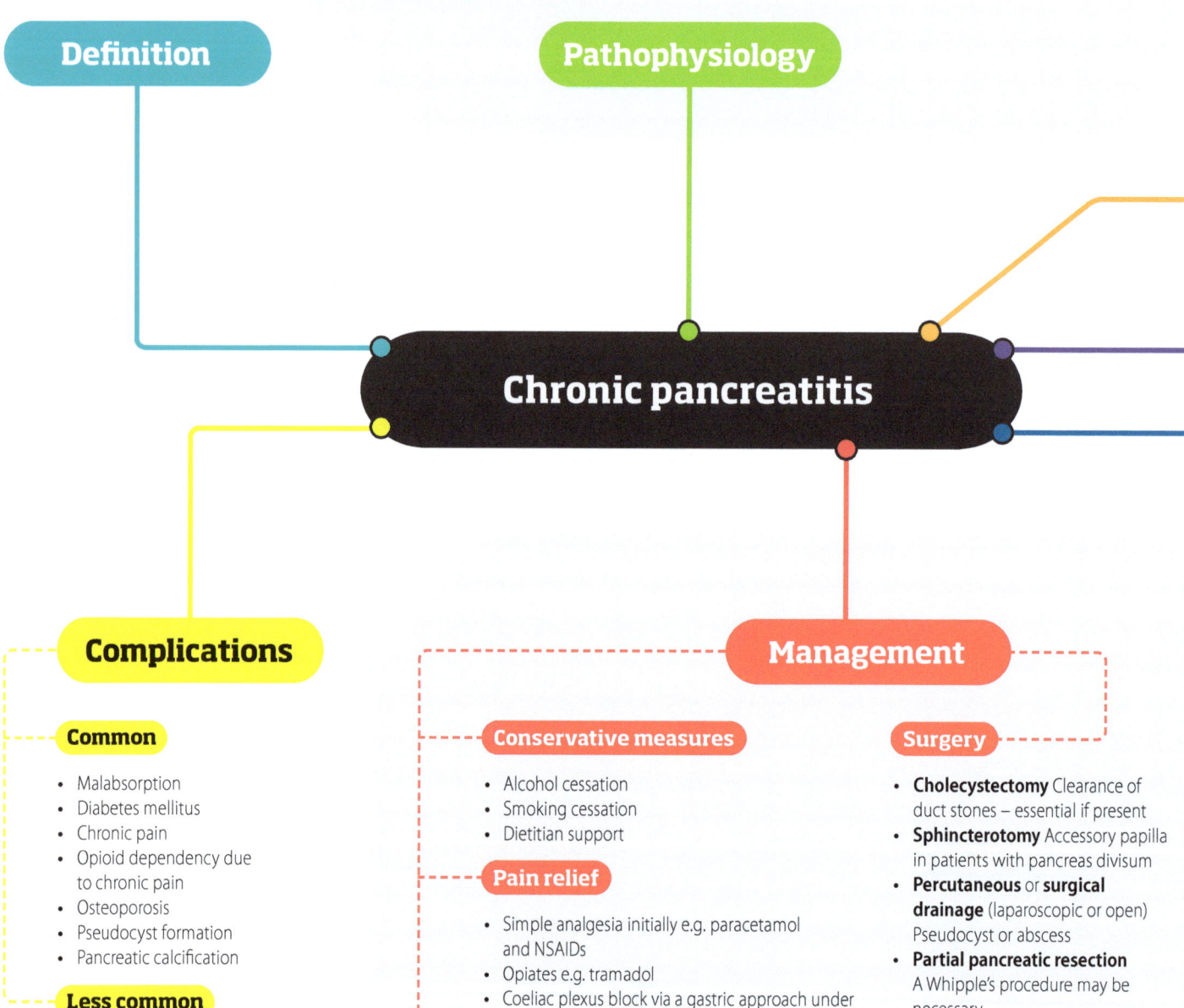

Definition

Pathophysiology

Chronic pancreatitis

Complications

Common

- Malabsorption
- Diabetes mellitus
- Chronic pain
- Opioid dependency due to chronic pain
- Osteoporosis
- Pseudocyst formation
- Pancreatic calcification

Less common

- Duodenal/gastric outlet obstruction
- Biliary obstruction
- Pancreatic cancer
- Fistulae
- Splenic or portal vein thrombosis
- Pseudoaneurysm

Management

Conservative measures

- Alcohol cessation
- Smoking cessation
- Dietitian support

Pain relief

- Simple analgesia initially e.g. paracetamol and NSAIDs
- Opiates e.g. tramadol
- Coeliac plexus block via a gastric approach under endoscopic US guidance
- ERCP may help to reduce pain by dilating strictures of the pancreatic ducts

Managing pancreatic insufficiency

- Replacement of pancreatic enzymes can help malabsorption and also reduce pain e.g. Creon®
- Fat-soluble vitamins (A, D, E, K)
- Treat diabetes mellitus accordingly e.g. insulin

Surgery

- **Cholecystectomy** Clearance of duct stones – essential if present
- **Sphincterotomy** Accessory papilla in patients with pancreas divisum
- **Percutaneous** or **surgical drainage** (laparoscopic or open) Pseudocyst or abscess
- **Partial pancreatic resection** A Whipple's procedure may be necessary
- **Extracorporeal shockwave lithotripsy** For adults with pancreatic duct obstruction caused by a dominant stone if surgery is unsuitable
- **Total pancreatectomy** A last resort for relief of intractable pain not responding to other methods

- **Alcohol** Approx. 70–80% of cases
- **Idiopathic** Approx. 25% of cases
- **Smoking** An independent risk factor
- **Congenital** Pancreas divisum, annular pancreas
- **Familial** Hereditary pancreatitis, cystic fibrosis
- **Metabolic** Hypercalcaemia, hyperlipidaemia
- **Iatrogenic** e.g. ERCP, abdominal radiotherapy

- **Drugs** e.g. Thiazide diuretics, azathioprine, tetracyclines, valproic acid and DDP-4 inhibitors
- **Trauma**
- **Obstruction of the pancreatic duct** e.g. Pseudocysts, ductal strictures, periampullary tumours, gallstones (uncommon)
- **Autoimmune disease** Sjögren syndrome, IBD and primary biliary cirrhosis

Clinical features

- Abdominal pain: classically epigastric pain radiating into the back
- Nausea and vomiting
- Decreased appetite
- Malabsorption with weight loss, diarrhoea, steatorrhea and protein deficiency
- Diabetes mellitus (see *Ch5: Diabetes mellitus*)

Investigations

Bloods

Serum amylase (usually normal but may be mildly raised in an acute on chronic attack), **albumin** and **clotting studies** (may be deranged in liver disease), **low calcium** and **B₁₂** (suggests malabsorption), **ALP** (raised levels suggests biliary tract obstruction if gamma-glutamyltransferase is also raised), raised **glucose/HbA1c** (in endocrine dysfunction), **serum trypsinogen** (low)

Imaging

- **AXR** 30% show pancreatic calcification in later stages (see *Fig. 1*).
- **Abdominal US** Reveals gallstones, duct dilatation, pancreatic morphology
- **Abdominal CT** 1st-line imaging modality for people with a history and symptoms suggestive of chronic alcohol-related pancreatitis
- **MRCP/ERCP** Useful to look for treatable strictures, tumours, stones or pseudocysts
- **Endoscopic US** Irregular duct walls, duct dilatation and cysts can be detected

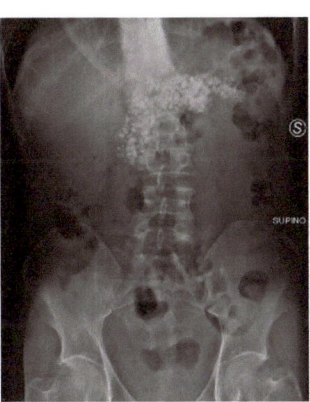

Fig. 1 Calcification of pancreas on AXR

Stool

- Faecal elastase (reduced if malabsorption present)

Cirrhosis results from necrosis of liver cells followed by fibrosis and nodule formation. This results in impairment of liver cell function and gross distortion of the liver architecture, leading to complications such as portal hypertension.

Cirrhosis can be described as:

- **Compensated** The liver can still function effectively with few or no clinical symptoms
- **Decompensated** The liver is damaged to the point that it cannot function adequately with evident clinical complications (see *Clinical features*)

- Liver fibrosis results from chronic insult (due to causes listed) resulting in abnormal connective tissue production and deposition
- Cirrhosis is an advanced stage of liver fibrosis that is accompanied by distortion of the hepatic architecture
- Historically, cirrhosis can be divided into 2 types histologically:
  - **Micronodular** (often caused by alcohol excess or biliary tract disease) *or*

- **Macronodular** (often seen in chronic viral hepatitis) depending on the size of nodules, although a mixed picture is also seen
- The major clinical consequences of cirrhosis are impaired hepatocyte function, increased intrahepatic resistance and the development of hepatocellular carcinoma
- Multiple circulatory abnormalities in cirrhosis are closely linked to the hepatic vascular alterations resulting in portal hypertension

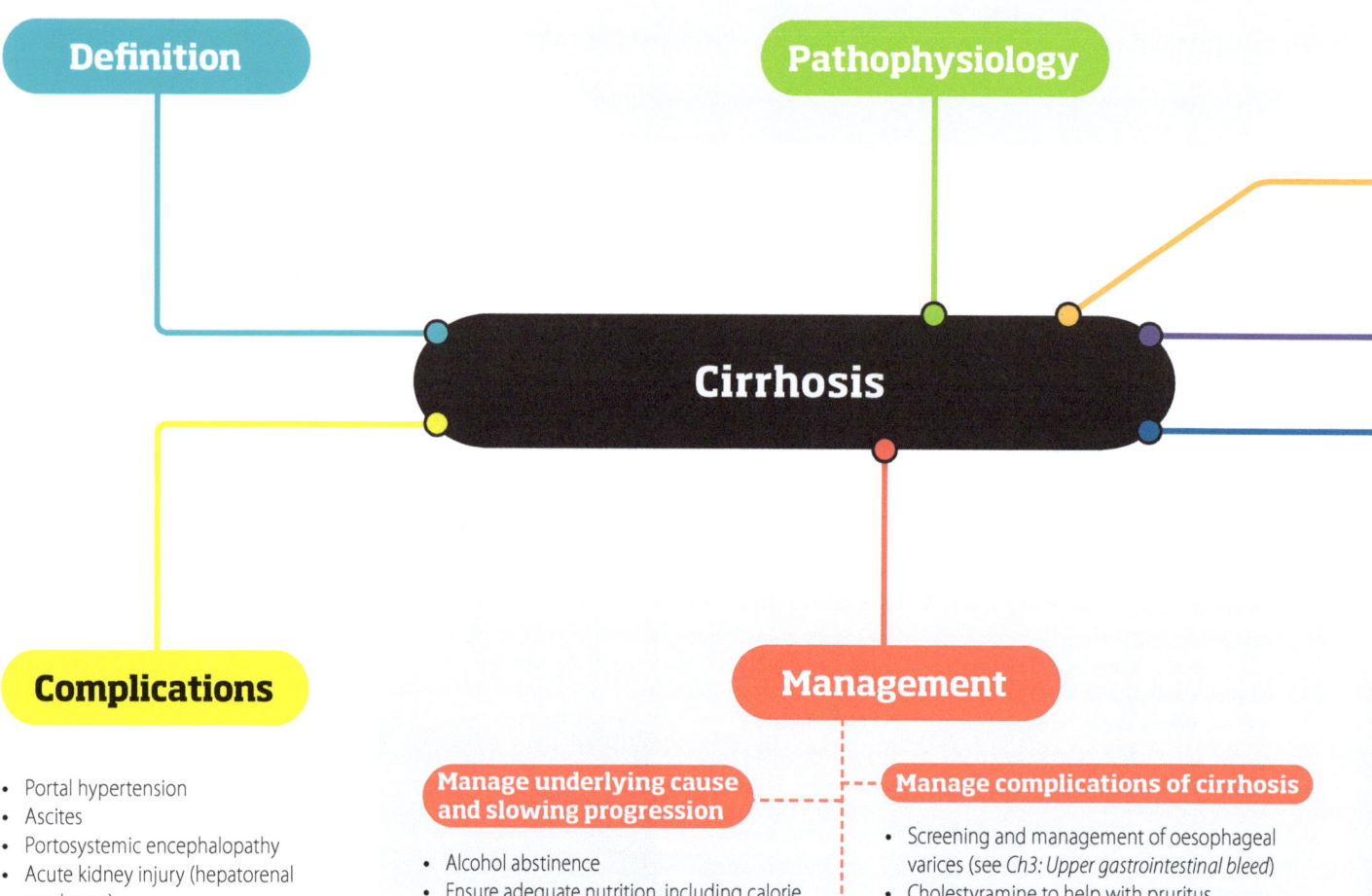

Definition

Pathophysiology

Cirrhosis

Complications

- Portal hypertension
- Ascites
- Portosystemic encephalopathy
- Acute kidney injury (hepatorenal syndrome)
- Hepatopulmonary syndrome
- HCC
- Bacteraemia, infection
- Malnutrition
- Osteoporosis

Management

Manage underlying cause and slowing progression

- Alcohol abstinence
- Ensure adequate nutrition, including calorie and protein intake
- Treat haemochromatosis accordingly e.g. venesection (see *Ch3: Haemochromatosis*)
- Treat viral hepatitis accordingly (see *Ch8: Hepatitis* sections)
- Steroids for autoimmune chronic active hepatitis
- Avoid hepatotoxic drugs

Manage complications of cirrhosis

- Screening and management of oesophageal varices (see *Ch3: Upper gastrointestinal bleed*)
- Cholestyramine to help with pruritus
- Manage hepatic encephalopathy appropriately e.g. with oral lactulose
- Management of ascites (see *Notes*)
- Screening and management of osteoporosis (see *Ch7: Osteoporosis*)

Monitoring and screening for hepatocellular carcinoma (HCC)

US liver ± alpha-fetoprotein every 6 months as surveillance for HCC

Liver transplantation

The only definitive treatment for cirrhosis

- **Alcohol** Excess
- **Viral hepatitis** Approx. 10% of cases (types B, C and D) ⎫ Most common causes
- **Non-alcoholic fatty liver disease (NAFLD)** ⎭
- **Genetic:**
  - Haemochromatosis
  - Alpha-1 antitrypsin deficiency
  - Wilson's disease
  - Galactosaemia (rare)
  - Congenital tyrosinaemia
  - Glycogen storage disease type IV
  - Cystic fibrosis
- **Autoimmune:**
  - Primary biliary cholangitis (PBC)
  - Primary sclerosing cholangitis (PSC)
  - Autoimmune hepatitis
  - Sarcoidosis
- **Hepatic venous outflow obstruction:**
  - Hepatic veno-occlusive disease
  - Budd–Chiari syndrome
  - Congestive hepatopathy (from constrictive pericarditis)
- **Drugs** e.g. Methotrexate, amiodarone, methyldopa

Causes

(Compensated cirrhosis may be asymptomatic)

Decompensated clinical features

- Jaundice
- Signs of portal hypertension: ascites, caput medusae, splenomegaly, variceal haemorrhage
- Signs of hepatic encephalopathy

Features of chronic liver disease

- Nails: leuconychia, Terry's nails, clubbing
- Palmar erythema
- Dupuytren's contracture
- Spider naevi (see *Fig. 1*)
- Xanthelasma
- Hepatomegaly
- Gynaecomastia (see *Fig. 2*), atrophic testes, loss of body hair
- Parotid enlargement

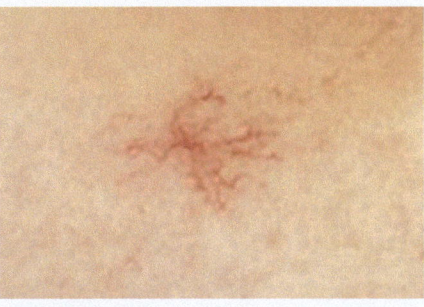

Fig. 1 Spider naevi

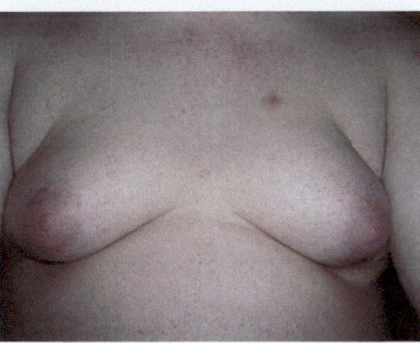

Fig. 2 Gynaecomastia

Clinical features

Investigations

- **Bloods:**
  - FBC (occult bleeding may cause anaemia, macrocytic anaemia in alcohol misuse, ↓WCC and platelets may indicate hypersplenism)
  - Biochemistry: LFTs (may show ↑bilirubin, ALT, AST, gamma-GT), clotting and albumin (↓albumin and ↑INR if synthetic function affected), U&Es (may show ↓Na⁺ and renal function deranged in hepatorenal syndrome), glucose (may be deranged)
  - Specific tests for underlying cause: serum alpha-fetoprotein (↓ in alpha-1 antitrypsin deficiency), ceruloplasmin (if suspected Wilson's disease); iron studies and *HFE* gene mutation analysis (in suspected haemochromatosis); viral hepatitis screen (if suspected viral hepatitis cause); enhanced liver fibrosis (ELF) test in people with NAFLD to test for advanced liver fibrosis; autoantibodies (ANA, AMA, SMA) to rule out autoimmune hepatitis and PBC
- **US abdomen** To detect cirrhosis and hepatocellular carcinoma (HCC) and also to assess for splenomegaly and ascites
- **Liver duplex** To assess for hepatic venous outflow obstruction
- **CT/MRI liver** To detect complications of cirrhosis, such as splenomegaly, ascites or HCC
- **Ascitic tap** For ascites to identify cause and rule out infection
- **Liver biopsy** Confirms diagnosis

Assessing severity of cirrhosis: Child-Pugh score (ABCDE)

Child–Pugh score is used to assess the prognosis of chronic liver disease, mainly cirrhosis:

- **A**lbumin (serum, mmol/L): <34 (1 point), 34–50 (2 points), >50 (3 points)
- **B**ilirubin (total, g/L): <34 (1 point), 34–50 (2 points), >50 (3 points)
- **C**oagulation INR: <1.7 (1 point), 1.7–2.3 (2 points), >2.3 (3 points)
- '**D**rum' abdomen (**Ascites**): none (1 point), mild (2 points), severe (3 points)
- **E**ncephalopathy (hepatic): none (1 point), grade I–II (2 points), grade III–IV or refractory (3 points)

Interpretation:
- **Class A** (5–6 points) = 1-year survival (100%), 2-year survival (85%)
- **Class B** (7–9 points) = 1-year survival (80%), 2-year survival (60%)
- **Class C** (10–15 points) = 1-year survival (45%), 2-year survival (35%)

Ascites

Definition

An abnormal accumulation of fluid within the peritoneal cavity.

Pathophysiology

- Ascitic fluid can accumulate as a **transudate** or an **exudate**
- Broadly speaking, transudates are a result of increased pressure in the hepatic portal vein, e.g. due to cirrhosis, while exudates are actively secreted fluid due to infection, inflammation or malignancy
- In cirrhosis, vasodilators are locally released due to portal hypertension; these affect the splanchnic arteries causing reduced arterial blood flow and arterial pressures leading to activation of mechanisms including the renin–angiotensin–aldosterone system, sympathetic nervous system and ADH which results in Na^+ and water retention
- The formation of oedema is also further exacerbated by hypoalbuminaemia

Causes

Transudate	Exudate
Portal hypertension e.g. cirrhosis	Cancer: metastasis or primary carcinomatosis
Hepatic veno-occlusive disease	Infection: including peritoneal TB
Budd–Chiari syndrome	Nephrotic syndrome
Cardiac failure	Lymphatic obstruction
Meigs syndrome	Serositis
Constrictive pericarditis	

Clinical features

- Abdominal swelling/fullness
- Shifting dullness
- Pleural effusion and peripheral oedema may also be present
- Other signs of underlying cause may also be present.

Diagnosis

- **Bloods** LFTs including serum albumin, specific tests (*see above*) depending on clinical features
- **Ascitic tap:**
  - Ascitic albumin to help differentiate between transudate and exudate (≥11g/L suggests exudate and <11g/L suggests transudate)
  - WCC, Gram stain and culture; neutrophil count >250cells/mm³ suggests bacterial (usually spontaneous peritonitis)
  - Cytology for malignant cells
  - Amylase to exclude pancreatitis

The serum-ascites albumin gradient (SAAG) is a formula which can further help to determine the cause of ascites:

SAAG = (albumin concentration of serum) – (albumin concentration of ascitic fluid)

A high gradient (>1.1g/dL) indicates the ascites is due to portal hypertension with 97% accuracy.

Management

- Treat underlying cause
- Bed rest, fluid and salt restriction
- **Diuretics** e.g. Spironolactone (50–100mg/day); furosemide can also be added
- **Paracentesis** Used in patients with tense ascites or those who are resistant to above treatments; provides rapid symptomatic relief; IV infusion of albumin is administered immediately afterwards
- **Transjugular intrahepatic portosystemic shunt (TIPS)** Occasionally used for resistant ascites caused by portal hypertension
- Treat spontaneous bacterial peritonitis accordingly with antibiotics according to local antimicrobial guidelines after diagnostic aspiration

Coeliac disease is an immune-mediated, inflammatory systemic disorder provoked by **gluten** and related prolamins in genetically susceptible individuals. This can result in malabsorption of nutrients due to chronic inflammation and damage (villous atrophy) to the lining of the small intestine. Coeliac disease is associated with dermatitis herpetiformis and other autoimmune disorders.

- Coeliac disease is strongly associated with **HLA-DQ2** (95% of patients) and **HLA-DQ8** (80%)
- The toxin **alpha-gliadin** is the toxic portion of the gluten which is contained in **wheat**, **rye** and **barley**
- Gliadin is deaminated by **tissue transglutaminase** (TTG); it then interacts with antigen-presenting cells in the lamina propria via HLA-DQ2 and -DQ8 and activates gluten-sensitive T cells
- The resultant inflammatory reaction and release of mediators causes **villous atrophy** and **crypt hyperplasia** (see *Fig. 1*)

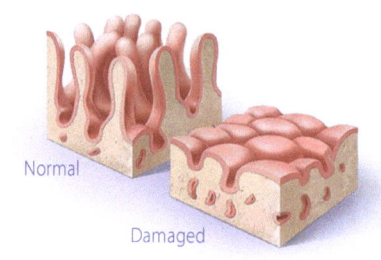

Normal

Damaged

Fig. 1 Lining of small bowel vs lining of small bowel with coeliac disease

Definition

Pathophysiology

Coeliac disease

Notes

Coeliac disease

Complications

- Anaemia (iron, folate and vitamin B_{12} deficiency)
- Hyposplenism
- Osteoporosis, osteomalacia
- Lactose intolerance
- Malignancy: enteropathy-associated T-cell lymphoma of small intestine, oesophageal cancer
- Subfertility, unfavourable pregnancy outcomes

- Chronic or intermittent diarrhoea
- Recurrent abdominal pain, cramping or distension
- Failure to thrive (in children)
- Nausea and vomiting
- Fatigue
- Sudden or unexpected weight loss
- Unexplained iron-deficiency anaemia, or other unspecified anaemia
- Dermatitis herpetiformis (see *Fig. 2*)

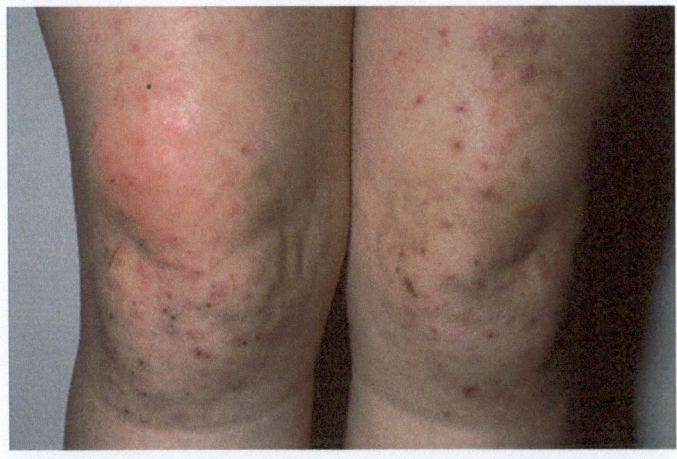

Fig. 2 Dermatitis herpetiformis: itchy symmetrical eruption of vesicles and crusts over the extensor surfaces of the body associated with coeliac disease; it is caused by deposition of IgA in the dermis

Clinical features

Investigations

- If patient is already taking a gluten-free diet they should be asked, if possible, to reintroduce gluten for at least 6 weeks prior to testing:
- **Routine bloods** FBC (anaemia), iron studies (iron deficiency), vitamin B_{12} (↓), folate (↓), LFTs, calcium, albumin
- **Immunology** TTG antibodies (IgA) are 1st line for diagnosis according to NICE, endomyseal antibody (IgA), anti-gliadin antibody (IgA or IgG) (not recommended by NICE), anti-casein antibodies are also found in some patients
- **Duodenal/jejunal biopsy** (see *Fig. 3*) Villous atrophy, crypt hyperplasia, ↑intraepithelial lymphocytes, lamina propria infiltration with lymphocytes
- **Dual energy X-ray absorptiometry (DEXA) scan** Performed at diagnosis due to increased risk of osteoporosis

Management

- The following patients should be screened for coeliac disease: autoimmune thyroid disease, dermatitis herpetiformis, irritable bowel syndrome, type 1 diabetes mellitus, 1st-degree relatives of patients with coeliac disease
- Lifelong strict gluten-free diet (GFD) is the only known effective treatment

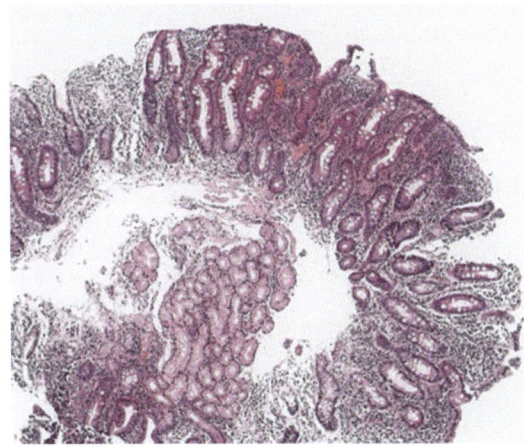

Fig. 3 Duodenal biopsy showing complete villous atrophy, marked crypt hyperplasia, intraepithelial lymphocytosis and inflammatory infiltrate in the lamina propria

Crohn's disease is a form of **inflammatory bowel disease (IBD)**. It is characterised by a **transmural granulomatous inflammation** which commonly affects the **terminal ileum** and colon but may be seen anywhere from the mouth to the anus. Unlike ulcerative colitis (UC), there may be unaffected bowel between areas of active disease (skip lesions). There may also be a number of extra-intestinal features present.

- The cause of Crohn's disease is unknown but it is generally accepted to be caused by an abnormal immune response to luminal antigens in genetically susceptible individuals
- **Microscopically**, the initial lesion starts as a focal inflammatory infiltrate around the crypts, followed by ulceration of superficial mucosa; later, inflammatory cells invade the deep mucosal layers and, in that process, begin to organise into non-caseating granulomas
- **Macroscopically**, the initial abnormality consists of hyperaemia and oedema of the involved mucosa; later, discrete superficial ulcers form over lymphoid aggregates and are seen as red spots or mucosal depressions
- Transmural inflammation results in thickening of the bowel wall and narrowing of the lumen; as the disease progresses, it is complicated by obstruction or deep ulceration leading to fistulisation by way of the sinus tracts penetrating the serosa, microperforation, abscess formation, adhesions and malabsorption

Definition

Pathophysiology

Crohn's disease

Complications

- Psychosocial impact
- Abscesses (intestinal wall or adjacent structures)
- Intestinal strictures
- Fistulas
- Anaemia: iron deficiency (blood loss or nutritional deficiency), vitamin B_{12} or folate deficiency (↓absorption), or anaemia of chronic disease
- Malnutrition, failure to thrive and delayed puberty (in children)
- Colorectal and small bowel cancer

Management

Conservative

- **Smoking cessation:** patient should be encouraged to stop smoking as smokers more likely to have significant symptoms, higher chance of relapse and more likely to have complications post surgery
- **Specialist nurse** advice and support
- **Dietary advice:** there are no specific foods that patients should avoid; patients should be encouraged to have a balanced diet; they may require supplements such as iron, B_{12}, folate or calcium
- **Psychological support:** assess the impact of symptoms on daily functioning, and assess for associated anxiety and/or depression

Medical (see *Table 2*)

- **Glucocorticoids** are generally used to induce remission
- **Aminosalicylates (5-ASAS)**, e.g. mesalazine, are used 2nd line to glucocorticoids to induce remission but are not as effective
- **Immunosuppressant**, e.g. azathioprine or mercaptopurine, may be used as an add-on medication to induce remission and are often used 1st line to maintain remission

Surgical

- Around 80% of patients with Crohn's disease will eventually have surgery
- Often indicated if there is failure of medical therapy or to manage complications e.g. intestinal obstruction, strictures, fistulas and perianal disease
- In patients who have isolated terminal ileum disease, however, an **ileocaecal resection** can be preferred to medication in the early stages to prolong and maintain remission

Other treatments

- **Enteral feeding** with an elemental diet or polymeric can be used to induce remission in addition to or instead of other measures, particularly if there is concern regarding the side effects of steroids e.g. in young children; it is not effective in maintaining remission
- **Total parenteral nutrition** is appropriate adjunctive therapy in complex, fistulating disease

- **Smoking** Risk is increased in smokers
- **Family history** Family history is present in about 25–40% of children
- **Infectious gastroenteritis** Risk is increased 4-fold following an episode of infectious gastroenteritis
- **CARD15 gene mutation** *CARD15* gene encodes NOD2, a protein which is produced by intestinal epithelial cells and triggers a protective inflammatory response which maintains intestinal homeostasis; mutations of this gene significantly increase the risk
- **Appendectomy** Risk increases early after an appendectomy and decreases to that of the general population about 5 years postoperatively
- **Drugs** NSAIDs and COCP may increase the risk of relapse or exacerbation of IBD, but the absolute risk is low

Risk factors

Intestinal
- Diarrhoea (most common symptom overall): can be bloody but less common
- Abdominal pain: most prominent symptom in children
- Weight loss and lethargy
- Perianal disease: e.g. skin tags or ulcers

Extra-intestinal
- Clubbing
- Skin: erythema nodosum, pyoderma gangrenosum

- Eyes: conjunctivitis, episcleritis, iritis
- Joints: large joint arthritis, sacroiliitis, ankylosing spondylitis
- Liver: fatty liver, primary sclerosing cholangitis (rare), cholangiocarcinoma (rare)
- Renal stones (oxalate)
- Osteomalacia
- Malnutrition
- Amyloidosis

Clinical features

Investigations

- **Bloods** FBC, CRP/ESR (↑ in active disease), U&Es, LFTs, vitamin B_{12}, folate, ferritin, vitamin D
- **Stool** Culture and microscopy, faecal calprotectin (a small calcium-binding protein) – the concentration in faeces has been shown to correlate well with the severity of intestinal inflammation and can therefore be used for diagnosis and monitoring
- **AXR** Used in patients with acute severe colitis; helps to rule out toxic megacolon or bowel obstruction
- **Ileocolonoscopy** Identifies macroscopic features and also biopsies from the terminal ileum to look for microscopic evidence of Crohn's disease are 1st line to establish diagnosis (contraindicated in an acute flare)
- **Barium enema** High sensitivity and specificity for examination of the terminal ileum, strictures ('Kantor's string sign'), proximal bowel dilatation, 'rose thorn' ulcers and fistulae
- **CT colon** To assess both mural and extramural manifestations of IBD
- **MRI colon** To assess both mural and extramural manifestations of IBD
- **Pelvic MRI** For perianal disease
- **Oesophagogastroduodenoscopy (OGD)** Recommended for patients with upper GI symptoms

Notes

Crohn's disease

Crohn's disease notes

Table 1 Ulcerative colitis vs Crohn's disease

	Ulcerative colitis	Crohn's disease
Site	Inflammation starts at the rectum and never spreads beyond ileocaecal valve	Can occur anywhere in the GI tract from the mouth to the anus but most commonly affects the terminal ileum
Macroscopic pathology	• No inflammation beyond the submucosa • Continuous pattern of inflammation	• Can extend through all layers of the bowel wall • Intermittent pattern of inflammation (skip lesions)
Microscopic pathology	• No inflammation beyond submucosa • Goblet cell depletion and crypt abscesses	• Transmural inflammation • Granulomas present • Increased goblet cells
Clinical features	• Usually causes bloody diarrhoea • Abdominal pain typically in left lower quadrant, tenesmus and urgency	• Does not usually cause bloody diarrhoea • Weight loss and upper GI symptoms more prominent • Mouth ulcers, perianal disease
Risk factors	Smoking reduces risk of disease	Smoking increases risk of disease
Endoscopy findings	Ulcers and pseudopolyps	Deep ulcers, skip lesions – 'cobble-stone' appearance
Complications	Complications include haemorrhage and toxic megacolon	Complications include bowel obstruction, abscess and fistulas
Extra-intestinal features	Primary sclerosing cholangitis is more common in UC	Gallstones are more common in Crohn's disease

Table 2 Pharmacological agents used in Crohn's disease

Glucocorticosteroids	• e.g. Prednisolone (oral), hydrocortisone (IV), budesonide (oral) • Usually reserved for active Crohn's disease to help induce remission • They should not routinely be used for maintenance
Aminosalicylates (5-ASAS)	• e.g. Mesalazine, sulfasalazine • These are used 2nd line to glucocorticoids to induce remission but are not as effective • They can be considered for maintaining remission in patients with previous surgery
Immunosuppressants	• e.g. Azathioprine, mercaptopurine, methotrexate, ciclosporin • Can be used with glucocorticosteroids to induce remission and can be useful as steroid-sparing agents to maintain remission • Azathioprine or mercaptopurine used 1st line to maintain remission with methotrexate 2nd line • Can be used long term but require frequent monitoring particularly for liver and bone marrow toxicity
Biological agents	• e.g. Infliximab, adalimumab, vedolizumab • Infliximab is an anti-TNF-alpha drug used in refractory disease and fistulating Crohn's disease • Adalimumab is another anti-TNF-alpha drug that can be used if there is intolerance to infliximab • Vedolizumab is an anti-integrin biological agent that is more gastrointestinally targeted; it is recommended by NICE as an option for treating moderate to severe active Crohn's disease only if a TNF-alpha inhibitor has failed, cannot be tolerated or is contraindicated
Metronidazole	Often used for isolated peri-anal disease

Gastric cancer refers to a neoplasm that can develop in any portion of the stomach and may spread to the lymph nodes and other organs.

Definition

Pathophysiology

- 95% of gastric carcinomas are adenocarcinomas; 64% of carcinomas are situated in the prepyloric region
- There are 3 morphological forms:
  - **Fungating tumours** Usually polypoid and may grow to be very large; tend to have a better prognosis
  - **Malignant ulcers** Broad-based tumours with a necrotic centre
  - **Infiltrating carcinoma** Spread widely beneath the mucosa and invade the muscular layer; large mucin droplets displace the nuclei laterally producing the so-called 'signet ring appearance'; very poor prognosis
- Metastatic spread can occur directly to adjacent structures, lymphatically via coeliac nodes, transcoelomically and haematogenously (via the portal or systemic vessels)

Gastric cancer

Management

Surgery

- Surgery is the treatment of choice for gastric cancer and the only potentially curative treatment modality
- Distal (antral) tumours should be treated by subtotal gastrectomy and proximal tumours by total gastrectomy

Chemotherapy and radiotherapy

- Perioperative combination chemotherapy is the treatment of choice for localised gastric cancer throughout the UK and most of Europe
- Adjuvant chemotherapy without radiotherapy after surgery is not currently standard procedure in the UK but may be helpful in high-risk patients
- 5-fluorouracil (5-FU) is the most effective chemotherapeutic agent; a combination of 5-FU with other agents is superior to single-agent treatment

Prognosis and staging

- **TNM staging** is used to stage gastric cancer
- Overall survival rate is 15% in the UK
- 11% of people live for at least 10 years
- Younger people tend to survive longer

Investigations

Bloods FBC (iron-deficiency anaemia is common), LFTs (may be deranged in liver metastases)
Upper GI endoscopy Investigation of choice to identify tumour(s); biopsies can be taken and small lesions evaluated more fully than radiological studies
Barium meal Rarely used in UK as superseded by endoscopy but it is less invasive
CT abdomen Mainly used for staging
Stool testing Faecal occult blood test positive in the vast majority of subjects

Risk factors

- Gastric cancer is the fourth most common cancer worldwide and the leading cause of cancer death in Japan
- It is only the 15th most common cancer in the UK but the 4th commonest cause of death from cancer in the UK

Epidemiology

- Increasing age (95% of gastric cancers occur in those aged >55 years)
- More common in men than women (UK ratio is 1.8:1)
- It is strongly associated with poor socio-economic status
- *Helicobacter pylori* can double the risk of gastric cancer in infected individuals
- Diet: low levels of fresh fruit and vegetable consumption, high salt and consumption of preserved foods increases the risk of gastric cancer
- Smoking
- Atrophic gastritis, pernicious anaemia, post partial-gastrectomy
- Ménétrier's disease
- Familial risk: a 2- to 3-fold increased risk to 1st-degree relatives of gastric cancer patients; link between E-cadherin gene mutations and some familial gastric cancers
- Blood group A
- Hypogammaglobulinaemia

Risk factors and epidemiology

Symptoms

- Epigastric pain
- Dyspepsia
- Nausea/vomiting
- Haematemesis
- Weight loss
- Anorexia
- Dysphagia
- Symptoms of anaemia

Signs

- Epigastric mass
- Troisier's sign: the clinical finding of a hard and enlarged left supraclavicular node (Virchow node), considered a sign of metastatic abdominal malignancy (see *Fig. 1*)
- Hepatomegaly, jaundice ascites (liver spread)
- Acanthosis nigricans: brown, poorly defined, velvety hyperpigmentation of the skin (see *Fig. 2*)
- Dermatomyositis
- Signs of anaemia

Clinical features

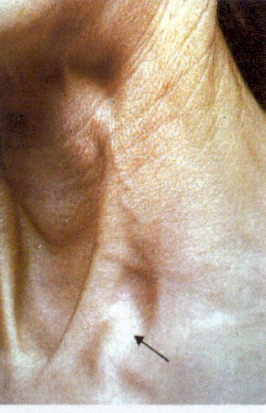

Fig. 1 Troisier's sign

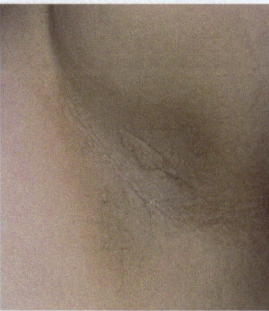

Fig. 2 Acanthosis nigricans

Notes

Gastric cancer

'**Dyspepsia**' is used to describe a complex of upper gastrointestinal (GI) tract symptoms which are typically present for ≥4 weeks, including upper abdominal pain or discomfort, heartburn, acid reflux, nausea and/or vomiting.

Gastro-oesophageal reflux disease (**GORD**) is usually a chronic condition where there is reflux of gastric contents (particularly acid, bile and pepsin) back into the oesophagus, causing predominant symptoms of heartburn and acid regurgitation.

- GORD includes all the consequences of reflux of acid or other irritants from the stomach into the oesophagus
- The main cause of GORD is incompetence of the antireflux barriers at the oesophagogastric junction; the antireflux barriers include two 'sphincter' mechanisms: the lower oesophageal sphincter (LOS), and the crural diaphragm that functions as an external sphincter
- Reflux occurs when LOS pressure is lower than the intragastric pressure
- Mucosal defence mechanisms may be overcome by prolonged exposure of the oesophageal mucosa to acid which may lead to severe and complicated oesophagitis

Pathophysiology

Definition

Gastro-oesophageal reflux disease

Management

Conservative

- Weight loss
- Smoking cessation
- Reduce alcohol intake
- Elevated head of the bed at night
- Take small, regular meals
- Avoid hot drinks, alcohol and eating 3 or 4h before bed
- Avoid offending drugs

Pharmacological

- **Antacids** e.g. Aluminium hydroxide, sodium bicarbonate, calcium carbonate
- **H_2 receptor antagonists** e.g. Ranitidine or cimetidine
- **PPIs** e.g. Omeprazole, lansoprazole and pantoprazole

Surgical

- **Fundoplication surgery** Strengthening the LOS by wrapping the gastric fundus around it
- **Laparoscopic insertion of a magnetic bead band** Involves putting a small flexible band of interlinked magnetic beads around the outside of the lower oesophagus, just above the stomach

Investigations

- **FBC** To exclude anaemia
- **Endoscopy** Investigation of choice
- **CXR** Hiatus hernias may be seen as a soft tissue opacity with or without an air-fluid level
- **Barium swallow** Useful for diagnosing hiatus hernia
- **Oesophageal pH monitoring** To assess if symptoms coincide with acid in the oesophagus

Complications

- Oesophageal ulcers
- Oesophageal haemorrhage
- Anaemia (usually 2° to chronic blood loss from severe oesophagitis)
- Oesophageal stricture
- Aspiration pneumonia
- Barrett's oesophagus
- Oesophageal adenocarcinoma
- Oral problems: dental erosions, gingivitis and halitosis

- Stress and anxiety
- Smoking
- Alcohol excess
- Fatty foods and coffee
- Drugs that decrease LOS pressure e.g. tricyclic antidepressants, anticholinergics, nitrates and calcium-channel blockers
- Pregnancy
- Hiatus hernia (see *Fig. 1*)
- Family history

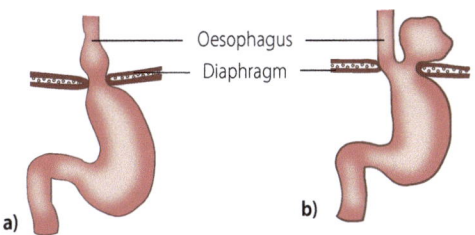

Oesophagus
Diaphragm

a)   b)

Fig. 1 There are two types of hiatus hernia:
(a) Sliding hiatus hernia The gastro-oesophageal junction slides up into the thoracic cavity (85–95% of cases)
(b) Rolling hiatus hernia (paraoesophageal) The gastro-oesophageal junction remains in place but a part of the stomach herniates into the chest next to the oesophagus (5–15% of cases); many are mixed, with a sliding component also

- **Heartburn** Related to meals, lying down, stooping and straining; relieved by antacids
- **Retrosternal discomfort**
- **Acid brash** Regurgitation of acid or bile
- **Water brash** (excessive salivation)
- **Odynophagia** (pain on swallowing)
- **Chest pain/epigastric pain**
- **Bloating**
- **Chronic hoarseness, chronic cough and asthmatic symptoms** (atypical symptoms)

Clinical features

Risk factors

Notes

Gastro-oesophageal reflux disease

Hereditary haemochromatosis (HH) is a multi-organ **autosomal recessive disorder** of iron absorption and metabolism resulting in iron accumulation.

Definition

- In most cases HH is caused by a mutation of the *HFE* **gene** on the short arm of chromosome 6
- The known mutations of *HFE* are C282Y and H63D; the C282Y mutation is most common in White populations
- HFE protein is responsible for regulation of the primary iron regulatory hormone, hepcidin
- Mutation of *HFE* results in decreased hepcidin production in response to elevated iron levels resulting in unregulated control of iron levels
- Increased intestinal absorption of iron causes accumulation of iron in tissues, especially the liver, which may lead to organ damage; other organs that may be affected by iron deposits include the pituitary gland, pancreas, joints, heart, skin and gonads

Pathophysiology

Hereditary haemochromatosis

Management

- **Phlebotomy** Should be carried out by removing 400–500ml of blood (200–250mg iron) weekly or every 2 weeks
- **Monitoring** C282Y homozygotes without evidence for iron overload could have ferritin monitored annually and treatment instituted when the ferritin rises above normal; haemoglobin and ferritin levels must be monitored regularly
- **Diet** Iron-containing vitamin preparations and iron-supplemented foods such as breakfast cereals should be avoided
- **Iron chelation therapy** Can be used as a 2nd-line option in patients who are intolerant of phlebotomy e.g. deferoxamine or deferasirox
- **Genetic testing of family members** Genotyping to detect the *HFE* gene mutations and iron studies should be performed on 1st-degree relatives of affected individuals
- **Immunisation** Patients with HFE-HC could be immunised against hepatitis A and B while iron-overloaded

Investigations

Screening tests

- **Iron studies** Transferrin saturation (>55% in men or >50% in women), ferritin (raised) and iron (raised), TIBC (low)
- **LFTs** May be deranged but often normal even with cirrhosis
- **CRP** Helps exclude inflammation as a cause for raised ferritin as ferritin is also an acute-phase reactant
- **Joint X-ray** Characteristically shows chondrocalcinosis

Further investigations

- **Molecular genetic testing** This is for C282Y and H63D mutations, but now rarely required because genetic testing for *HFE* mutations is very reliable
- **Liver biopsy** With Perl's stain, now rarely required because genetic testing for *HFE* mutations is very reliable
- **MRI liver** Useful non-invasive method to detect and quantify hepatic iron excess
- **Fasting glucose/HbA1c** To detect diabetes
- **ECG/ECHO** Detect arrhythmias and heart failure

- **Pituitary** Fatigue, loss of libido, erectile dysfunction, testicular atrophy
- **Pancreas** Diabetes mellitus
- **Skin** 'Bronze' skin pigmentation (*see Fig. 2*)
- **Joints** Arthritis (especially of the hands)
- **Cardiac** Arrhythmias, cardiomyopathy, heart failure
- **Liver** Stigmata of chronic liver disease, hepatomegaly, cirrhosis, hepatocellular deposition

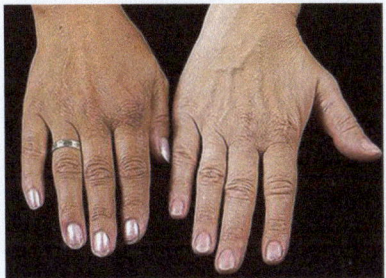

Fig. 2 'Bronze' skin pigmentation in HH

Clinical features (see *Fig. 1*)

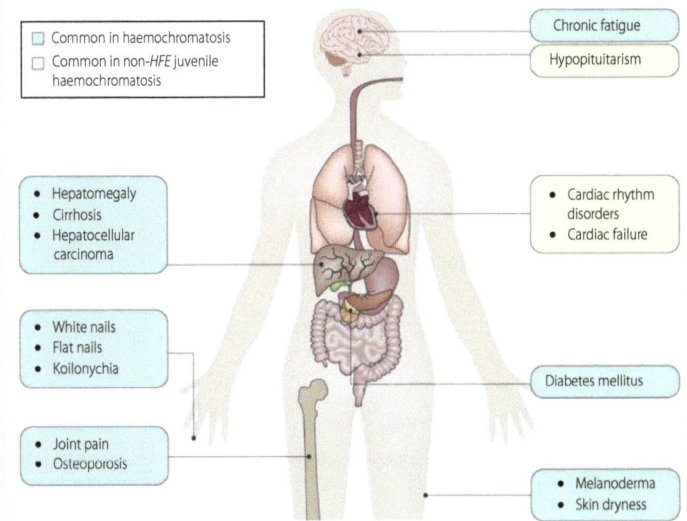

- ☐ Common in haemochromatosis
- ☐ Common in non-*HFE* juvenile haemochromatosis

Chronic fatigue

Hypopituitarism

- Hepatomegaly
- Cirrhosis
- Hepatocellular carcinoma

- Cardiac rhythm disorders
- Cardiac failure

- White nails
- Flat nails
- Koilonychia

Diabetes mellitus

- Joint pain
- Osteoporosis

- Melanoderma
- Skin dryness

Fig. 1 Clinical manifestations of HH

Notes

Irritable bowel syndrome (IBS) is a chronic, relapsing, and often lifelong disorder of the lower GI tract, with no apparent structural or biochemical cause.

Definition

- There is no structural lesion or organic cause for IBS; however, it is thought to be associated with abnormal smooth muscle activity ± visceral hypersensitivity, and abnormal central processing of painful stimuli
- Furthermore, there is evidence of abnormal bowel transit time in affected individuals, suggesting possible disturbed GI motility
- Balloon distension of the bowel in affected individuals leads to perception of pain at lower thresholds than those without it, suggesting some role of the central pain processing system
- IBS has been linked with increased levels of psychiatric distress and poor coping strategies
- There may be a genetic component to IBS as there can be aggregation of the condition in families

Pathophysiology

Irritable bowel syndrome

Management

Conservative

Diet:

- Regular meals, avoiding long gaps between meals and avoid rushing meals
- Drink plenty of fluids (at least 8 cups/day) but restrict tea/coffee
- Reduce intake of alcohol and fizzy drinks
- Limitation of high-fibre foods (e.g. wholemeal flour or bran) and resistant starches and limit fresh fruits to 3 portions per day; those with constipation as a predominant symptom may need to increase fibre intake however
- Avoid sorbitol with diarrhoea
- Consider increasing oats and linseeds for wind
- Consider referral to dietitian for those who find diet plays a significant role in their symptoms for advice about exclusion diets

Lifestyle and physical activity:

- Approx. 75% of patients are helped by explanation and symptomatic relief
- Encourage increased physical activity, exercise and time for relaxation

Pharmacological treatments

- **Loperamide** 1st-line treatment for diarrhoea
- **Antispasmodics** e.g. Mebeverine should be used as required for abdominal pain and spasms
- **Peppermint oil** Shown to be effective as an antispasmodic and for bloating, with very few adverse effects
- **Laxatives** May be used as required for constipation; linaclotide can be used as an alternative when other laxatives have not worked; lactulose should be avoided
- **Antidepressants** TCAs and SSRIs; NICE guidelines support the use of an SSRI only if a low-dose TCA has not been effective; treatment should be started at a low dose e.g. 10mg amitriptyline and increased if necessary
- **Antibiotics** May have a role in IBS by altering the bacterial composition of the GI tract e.g. short-course therapy with rifaximin or neomycin

Other therapies

- **Psychological intervention** If symptoms do not respond to pharmacological treatments after 12 months and for those who develop refractory IBS: consider referral for cognitive behavioural therapy (CBT) or hypnotherapy

- **Genetic** Twin studies and family studies confirm familial aggregation of IBS
- **Enteric infection** e.g. Following gastroenteritis
- **Gastrointestinal inflammation** e.g. Secondary to inflammatory bowel disease
- **Dietary factors** e.g. Excessive alcohol, caffeine, spicy and fatty foods (up to 90% of people report that food triggers symptoms)
- **Drugs** e.g. Antibiotics
- **Psychosocial** e.g. Associated stress, anxiety and/or depression

Risk factors

- **Abdominal pain** Often relieved by defecation or passage of wind
- **Abdominal bloating and distension**
- **Excess flatus**
- **Change in bowel habit**
- **Altered stool passage** Subtypes of IBS can be classified according to the predominant stool pattern: IBS with constipation, IBS with diarrhoea, and mixed IBS with alternating diarrhoea and constipation
- **Sensation of incomplete evacuation of stool**
- **Rectal passage of mucus**

Clinical features

Investigations

All investigations in IBS are normal. The following investigations should be carried out in all patients:
- **FBC, ESR, CRP, LFTs** Useful tests to screen for inflammation and other pathology
- **Coeliac disease screening** e.g. Tissue transglutaminase
- **CA-125** For women with symptoms which could be ovarian cancer
- **Faecal calprotectin** For those with symptoms which could be IBD

The following tests are NOT required to confirm IBS in those who meet the diagnostic criteria but should be done if diagnosis unclear:
- TFTs
- US abdomen
- Colonoscopy/sigmoidoscopy/barium enema
- Faecal occult blood
- Faecal ova and parasite tests
- *Helicobacter pylori* screening e.g. through a stool test

Diagnostic criteria (NICE, CG61)

The diagnosis should be considered if the patient has had the following for at least 6 months:
- Abdominal pain *and/or*
- Bloating *and/or*
- Change in bowel habit

A positive diagnosis of IBS should be made if the patient has abdominal pain relieved by defecation or associated with altered bowel frequency or stool form, in addition to 2 of the following 4 symptoms:
- Altered stool passage (straining, urgency, incomplete evacuation)
- Abdominal bloating, distension, tension or hardness
- Symptoms made worse by eating
- Passage of mucus

(Features such as lethargy, nausea, backache and bladder symptoms may also support the diagnosis)

Jaundice (also known as **icterus**) describes the yellow pigmentation of the skin, sclera, and mucous membranes as a result of **raised plasma bilirubin** (see *Fig. 1*). Normal serum bilirubin is approx. 3–20μmol/L; clinical jaundice may not become apparent until serum bilirubin is >35μmol/L.

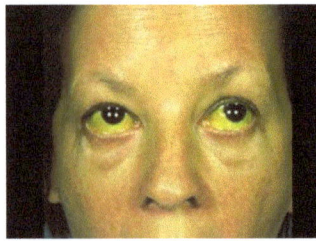

Fig. 1 Jaundiced patient

Causes

Pre-hepatic

- Haemolytic anaemias: sickle cell, thalassaemia, hereditary spherocytosis, glucose-6-phosphate dehydrogenase deficiency, haemolytic uraemic syndrome
- Drugs: e.g. methyldopa and sulfasalazine
- Severe rhabdomyolysis
- Malaria
- Gilbert syndrome: an autosomal recessive condition of defective bilirubin conjugation due to a deficiency of UDP glucuronyl transferase; no treatment is required
- Crigler–Najjar syndrome

Hepatic

- Viral hepatitis: including hepatitis A–E, CMV and EBV
- Alcohol
- Cirrhosis
- Non-alcoholic fatty liver disease (NAFLD)
- Autoimmune liver disorders: e.g. primary biliary cholangitis (PBC), autoimmune hepatitis
- Metabolic causes of intra-hepatic jaundice
- Drugs: e.g. paracetamol overdose, pyrazinamide, rifampicin and isoniazid
- Leptospirosis
- Liver malignancy
- Wilson's disease

Post-hepatic

- Gallstones
- Surgical strictures
- Biliary atresia
- Cholangiocarcinoma
- Extra-hepatic malignancy: e.g. pancreatic cancer
- Pancreatitis
- Parasitic infection: including hydatid disease, liver fluke and roundworms
- Primary sclerosing cholangitis
- Cholestasis of pregnancy
- Drugs: e.g. co-amoxiclav, flucloxacillin, oral contraceptives, hormone replacement therapy and corticosteroids

Definition

Management

Treat underlying cause

Jaundice

Diagnosis (see *Table 1*)

Bloods

- ALT, AST, bilirubin (including bilirubin split, see *Table 1*), gamma-GT, ALP, albumin, clotting, FBC including reticulocyte count and blood smear (to detect haemolysis), LDH (↑ in haemolysis)

Table 1 Distinguishing between pre-hepatic, hepatic and post-hepatic jaundice

Clinical features/LFTs	Pre-hepatic	Hepatic	Post-hepatic
Urine appearance	Normal	Dark	Dark
Stool appearance	Normal	Pale	Pale
Total bilirubin	↑	↑	↑
Conjugated bilirubin	↑	↑	↑
Unconjugated bilirubin	↑	↑	→
ALP	Normal	↑	↑

- Hepatitis serology, ANA (+ve in 20–50% of patients with PBC), ASMA (+ve in autoimmune hepatitis), AMA (+ve in 90–95% of PBC), serum immunoglobulins (↑IgG in acute hepatitis, ↑IgM in autoimmune disease, PBC or chronic infection)
- Viral serology for hepatitis A, B, C, E; CMV
- Monospot test for EBV
- Alpha fetoprotein: ↑ in hepatocellular carcinoma
- Caeruloplasmin: ↓ in Wilson's disease
- Alpha-1 antitrypsin (↓ in alpha-1 antitrypsin deficiency)

Urine

Urinary bilirubin and urobilinogen:

- ↑Urinary bilirubin ↓urobilinogen is suggestive of obstructive jaundice
- → or ↑urinary bilirubin with ↑urobilinogen suggests hepatocellular failure or increased red cell breakdown

Imaging

- Abdominal US: to detect liver abnormalities, hepatosplenomegaly and gallstones
- CT abdomen (as with US but more detailed)
- Magnetic resonance cholangiopancreatography (MRCP): test of choice in obstructive jaundice
- Liver biopsy, laparotomy: may ultimately be required to make the diagnosis in some cases of jaundice

- Jaundice can be caused by a wide variety of disorders which range from benign to life-threatening conditions
- Bilirubin is a breakdown product of haem molecules in red blood cells and other proteins such as myoglobin
- The causes of jaundice can be broadly classified by the stages of bilirubin metabolism (see *Fig. 2*); dysfunction at any of these 3 phases can lead to jaundice:
  - **Pre-hepatic** Haem molecules are degraded in macrophages via biliverdin to bilirubin; this occurs mainly in the spleen and liver; bilirubin is then bound to plasma albumin and transported to the liver for conjugation
  - **Intra-hepatic** In the liver, unconjugated bilirubin is then conjugated and can be excreted in bile
  - **Post-hepatic** Soluble bilirubin is transported through the liver and cystic ducts in bile and then stored in the gallbladder or passes into the duodenum; in the intestine, some bilirubin is excreted in the stool (as stercobilinogen) and the rest is metabolised by gut flora into urobilinogen which is reabsorbed and excreted by the kidneys

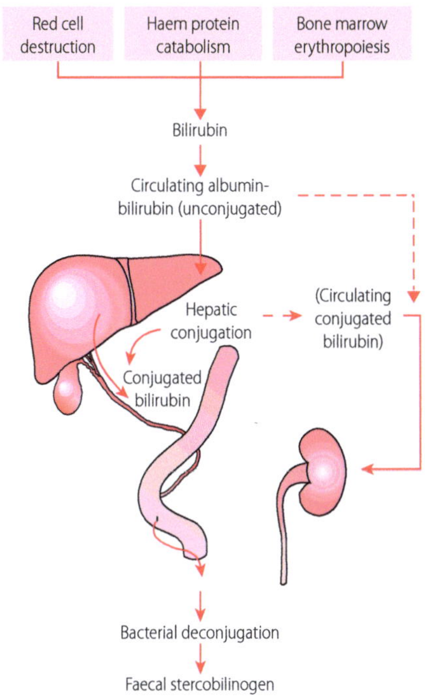

Pathophysiology

Fig. 2 Metabolism of bilirubin

Notes

Jaundice

- Over 8000 new oesophageal cancers are diagnosed each year in the UK
- The incidence of oesophageal carcinoma varies considerably with geographical location; high rates in China and Iran (SCC) have been directly linked to the preservation of food using nitrosamines
- Adenocarcinoma is seen more frequently in Caucasian populations

- Smoking
- Alcohol
- GORD
- Barrett's oesophagus
- Achalasia
- Plummer–Vinson syndrome
- Tylosis and Paterson–Brown–Kelly syndrome (SCC)
- Diets rich in nitrosamines (SCC)
- Coeliac disease, scleroderma (rare)

Oesophageal cancer is cancer of the oesophagus with the two main types being **squamous cell carcinoma** (SCC) and **adenocarcinoma**.

Epidemiology

Risk factors

Definition

Oesophageal cancer and other causes of dysphagia

Notes

Oesophageal cancer and other causes of dysphagia

Management

- Involvement of a **multidisciplinary team** including a gastroenterologist, specialist nurse, dietitian, speech and language therapy
- Operable disease is best managed by surgical resection
- The two most commonly performed surgeries are the **transhiatal oesophagectomy** and the **transthoracic oesophagectomy**, also known as the **Ivor Lewis procedure**
- In addition to surgical resection many patients will be treated with **adjuvant chemotherapy**
- For non-operable tumours, treatment is mostly palliative
- **Palliative** options include **stent insertion**, **radiotherapy**, **chemotherapy**, **laser therapy** or a combination of these
- **Nutritional support** in the form of **nasogastric tube**, **percutaneous endoscopic gastrostomy (PEG)** or **radiologically inserted gastrostomy (RIG)** insertion

- **SCC** Mainly found in the **upper two-thirds** of the oesophagus and thought to develop from **squamous dysplasia/intraepithelial neoplasia**
- **Dysplastic squamous epithelium** Characterised by cytological abnormalities which are usually confined to the epithelium; invasion of these neoplastic squamous cells into lamina propria and deeper layers results in invasive oesophageal SCC
- **Adenocarcinoma** usually arises from **Barrett's oesophagus** in the **lower third of the oesophagus** where **normal distal squamous epithelial lining** has been replaced by **metaplastic columnar epithelium** (see *Fig. 1*).

- Dissemination of the tumour may occur in 3 ways:
  - **Direct spread** Occurs both laterally, through the component layers of the oesophageal wall, and longitudinally within the oesophageal wall
  - **Via lymphatics** Common
  - **Haematogenous spread** May involve a variety of different organs e.g. liver, lungs, brain and bones

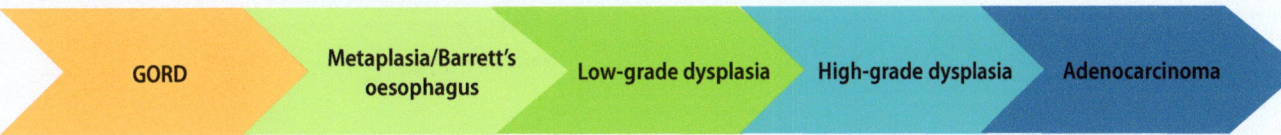

| GORD | Metaplasia/Barrett's oesophagus | Low-grade dysplasia | High-grade dysplasia | Adenocarcinoma |

Fig. 1 Stages of oesophageal adenocarcinoma

Pathophysiology

Investigations

- **Bloods** FBC, U&Es, LFT, glucose, CRP
- **Upper GI endoscopy and biopsies** The gold standard for diagnosis (see *Fig. 2*)
- **Barium swallow** Useful in diagnosing benign motility disorders but has no place in the assessment of tumours
- **CT** Chest, abdomen and pelvis for staging
- **Endoscopic US** For local staging if CT does not show metastatic disease
- **Staging laparoscopy** To detect occult peritoneal disease
- **PET CT** Performed in those with negative laparoscopy

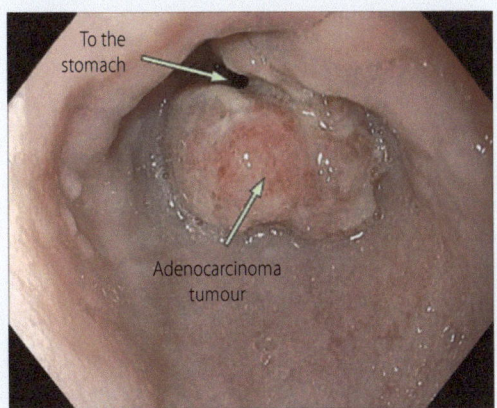

To the stomach

Adenocarcinoma tumour

Fig. 2 Oesophageal adenocarcinoma on endoscopy

Clinical features (VBAD)

- **V**omiting
- **B**lood loss Melaena, haematemesis
- **A**norexia Plus weight loss
- **D**ysphagia Most common presenting symptom
- Other symptoms: odynophagia, hoarseness, cough, retrosternal pain, intractable hiccups, lymphadenopathy

Staging and prognosis

- **TNM staging** is used for oesophageal cancer
- The prognosis for oesophageal carcinoma varies depending on the stage at presentation
- The overall 5-year survival rate is 20–25% for all stages
- The survival rates for adenocarcinoma and squamous cell carcinoma are roughly the same

Causes of dysphagia by classification

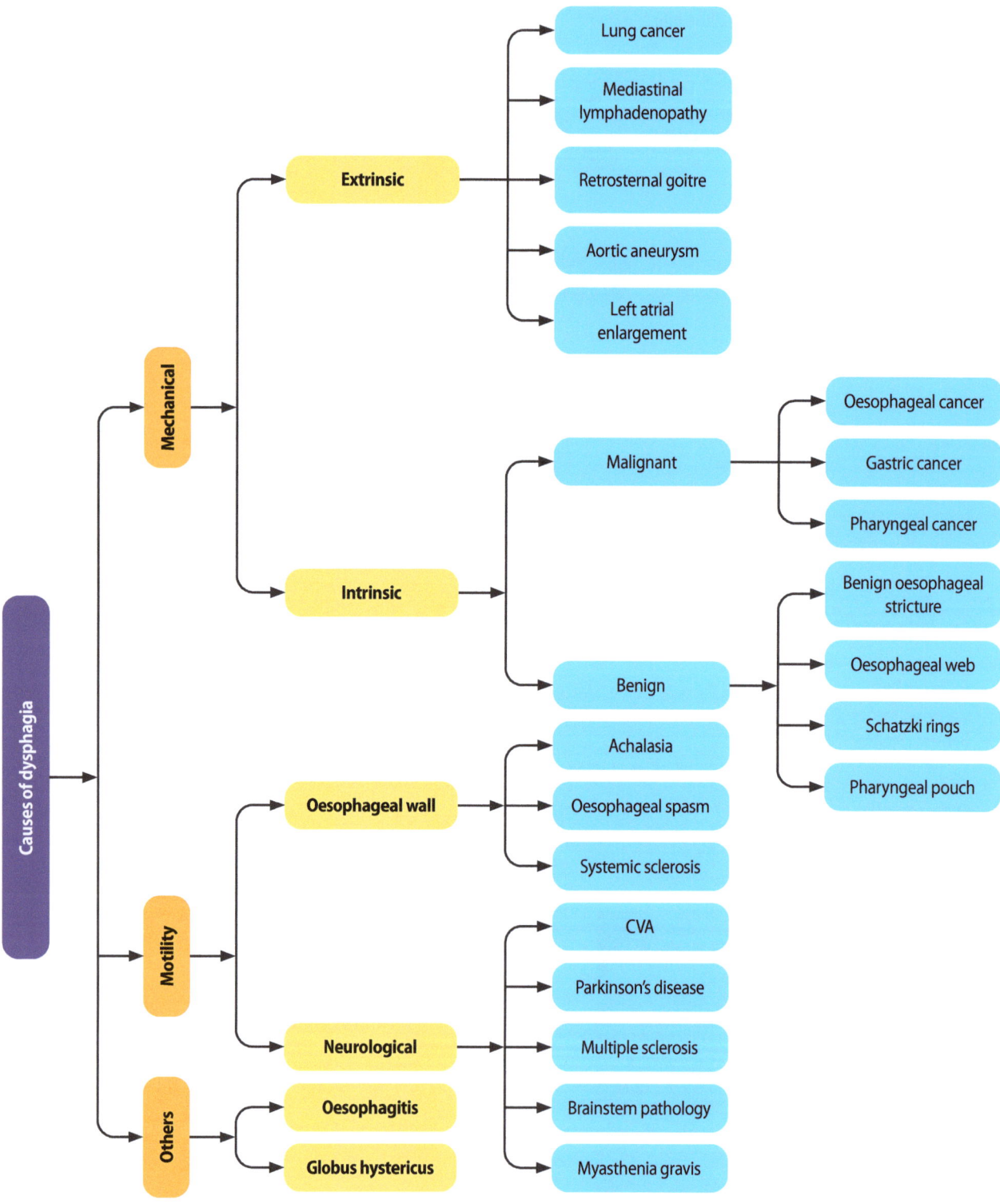

Fig. 3 Causes of dysphagia

Specific causes of dysphagia

Achalasia

- Primarily a disorder of motility of the lower oesophageal or cardiac sphincter
- Dysphagia of both liquids and solids from the start; usually causes heartburn and regurgitation of food
- Diagnosis:
  - **Oesophageal manometry** Excessive lower oesophageal sphincter tone which doesn't relax on swallowing
  - **Barium swallow** Shows grossly expanded oesophagus, fluid level, 'bird's beak' appearance
  - **CXR** Wide mediastinum, fluid level
- Management options include intrasphincteric injection of botulinum toxin, Heller cardiomyotomy and pneumatic (balloon) dilatation

Oesophagitis

- This may be caused by reflux (reflux oesophagitis) or infection such as candida (oesophageal candidiasis)
- Odynophagia often present but no weight loss and systemically well
- In oesophageal candidiasis there may be a history of HIV/AIDS or other risk factors such as chemotherapy or inhaled steroid use

Notes

Oesophageal cancer and other causes of dysphagia

Pathophysiology

- In both types of peptic ulceration, gastric and duodenal, there is an imbalance between secretion and neutralisation of secreted acid
- Most ulcers occur when the normal mechanisms are disrupted by superimposed processes e.g. *Helicobacter pylori* infection and the ingestion of NSAIDs (see *Risk factors*)

Definition

A **peptic ulcer** describes a breach in the epithelium of the **gastric** or **duodenal mucosa** that penetrates the muscularis mucosae; it is confirmed on endoscopy.

Risk factors

- *H. pylori* **infection:** 95% of duodenal and 70–80% of gastric ulcers are associated with *H. pylori* infection
- **Drugs:** NSAIDs (most common), aspirin, bisphosphonates, corticosteroids, potassium supplements, SSRIs and recreational drugs e.g. crack cocaine
- **Smoking**
- **Excessive alcohol** consumption
- Stress
- **Zollinger–Ellison syndrome** (rare): this hypersecretory state may be associated with multiple peptic ulcers, diarrhoea, weight loss and hypercalcaemia

Peptic ulcer disease

Management

Conservative

- Smoking cessation
- Reducing alcohol intake
- Stop offending drugs e.g. NSAIDs

Medical

- **Antacids** e.g. Aluminium hydroxide, sodium bicarbonate
- **H$_2$ antagonists** e.g. Ranitidine, cimetidine
- **PPIs** e.g. Lansoprazole, omeprazole, pantoprazole
- *H. pylori* **triple eradication therapy** – offer people who test positive for *H. pylori* a 7-day, twice-daily course of treatment with:
  - A PPI, e.g. omeprazole 20mg BD, *and*
  - Amoxicillin 1g, *and*
  - Either clarithromycin 500mg or metronidazole 400mg

Surgical

Indications:

- Failure of medical treatment
- Complications, e.g. recurrent haemorrhage, perforation, outflow obstruction
- A possibility of malignancy

Possible interventions:

- **Vagotomy** Removal of all or some of the branches of the vagus nerve in order to prevent excessive acid secretion; it is the surgical treatment of choice for chronic duodenal ulceration
- **Partial gastrectomy** Remove an ulcer, or remove a gastrin-secreting mucosa; a Billroth I type of partial gastrectomy is the standard type of operation for a chronic gastric ulcer

Complications

- **Haemorrhage:** acute massive haemorrhage may be life-threatening
- **Perforation:** this may cause peritonitis which may be life-threatening
- **Gastric outlet obstruction:** this may result from strictures and stenosis of the pylorus and/or duodenum due to chronic inflammation and scarring
- **Gastric malignancy:** there is an increased risk in *H. pylori* positive gastric ulcer disease

- May be asymptomatic
- Epigastric pain: gastric ulcers typically give rise to pain 15–20min after meals, whereas duodenal ulceration typically causes pain 1–3h after a meal and may be relieved by food
- Epigastric tenderness
- Nausea ± vomiting
- Oral flatulence, bloating, distension and intolerance of fatty food
- Heartburn (although more typically associated with GORD)
- Pain radiating to back (posterior ulcer)
- Symptoms are relieved by antacids (not specific)
- Haematemesis and melaena (if ulcer bleeding)

Clinical features

- **Bloods** FBC, U&Es, LFTs, iron studies
- ***H. pylori* testing** Using a carbon-13 urea breath test or a stool antigen test, or laboratory-based serology (not recommended)
- **Faecal occult blood** To exclude blood loss
- **Upper GI endoscopy** Diagnostic of peptic ulcers; endoscopy is required if the patient is presenting for the first time and is above the age of 55 years or if there are any red flag features:
  - Anaemia (iron deficiency)
  - Weight loss
  - Progressive dysphagia
  - Persistent vomiting
  - Epigastric mass
  - Chronic blood loss

Investigations

Notes

Peptic ulcer disease

Definition

Primary biliary cholangitis (PBC; previously known as **primary biliary cirrhosis**) is an autoimmune disease characterised by chronic progressive destruction of intrahepatic bile ducts, resulting in chronic cholestasis, portal inflammation and fibrosis which will eventually lead to cirrhosis and liver failure.

Clinical features

- The typical patient is a woman aged 30–65 years
- Presentation of PBC may vary greatly from asymptomatic and slowly progressive to symptomatic and rapidly evolving
- Jaundice (cholestatic) with pale stool, dark urine

Symptoms

- Fatigue
- Pruritus
- Right upper quadrant pain/discomfort

Signs

- Hepatomegaly (25%)
- Hyperpigmentation (25%)
- Splenomegaly (15%)
- Jaundice (10%)
- Xanthelasma (later stages due to hypercholesterolaemia)

Primary biliary cholangitis

Complications

- Renal tubular acidosis
- Hypothyroidism (in approx. 20%)
- Hepatocellular carcinoma
- Steatorrhoea and fat-soluble vitamin deficiency
- Complications of cirrhosis

Staging

1. **Portal stage:** portal inflammation and bile duct abnormalities
2. **Periportal stage:** periportal fibrosis, with or without periportal inflammation
3. **Septal stage:** septal fibrosis and active inflammation
4. **Cirrhotic stage:** nodules with various degrees of inflammation

Management

- **Cholestyramine:** for itching
- **Fat-soluble vitamin supplementation:** A, D, E, K
- **Ursodeoxycholic acid:** to slow disease progression and reduce need for liver transplantation
- **Liver transplantation:** e.g. if bilirubin >100 (PBC is a major indication); recurrence in graft can occur

- Sjögren syndrome (seen in up to 80% of patients)
- Rheumatoid arthritis
- Seronegative arthritis
- Systemic sclerosis
- Thyroid disease
- Coeliac disease
- Hyperlipidaemia
- Gallstones
- Osteoporosis
- Hepatocellular malignancy

Diagnosis is based on 2 of the following 3 criteria being met:
1. Biochemical evidence of cholestasis with evidence of increased **ALP activity**
2. Presence of **AMAs**
3. **Histological evidence** of nonsuppurative destructive cholangitis and destruction of interlobular bile ducts

Associations

Diagnostic criteria

Notes

Primary biliary cholangitis

Investigations

Bloods

- FBC (usually normal), ESR (may be raised), LFTs (ALP characteristically raised, ALT/AST variable, bilirubin usually normal but rises with disease progression)
- Lipids: cholesterol often raised
- Autoantibodies: **anti-mitochondrial antibodies (AMA) M2 subtype** are present in 98% of patients and are highly specific; smooth muscle antibodies present in 30% of patients; anti-nuclear antibodies (ANA) are present in about 35% of patients
- Serum IgM (raised in >80%)
- TFTs often reveal a lowered T4

Imaging

- US abdomen: to help detect extrahepatic obstructive causes e.g. gallstones
- MRI or endoscopic retrograde cholangiography: to exclude primary sclerosing cholangitis or other disorders that might lead to chronic cholestasis
- Transient elastography: to evaluate the degree of liver fibrosis
- Liver biopsy: confirms the diagnosis but not mandatory to make the diagnosis (see *Diagnostic criteria*)

Definition

Primary sclerosing cholangitis (PSC) is a rare chronic cholestatic disorder of unknown cause characterised by inflammation and fibrosis of intrahepatic and extrahepatic bile ducts, resulting in multifocal biliary strictures.

Pathophysiology

- The aetiology of PSC remains unknown, but it is thought to be multifactorial, including genetic predisposition, exposure to an environmental antigen and subsequent immunologic response
- There is also an increased prevalence of HLA alleles A1, B8 and DR3 in PSC
- An autoimmune mechanism is also suggested as there is a significant overlap between IBD and PSC
- There is also a marked increase in serum autoantibody levels in patients with PSC including **anti-neutrophil cytoplasmic antibodies (ANCA)**, **anti-cardiolipin (ACL) antibodies** and **anti-nuclear antibodies (ANA)**.

Primary sclerosing cholangitis

Complications

Biliary complications

- Biliary obstruction due to stones or strictures
- Acute or chronic cholangitis

Cirrhosis and associated complications

- Ascites
- Portal hypertension
- Oesophageal varices
- Liver failure

Increased risk of cancers

- Cholangiocarcinoma
- Colorectal cancer

Management

Medical

- **Ursodeoxycholic acid** may improve liver function and the patient's symptoms but no definitive improvement in histology or mortality
- **Cholestyramine** helps to relieve pruritus; rifampicin, naltrexone and sertraline may also be used for pruritus
- Treat **fat-soluble vitamin (A, D, E, K)** deficiencies

Surgical

- **Percutaneous transhepatic balloon dilatation** May be of benefit for dominant strictures
- **Liver transplantation** Potentially curative and is indicated where there is hepatic failure, ascites or oesophageal varices

- PSC is a rare condition with a prevalence of 1–16 per 100 000
- More common in males (2:1)
- Typical age of diagnosis is 4–5th decade of life
- Approx. 80% of patients with PSC have inflammatory bowel disease (IBD) but only approx. 5% of patients with IBD have PSC

Epidemiology/risk factors

Symptoms

- May be asymptomatic (presenting with abnormal LFTs or hepatomegaly)
- Jaundice and pruritus
- Right upper quadrant abdominal pain
- Fatigue, weight loss, fevers and sweats

Signs

- Jaundice
- Hepatomegaly and splenomegaly
- Signs of cirrhosis, portal hypertension or hepatic failure (advanced stage)

Clinical features

Staging (histological)

- **Stage 1** Bile duct injury and portal inflammation with minimal fibrosis
- **Stage 2** Expansion of portal tracts, periportal fibrosis, and inflammation
- **Stage 3** Fibrous septa, bridging fibrosis, more prominent ductopenia
- **Stage 4** End-stage disease with secondary biliary cirrhosis

Investigations

Bloods

- LFTs: often abnormal, ↑ALP and gamma-glutamyltransferase (GGT) is most common; ALT and AST may be normal or elevated; bilirubin is raised in advanced PSC
- Serum albumin (may be low) and prothrombin time may rise as the disease progresses
- IG, IgM and the serum globulin fraction levels may be elevated
- There may also be hypergammaglobulinaemia, raised IgM levels, raised antibodies: perinuclear ANCA (p-ANCA), ACL antibodies and ANA

Imaging and other tests

- **US abdomen** Useful initial investigation and may show bile duct dilatation and liver and splenic changes (not diagnostic however)
- **MRCP** The gold standard to visualise the intrahepatic and extrahepatic bile ducts
- **ERCP** or **transhepatic cholangiography** May also have a role (though both are invasive)
- **MRI abdomen** May help to exclude other disease and evaluate the biliary system
- **Liver biopsy** Rarely diagnostic but may be useful for staging PSC (see below)
- **Colonoscopy and biopsies** Should be performed in patients diagnosed with PSC without known IBD and then repeated annually in PSC patients with colitis

Notes

Primary sclerosing cholangitis

Definition

Ulcerative colitis (UC) is a chronic, relapsing-remitting, non-infectious inflammatory disease of the GI tract. In addition, UC has a number of extra-intestinal manifestations. It is sometimes difficult to distinguish between UC and **isolated colonic Crohn's disease**. These patients can be described as having **indeterminate colitis**.

Pathophysiology

- Microscopically, acute and chronic inflammatory cells infiltrate the lamina propria, crypt branching and villous atrophy are present in UC; neutrophils migrate through the walls of glands to form crypt abscesses; there is depletion of goblet cells and mucin from gland epithelium
- Unlike Crohn's disease, there is no inflammation beyond submucosa
- There is widespread ulceration with preservation of adjacent mucosa which has the appearance of polyps ('pseudopolyps')
- The extent of colitis can be classified into 3 types (see Fig. 1)

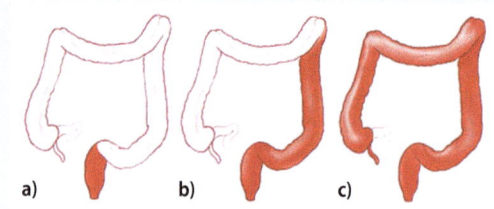

Fig. 1 (a) Ulcerative proctitis (inflammation is limited to the rectum), **(b) left-sided colitis** (inflammation does not extend proximally beyond the splenic flexure), **(c) pancolitis** (inflammation extends proximally beyond the splenic flexure to involve the entire colon)

Ulcerative colitis

Management

Inducing remission

- Rectal (topical) aminosalicylates or steroids: for distal colitis rectal mesalazine has been shown to be superior to rectal steroids and oral aminosalicylates
- Oral aminosalicylates
- Oral prednisolone is usually used 2nd line for patients who fail to respond to aminosalicylates
- IV steroids for severe colitis
- Infliximab for moderate-to-severe UC, when disease is refractory to conventional treatment using corticosteroids and/or immunosuppressive agents

Maintaining remission

- Oral aminosalicylates e.g. mesalazine
- Azathioprine and mercaptopurine
- Probiotics may prevent relapse in patients with mild-to-moderate disease

Surgical

- Surgery is required in approx. 20% of patients with UC
- Colectomy is a curative option for patients who fail to respond to, or are intolerant of, medical treatment, or in those with complications such as colorectal cancer

Investigations

- **Bloods** FBC, CRP ($\uparrow$ in active disease), U&Es, LFTs
- **Stool** Culture and microscopy, faecal calprotectin (a small calcium-binding protein; the concentration of calprotectin in faeces has been shown to correlate well with the severity of intestinal inflammation)
- **AXR** Useful for acute severe colitis to assess extent of colonic involvement; may show lack of faecal shadows, mucosal thickening or toxic megacolon
- **Erect CXR** To rule out perforation in acute severe colitis
- **Barium enema** Loss of haustrations, superficial ulceration, 'pseudopolyps', 'drainpipe colon' (colon is narrow and short)
- **Rigid or flexible sigmoidoscopy** With biopsy
- **Colonoscopy with multiple biopsies** 1st-line procedure for diagnosing colitis

- Family history: 1st-degree relatives of people with UC have a 10–15% increased risk of developing the disease compared with people without a family history
- Oral contraceptives: there is an association between the use of oral contraceptives and the development of IBD
- Not smoking: the risk of UC is reduced in smokers (in contrast to Crohn's disease, where smoking increases the risk)

Risk factors

Intestinal

- Bloody diarrhoea
- Urgency
- Tenesmus
- Abdominal pain, particularly in the left lower quadrant
- Systemic upset: malaise, fever, weight loss

Extra-intestinal

▶Related to disease activity:

- Erythema nodosum
- Aphthous ulcers
- Episcleritis
- Arthritis: pauciarticular, asymmetric
- Osteoporosis

▶Unrelated to disease activity:

- Pyoderma gangrenosum
- Anterior uveitis
- Sacroiliitis
- Ankylosing spondylitis
- Clubbing
- Primary sclerosing cholangitis

Clinical features

Severity

Truelove and Witts' severity index

▶Mild:

- <4 stools/day
- Small amounts of bloody stool
- No anaemia
- Pulse rate <90
- No fever
- Normal ESR/CRP

▶Moderate:

- 4–6 stools/day
- Increased blood in stools compared with above
- No anaemia
- Pulse rate <90
- No fever
- Normal ESR/CRP

▶Severe:

- ≥6 stools/day
- Visible blood in stools
- At least one feature of systemic upset: temperature >37.8℃, pulse rate >90, anaemia, ESR >30

Complications

- Psychological effects
- Toxic megacolon
- Colorectal cancer
- Venous thromboembolism
- Osteoporosis (due to steroid use)

Upper gastrointestinal bleed

Definition

Acute upper gastrointestinal bleeding (UGIB) is a gastroenterological emergency with a mortality of 6–13%.

Causes

Common
- Peptic ulceration
- Mucosal inflammation (oesophagitis, gastritis or duodenitis)
- Oesophageal varices
- Mallory–Weiss tear
- Gastric carcinoma
- Coagulation disorders e.g. thrombocytopenia, warfarin

Rare
- Aortoenteric fistula (especially after aortic surgery)
- Benign tumours: e.g. leiomyoma, carcinoid tumour, angioma
- Congenital: e.g. Ehlers–Danlos, Osler–Weber–Rendu, pseudoxanthoma elasticum

Management

Resuscitation
- ABC approach, wide-bore IV cannula ×2
- IV fluids e.g. normal saline or Hartmann's solution while waiting for blood products
- Patients with massive bleeding should be transfused with blood, platelets and clotting factors in line with local massive haemorrhage protocols
- Red cells should be considered after loss of 30% of the circulating volume
- Fresh frozen plasma in those who have either a fibrinogen level <1g/L, or a PT (INR) or APTT >1.5× normal
- Platelets if actively bleeding and with platelet count of less than 50×10^9/L
- Prothrombin complex concentrate in patients who are taking warfarin and actively bleeding
- Terlipressin and prophylactic antibiotics should be given to patients at presentation for variceal bleeds

Endoscopy

Endoscopy should be offered immediately after resuscitation in patients with a severe bleed. All patients should have endoscopy within 24h. The subsequent management then depends on whether the bleed is non-variceal or variceal.

Non-variceal bleed:
- PPIs should not be routinely given but only to patients with stigmata of recent haemorrhage shown at endoscopy
- Bleeding during endoscopy should be stopped with a mechanical method (e.g. clips) with or without adrenaline, thermal coagulation with adrenaline, fibrin or thrombin with adrenaline
- Interventional radiology should be offered to unstable patients who re-bleed after endoscopic treatment and urgent surgery if interventional radiology is not readily available

Variceal bleed:
- Band ligation should be used for oesophageal varices and injections of N-butyl-2-cyanoacrylate for patients with gastric varices
- Transjugular intrahepatic portosystemic shunts (TIPS) should be offered if bleeding from varices is not controlled despite above measures

Assessment

History

- Abdominal pain
- Bleeding:
  - Haematemesis
  - Coffee-ground vomit
  - Melaena
  - Haematochezia
- Loss of blood: shock, syncope, presyncope
- Features of underlying cause e.g. dyspepsia, weight loss, jaundice
- Risk factors: alcohol, drugs (NSAIDs, corticosteroids)
- Past history of bleeding

Examination

- Pallor and other signs of anaemia
- Pulse: usually tachycardia
- Blood pressure: may be low
- Postural hypotension
- Cool extremities
- Chest pain
- Confusion
- Delirium
- Evidence of dehydration (dry mucosa, sunken eyes, skin turgor reduced)
- Stigmata of liver disease may be present e.g. jaundice, gynaecomastia, ascites, spider naevi, hepatic flap
- Signs of a tumour may be present e.g. nodular liver, abdominal mass, lymphadenopathy
- Subcutaneous emphysema and vomiting suggest Boerhaave syndrome (oesophageal perforation)
- Urine output should be monitored (oliguria is a sign of shock)

Investigations

Bloods

- **FBC** Haemoglobin to check for anaemia; often measured serially to help assess trend
- **Clotting** Partial thromboplastin time (PTT), INR, activated partial thromboplastin time (APTT)
- **Cross-match**
- **LFTs** To identify liver disease
- **U&Es** Urea is typically raised

Endoscopy

Endoscopy should be undertaken immediately after resuscitation for unstable patients with severe acute UGIB.

Imaging

- Erect CXR: may identify perforated viscus
- Erect and supine AXR: to exclude perforated viscus and ileus
- Abdominal CT or US: To identify underlying disease and haemorrhage
- Angiography may be useful if endoscopy fails to identify site of bleeding

Notes

Upper gastrointestinal bleed

Risk assessment

The following formal risk assessment scores are recommended NICE for all patients with acute UGIB:
- The **Blatchford score** at first assessment *and*
- **Rockall score** after endoscopy

Blatchford score (initial assessment)

Admission risk marker	Score component value
Blood urea (mmol/L)	
6.5–8.0	2
8.0–10.0	3
10.0–25	4
>25	6
Haemoglobin (g/dl) for men	
12.0–12.9	1
10.0–11.9	3
<10.0	6
Haemoglobin (g/dl) for women	
10.0–11.9	1
<10.0	6
Systolic blood pressure (mmHg)	
100–109	1
90–99	2
<90	3
Other markers	
Pulse ≥100 (per min)	1
Presentation with melaena	1
Presentation with syncope	2
Hepatic disease	2
Cardiac failure	2

Scores range from 0 to 23, with higher **scores** corresponding to increasing acuity and mortality

The Rockall score (post-endoscopy)

Variable	Score 0	Score 1	Score 2	Score 3
Age (years)	<60	60–79	≥80	
Shock	No shock	Pulse >100 SBP >100	SBP <100	
Comorbidity	Nil major		CHF, IHD, major morbidity	Renal failure, liver failure, metastatic cancer
Diagnosis	Mallory–Weiss	All other diagnoses	GI malignancy	
Evidence of bleeding	None		Blood, adherent clot, spurting vessel	

A score <3 carries good prognosis but total score >8 carries high risk of mortality

Definition

Wilson's disease is a rare **autosomal recessive disorder** characterised by excessive copper deposition in various parts of the body.

Pathophysiology

- Wilson's disease is an autosomal recessive disorder which involves mutation of the *ATP7B* gene on chromosome 13
- The fundamental defect is a failure of hepatic excretion of copper into bile: copper accumulates in the liver and secondarily suppresses the synthesis of caeruloplasmin (major copper-carrying protein in the blood)
- Eventually, copper spills over into the circulation and deposits in the basal ganglia and brain, liver, kidneys, cornea and other organs

Investigations

- Serum caeruloplasmin (↓)
- Serum copper (often ↓) is counter-intuitive, but 95% of plasma copper is carried by caeruloplasmin
- 24-h urinary copper excretion (↑)
- LFTs may be deranged in liver disease
- ECG may indicate cardiac involvement
- Liver biopsy is often diagnostic but only required if clinical signs and non-invasive tests are inconclusive or if there is suspicion of additional liver pathology
- MRI brain may show lesions in the brain compatible with the neurological features; it is common to find increased density in the basal ganglia

Wilson's disease

Management

Non-pharmacological

- Avoid foods containing high amount of copper e.g. chocolate, peanuts and mushrooms
- Monitor urinary copper level to indicate when the patient is back to within normal limits in response to treatment; hepatic and renal function, FBC and clotting should also be monitored
- Annual slit-lamp examination of Kayser–Fleischer rings should document fading or disappearance if copper is being adequately removed
- Genetic screening of all siblings of sufferers; treatment is required for all homozygotes, even if asymptomatic (but not for heterozygotes)

Pharmacological

- **Penicillamine** A copper-chelating agent that is often used 1st line; major side effects include skin disorders, nephrotic syndrome, lupus-like systemic inflammatory conditions and bone marrow suppression; some patients with neurological Wilson's disease experience severe (often transient) deterioration of neurological symptoms when starting treatment with penicillamine
- **Trientine hydrochloride** An alternative chelating agent which is often used as 1st-line therapy for patients with hepatic and neurological disease
- **Zinc** Prevents the absorption of copper but chelation treatment should continue for 2–3 weeks after it has been started, as the onset is slow

Surgical/other

- **Liver transplantation** Indicated for approximately 5% of patients with acute liver failure as the first presentation of disease; outcomes are usually excellent
- **Deep brain stimulation** May be effective in treating medically refractory residual neurological symptoms in a subgroup of patients

Clinical features

- **Liver** Hepatitis, cirrhosis, liver failure
- **Neurological** Basal ganglia degeneration, speech, behavioural and psychiatric problems, Parkinsonism, asterixis, chorea, dementia
- **Cornea** Kayser–Fleischer rings (dark rings that encircle the iris; *Fig. 1*)
- **Kidneys** Renal tubular acidosis (especially Fanconi syndrome)
- **Rheumatological** Osteopenia and osteoarthritis
- **Cardiac** Cardiac arrhythmias and cardiomyopathy
- Other features include pancreatitis, hypoparathyroidism, infertility, blue nails

Note: The onset of symptoms is usually between 10 and 25 years. Children usually present with liver disease whereas the first sign of disease in young adults is often neurological disease.

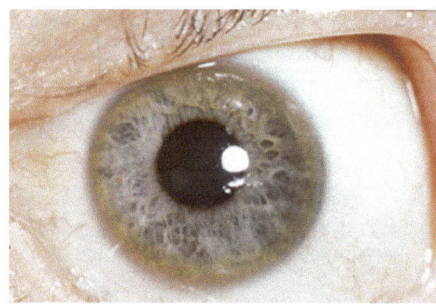

Fig. 1 Kayser–Fleischer rings, a pathognomonic sign of Wilson's disease

Chapter 4

Renal

Acute kidney injury (AKI) is the abrupt loss of kidney function, resulting in the retention of urea and other nitrogenous waste products and in the dysregulation of extracellular volume and electrolytes. This can occur in the setting of previously normal renal function or in patients with pre-existing renal disease (acute on chronic kidney disease). It is usually characterised by a rise in creatinine.

Definition

Diagnostic criteria

- **Stage 1** Creatinine rise of 1.5–1.9× baseline within 7 days or urine output <0.5ml/kg/h for >6h consecutively
- **Stage 2** Creatinine rise of 2.0–2.9× baseline within 7 days or <0.5ml/kg/h for >12h
- **Stage 3** Creatinine rise of more than 3× baseline within 7 days or <0.3ml/kg/h for >24h or anuria for 12h

Risk factors

- ≥65 years
- History of AKI
- Chronic kidney disease
- Symptoms or history of urological obstruction or conditions which may lead to obstruction
- Chronic conditions e.g. heart failure, liver disease and diabetes mellitus
- Neurological or cognitive impairment or disability
- Sepsis
- Hypovolaemia
- Oliguria
- Nephrotoxic drug use within the last week
- Exposure to iodinated contrast agents within the past week

Acute kidney injury

Management

Identify cause and treat

- Pre-renal: IV fluids, treat sepsis
- Renal: stop nephrotoxic drugs e.g. NSAIDs, ACE inhibitors

Monitoring

- Vital signs and fluid balance hourly
- Daily U&Es

Treat complications

- Treat hyperkalaemia: calcium gluconate, insulin/dextrose, salbutamol
- Treat pulmonary oedema
- Treat metabolic acidosis

Dialysis indications (**AEIOU$_2$**):

- **A**cidosis (metabolic): pH <7.2 or BE <10
- **E**lectrolyte disturbance: persistent hyperkalaemia (K$^+$ >7.0mmol/L)
- **I**ntoxication with drugs e.g. lithium and salicylates
- **O**edema-refractory pulmonary oedema
- **U**raemic pericarditis
- **U**raemic encephalopathy

Referral to nephrology:

If the criteria for dialysis are met as above, uncertainty about cause, management or prognosis, likely diagnosis will need specialist treatment (glomerulonephritis, vasculitis, tubulo-interstitial nephritis, myeloma), inadequate response to treatment, or complications, history of renal transplant or CKD stage 4 or 5, stage 3 AKI

Complications

- Pulmonary oedema
- Hyperkalaemia
- Other electrolyte disturbances, e.g. hyperphosphataemia, hyponatraemia, hypermagnesaemia, hypocalcaemia
- Metabolic acidosis
- Uraemic pericarditis

Causes

Pre-renal (most common)

- **Hypovolaemia** e.g. Haemorrhage, gastrointestinal losses, renal losses, burns, diuretic use
- **↓Cardiac output** e.g. Cardiac failure, liver failure, sepsis, drugs
- Drugs that reduce blood pressure, circulating volume, or renal blood flow (e.g. ACE inhibitors, ARBs, NSAIDs, loop diuretics)

Renal

- **Drugs** e.g. ACE inhibitors, NSAIDs, aminoglycosides e.g. gentamicin, cytotoxic drugs e.g. cisplastin
- **Vascular** e.g. Vasculitis, thrombosis, athero/thromboembolism, dissection
- **Glomerular** e.g. Glomerulonephritis, Goodpasture syndrome
- **Tubular** e.g. Ischaemia, rhabdomyolysis, myeloma, contrast-agent induced
- **Interstitial** e.g. Interstitial nephritis, e.g. ascending urinary tract infection

Post-renal (least common)

- **Obstruction** e.g. Renal stones, pyonephrosis, blocked catheter, pelvic mass, enlarged prostate, cervical carcinoma, retroperitoneal fibrosis

Clinical features

- The presentation will depend on the underlying cause and severity of AKI
- Usually accompanied by oliguria or anuria
- Nausea, vomiting
- Dehydration
- Confusion

Investigations

Urine

- **Dipstick** For blood, protein, leucocytes, nitrites and glucose in all patients; detects treatable conditions such as glomerulonephritis, acute pyelonephritis and interstitial nephritis
- **Microscopy, culture** and **sensitivity**
- **Electrolytes and osmolality**

Bloods

- **FBC** ↑Eosinophils in acute interstitial nephritis, cholesterol embolisation and vasculitis; ↓platelets and haemolytic anaemia suggest thrombotic microangiopathy
- **U&Es** ↑Urea, creatinine ± ↑K^+
- **LFTs, CK** ↑In rhabdomyolysis
- **CRP/ESR** ↑In infection/inflammation
- **Immunology** ANA (SLE), ANCA (Wegener's granulomatosis), anti-DsDNA (SLE), anti-GBM, ASOT (post-streptococcal glomerulonephritis), ↓C3, C4 (SLE)
- **Virology** Hepatitis B and C, HIV
- **ABG** Detect electrolyte disturbance and metabolic acidosis
- **Blood culture** For sepsis

Imaging

- **CXR** To rule out pulmonary oedema as a complication of AKI
- **US KUB** If no identified cause of AKI or patient at risk of urinary tract obstruction, offer urgent ultrasound of the urinary tract
- **Doppler US** Assessment of renal artery and veins for possible occlusion
- **MRA** For more accurate assessment of renal vascular occlusion

Notes

Acute kidney injury

Definition

Chronic kidney disease (CKD) is an abnormality of kidney function or structure that is present for more than 3 months, with implications for health.

Causes

- Diabetes
- Hypertension
- Glomerulonephritis
- Obstructive uropathy
- Drugs e.g. lithium, ciclosporin, mesalazine, aminoglycosides
- Polycystic kidney disease
- Alport syndrome
- Recurrent kidney stones
- Acute pyelonephritis/tubulointerstitial disease
- SLE
- Myeloma
- Vasculitis

Chronic kidney disease

Classification (see *Notes*)

Complications

- Cardiovascular disease
- Renal anaemia
- Renal bone disease
- Malnutrition
- Neuropathy
- Hypertension
- Metabolic acidosis
- Carpal tunnel syndrome
- Lipid abnormalities
- ↑Risk of infections

Management

Renoprotection

- Optimum control of BP <130/80mmHg
- ACE inhibitor or angiotensin 2 receptor blocker

Reduce cardiovascular risk

- Optimum control of BP
- Statins
- Smoking cessation
- Optimise diabetes control
- Low-salt diet

Correction of complications

- **Metabolic acidosis** → Sodium bicarbonate
- **Hyperphosphataemia** → Dietary phosphate restriction and phosphate binders
- **Anaemia** → Treat underlying cause e.g. iron deficiency, recombinant human erythropoietin
- **Hyperkalaemia** → Dietary restriction, diuretic use e.g. furosemide
- **Infection risk** → Influenza and pneumococcal vaccinations
- **Vitamin D deficiency** → Vitamin D supplementation

Renal replacement therapy (see *Notes*)

- Haemodialysis
- Peritoneal dialysis
- Renal transplant

Bloods

- **U&Es** ↑Creatinine, ↑urea ↑K^+
- **eGFR** Impaired (see *Notes*)
- **FBC** Normocytic anaemia (↓erythropoietin production)
- **Phosphate** ↑ (phosphate retention)
- **Vitamin D** ↓ Due to impaired production of 1,25-dihydroxyvitamin D
- **Calcium** Initially ↓ due to vitamin D deficiency but may be → or ↑ if 2° and 3° hyperparathyroidism develop
- **Bicarbonate** ↓ (metabolic acidosis)
- **PTH** ↑ In 2° and 3° hyperparathyroidism
- **Lipid profile** Dyslipidaemia is common
- **Autoimmune screen** ANA (SLE), ANCA (Wegener's), anti-GBM (Goodpasture syndrome)

Urine

- **Urinalysis** Haematuria and/or proteinuria
- **Urine ACR** See *Notes*

Imaging

- **Renal US** Renal size generally small in chronic renal failure; exclude presence of obstruction/hydronephrosis; kidney stones
- **AXR** May reveal calcium-containing kidney stones
- **Bone X-ray** May reveal renal osteodystrophy
- **Abdominal CT** May reveal kidney stones, renal masses or cysts
- **Abdominal MRI** May reveal mass lesions in the kidney

Renal biopsy

Helps to determine pathological diagnosis of CKD if diagnosis uncertain.

Investigations

Clinical features

- **Anaemia** Pallor, lethargy, breathlessness
- **Skin** Pigmentation, pruritus
- **GI tract** Anorexia, nausea, vomiting
- **Endocrine** Amenorrhoea, erectile dysfunction, infertility
- **Neurology** Confusion, coma, fits (severe uraemia), polyneuropathy
- **Cardiovascular system** Hypertension, uraemic pericarditis, peripheral vascular disease, heart failure
- **Renal** Nocturia, polyuria, oedema
- **Bone** Osteomalacia, muscle weakness, bone pain, osteosclerosis, hyperparathyroidism
- **Platelet abnormalities** Epistaxis, bruising

Notes

Classification of CKD

- CKD is classified based on the estimated glomerular filtration rate (eGFR) and the level of proteinuria; classifying helps to risk stratify patients
- Patients are classified as G1–G5, based on the eGFR, and A1–A3 based on the ACR (albumin : creatinine ratio); e.g. a person with an eGFR of 30ml/min/1.73m^2 and an ACR of 15mg/mmol has CKD G3bA2 as detailed below:
- It is important to note that patients with an eGFR of >60ml/min/1.73m^2 should not be classified as having CKD unless they have other markers of kidney disease:
  - persistent microalbuminuria
  - persistent proteinuria
  - persistent haematuria (after exclusion of other causes e.g. urological disease)
  - structural abnormalities of the kidneys demonstrated on US or other radiological tests e.g. polycystic kidney disease
  - reflux nephropathy
  - biopsy-proven chronic glomerulonephritis (most of these patients will have microalbuminuria or proteinuria, and/or haematuria)

AKI vs CKD

AKI	CKD
Short duration of symptoms	Long duration of symptoms
Sharp decline in renal function	Gradual decline in renal function
Anaemia of chronic disease not present	Anaemia of chronic disease may be present
Usually normal kidney size on ultrasound scan	Usually small kidney on ultrasound scan
Renal osteodystrophy not present	Renal osteodystrophy may be present

Referral to nephrologist

- Advanced chronic kidney disease (category G4 or G5)
- Rapidly deteriorating renal function
- High levels of proteinuria
- Proteinuria and haematuria
- Poorly controlled HTN, despite being on 4 or more agents
- Suspected rare or genetic cause of CKD
- Suspected renal artery stenosis

Classification of chronic kidney disease using GFR and ACR categories

GFR and ACR categories and risk of adverse outcomes			ACR categories (mg/mmol), description and range		
			<3 Normal to mildly increased	3–30 Moderately increased	>30 Severely increased
			A1	A2	A3
GFR categories (ml/min/1.73m^2), description and range	≥90 Normal and high	G1	No CKD in the absence of markers of kidney damage		
	60–89 Mild reduction related to normal range for a young adult	G2			
	45–59 Mild–moderate reduction	G3a			
	30–44 Moderate–severe reduction	G3b			
	15–29 Severe reduction	G4			
	<15 Kidney failure	G5			

Increasing risk

Haemodialysis

- Haemodialysis involves pumping blood from the body through an artificial kidney in which the blood is surrounded by a solution of electrolytes (the dialysate); solutes present in the blood at excessive concentrations, e.g. urea, potassium, creatinine, diffuse into the dialysate and are removed; blood is drawn from an arteriovenous fistula and then circulated through the dialyser and returned into the fistula
- Heparin is constantly infused to prevent contact of blood with foreign surfaces activating the clotting cascade
- Ultrafiltration is used to regulate the distribution of water between the blood and dialysate
- Haemodialysis requires the patient to have very good vascular access, which is attained by creating a fistula between a peripheral artery and vein (commonly radial or brachial), or a permanent catheter inserted into an internal jugular or subclavian vein; the fistula takes several weeks to mature and should ideally be fashioned 3–6 months before starting haemodialysis
- Haemodialysis can be carried out in a hospital setting or in the patient's home; it is usually performed 3×/week for about 4h
- **Complications** Access-related complications (local infection, endocarditis, osteomyelitis, stenosis, thrombosis or aneurysm), hypotension (common), cardiac arrhythmias, air embolism, nausea / vomiting, headache, cramps, infected central lines, dialyser reactions, heparin-induced thrombocytopenia, haemolysis, disequilibration syndrome (restlessness, headache, tremors, fits and coma), depression

Peritoneal dialysis

- Peritoneal dialysis should be considered as 1st choice of treatment for: children 2 years or younger, people with residual renal function and adults without significant associated comorbidities
- A dialysate is infused into the peritoneal cavity and the blood flowing through peritoneal capillaries acts as the blood source; ultrafiltration is controlled by altering the osmolality of the dialysate solution and thus drawing water out of the patient's blood; a permanent tube (Tenkoff catheter) is inserted into the patient's peritoneum (under local or general anaesthetic) through which dialysate is infused; the waste solutes are removed by exchanging the peritoneal fluid for a fresh solution
- The main advantage of peritoneal dialysis is that it can be performed at home, at work or while on holiday, therefore allows a high degree of independence and control although a great deal of support is still required
- **Complications** Peritonitis, sclerosing peritonitis, catheter problems (infection, blockage, kinking, leaks or slow drainage), constipation, fluid retention, hyperglycaemia, weight gain, hernias (incisional, inguinal, umbilical), back pain, malnutrition and depression

Renal transplant

- A kidney transplant provides the best long-term outcome for patients with end-stage kidney disease; the kidney may come from a cadaveric donor (85–90%) or from a living donor
- All patients with end-stage kidney disease should be considered for a transplant; age is not a major factor itself for outcome but the presence of comorbidities significantly affects survival
- To prevent rejection, the recipients receive induction at the time of transplant with monoclonal or polyclonal antibodies; maintenance immunosuppression is then required in the long term to prevent rejection
- Patients need to be followed up for life and this includes annual screening for cancers, drug toxicity and cardiovascular disease
- **Benefits of transplantation**: Can stop dialysis, improved quality of life with normal diet and activity, relaxation of fluid restriction, reversal of anaemia and renal bone disease
- **Complications** Postoperative problems e.g. deep vein thrombosis, pulmonary embolism and pneumonia; opportunistic infections: viral (especially herpes simplex and CMV), fungal and bacterial; malignancies (particularly lymphomas and skin cancers), drug toxicity, bone marrow suppression, recurrence of the original disease in the transplant, urinary tract obstruction, cardiovascular disease, hypertension, dyslipidaemia, graft rejection (hyperacute, accelerated, acute or chronic)

Nephritic syndrome refers to a group of clinical features that are caused by acute inflammation of the glomeruli (**glomerulonephritis**). It is characterised by haematuria, proteinuria, rise in serum creatinine and systemic hypertension.

- Nephritic syndrome occurs as a result of inflammatory damage to the renal endothelium
- The main causes of glomerulonephritis share intraglomerular inflammation and include vasculitis, antibody-mediated damage and immune-complex disease

- **Acute glomerulonephritis** When nephritic syndrome occurs acutely (most common form)
- **Rapidly progressive glomerulonephritis (RPGN)** When renal function (as measured by the glomerular filtration rate, GFR) deteriorates over a period of days to weeks; it is typically associated with crescents on renal biopsy; underlying causes include Goodpasture syndrome, SLE and granulomatosis with polyangiitis
- **Chronic glomerulonephritis** Nephritic syndrome occurring over months to years with no change in the renal function

Definition

Pathophysiology

Classification

Nephritic syndrome

Investigations

Management

- Treat underlying cause
- Inflammatory renal disorders should be treated with immunosuppressive agents, which typically include immunosuppression with steroids, mTOR inhibitors (e.g. sirolimus) and cytotoxic drugs e.g. cyclophosphamide
- Nephritic syndrome due to preformed antibodies may benefit from having those antibodies removed by plasmapheresis, especially in the setting of pulmonary haemorrhage
- Monitor fluid balance, weight, blood pressure and renal function
- Restrict Na^+ and K^+ as appropriate
- Fluid restriction
- Treat hypertension accordingly
- Consider prophylactic penicillin
- Consider dialysis for end-stage renal failure

Bloods

- **U&Es, eGFR**
- **Serum antistreptolysin-O titre**
- **Glucose**
- **Autoantibodies** ANA, anti-DsDNA and anti-Smith antibody (SLE), anti-GBM antibody (Goodpasture syndrome), ANCA (granulomatosis with polyangiitis)
- **Complement levels** (C3, C4) Usually low
- **Hepatitis and HIV screen**
- **Cryoglobulins** Raised in cryoglobulinaemia

Urine

- **Dipstick** Positive for protein and blood
- **Microscopy** Red cell casts (see *Fig. 2*)
- **Microalbumin** Raised but not in nephrotic range

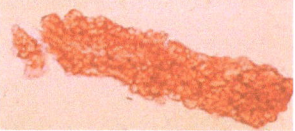

Fig. 2 Red cell cast on urine microscopy

Imaging

- **CXR** May show cavities in granulomatosis with polyangiitis or malignancy
- **US kidneys** To assess renal size and to look for renal vein thrombosis

Renal biopsy

Confirms diagnosis of glomerulonephritis

Other

Throat swab or skin swab for *Streptococcus* spp. if clinically indicated

- **Post-streptococcal glomerulonephritis** (see *Notes*)
- **IgA nephropathy** (see *Notes*)
- **Henoch–Schönlein purpura (HSP)** An IgA-mediated small vessel vasculitis usually seen in children following an infection; presents with palpable purpuric rash (over buttocks and extensor surfaces of arms and legs, see *Fig. 1*), abdominal pain, polyarthritis and features of IgA nephropathy

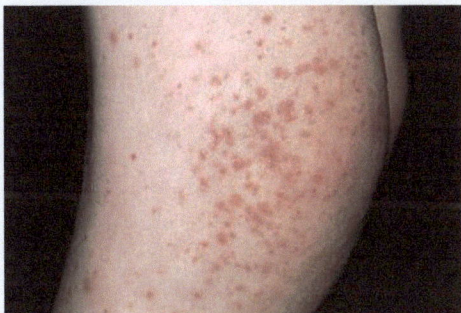

Fig. 1 Rash in Henoch–Schönlein purpura

- **Haemolytic uraemic syndrome** Most commonly associated with *E. coli* O157:H7 and causes a triad of microangiopathic haemolytic anaemia, thrombocytopenia and acute kidney injury

Common causes in adults

- **Non-streptococcal post-infectious glomerulonephritis** Viruses (e.g. HIV, hepatitis B and C, mumps), bacteria (e.g. staphylococci, legionella), fungi (e.g. candida and histoplasma), parasites (e.g. malaria and schistosomiasis)
- **Goodpasture syndrome** A rare autoimmune disease caused by a type II antigen–antibody reaction leading to diffuse pulmonary haemorrhage and glomerulonephritis; there are circulating antiglomerular basement membrane (anti-GBM) antibodies
- **Membranoproliferative glomerulonephritis**
- **Granulomatosis with polyangiitis** (see *Notes*)
- **Infective endocarditis**
- **SLE**
- **Cryoglobulinaemia**

Causes

Notes

Nephritic syndrome

Clinical features (PHAROH)

- **P**roteinuria (subnephrotic syndrome) and **P**yuria
- **H**aematuria: visible or non-visible
- **A**zotaemia: elevated urea and creatinine
- **R**ed cell casts: seen on urine microscopy
- **O**edema and **O**liguria
- **H**ypertension

Post-streptococcal glomerulonephritis

Post-streptococcal glomerulonephritis typically occurs 7–14 days following a **group A beta-haemolytic *Streptococcus* spp**. infection (usually *S. pyogenes* causing a throat infection or skin infection).

Pathophysiology

It is caused by immune complex (IgG, IgM and C3) deposition in the glomeruli

Clinical features

- Young children are most commonly affected
- General: headache, malaise, fever, nausea, anorexia
- Haematuria
- Oedema
- Oliguria
- Proteinuria
- Hypertension

Diagnostic features

- Low complement levels
- Raised ASO titre
- Renal biopsy features: diffuse proliferative glomerulonephritis, endothelial proliferation with neutrophils, subepithelial 'humps' caused by lumpy immune-complex deposits, immunofluorescence: granular or 'starry sky' appearance

Management

- Treatment is usually supportive and focuses on managing hypertension and oedema
- Patients should receive penicillin to eradicate the bacteria
- Carries a good prognosis

IgA nephropathy

IgA nephropathy (also known as Berger's disease) is the commonest cause of glomerulonephritis worldwide. It classically presents as **macroscopic haematuria** in young people following an upper respiratory tract infection.

Pathophysiology

- Thought to be caused by mesangial deposition of IgA immune complexes
- There is considerable pathological overlap with HSP

Clinical features

- Young males more commonly affected
- Causes recurrent episodes of macroscopic haematuria
- Typically associated with a recent upper respiratory tract infection
- Nephrotic range of proteinuria is rare
- Renal failure is unusual and seen in a minority of patients

Diagnostic features

- Plasma levels of IgA are raised in about half of cases
- Histology shows mesangial hypercellularity, segmental glomerulosclerosis, endocapillary hypercellularity and positive immunofluorescence for IgA and C3

Management

- Monitor renal function and blood pressure
- Treat hypertension with ACE inhibitors or ARBs
- Steroids reduce the progression of kidney disease
- Poor prognostic indicators include hypertension and heavy proteinuria

Granulomatosis with polyangiitis

Granulomatosis with polyangiitis (previously known as Wegener's granulomatosis) is a rare autoimmune condition associated with a necrotising granulomatous vasculitis, affecting both upper and lower respiratory tract as well as causing acute glomerulonephritis.

Pathophysiology

- There is an upregulation in the production of cytoplasmic **anti-neutrophil cytoplasmic antibodies (c-ANCA)**
- The c-ANCA autoantibodies interact with activated neutrophils and endothelial cells within blood vessel walls, causing vessel inflammation and damage
- This causes granulomatous inflammation within blood vessels, especially in the respiratory tract and the kidneys

Clinical features

- Upper respiratory tract: epistaxis, sinusitis, nasal crusting
- Lower respiratory tract: dyspnoea, haemoptysis
- Saddle-shape nose deformity
- Other features: vasculitic rash, eye involvement (e.g. proptosis) and cranial nerve lesions

Diagnostic features

- c-ANCA (positive in >90%), p-ANCA (positive in 25%)
- CXR: wide variety of presentations, including cavitating lesions
- Renal biopsy: epithelial crescents in Bowman's capsule

Management

- Treatment options include steroids, cyclophosphamide and plasma exchange
- Median survival is approximately 8–9 years

Nephrotic syndrome is a clinical syndrome showing specific features of:
- **PrOteinuria** (≥3.5g/day) causing
- **HypOalbuminaemia** (serum albumin ≤30g/L) causing
- **O**edema

It is caused by increased permeability of serum protein in the renal glomerulus.

Definition

Causes

Primary glomerular diseases
- **Minimal change glomerular disease** (accounts for 75% of cases in children and 25% in adults)
- **Focal segmental glomerulosclerosis:** the most common cause of idiopathic nephrotic syndrome in adults
- **Membranous glomerular disease**
- **Membranoproliferative glomerulonephritis**

Secondary glomerular diseases
- **Infection** e.g. HIV, hepatitis B and C, mycoplasma, syphilis, malaria
- **Collagen vascular diseases** e.g. SLE, RA, polyarteritis nodosa
- **Metabolic diseases** e.g. diabetes mellitus, amyloidosis
- **Inherited disease** e.g. Alport syndrome, hereditary nephritis
- **Malignant disease** e.g. myeloma, leukaemia, lymphoma, carcinoma
- **Drugs** e.g. NSAIDs, lithium, gold, penicillamine and toxins (e.g. bee sting, snake bite)
- **Pregnancy** e.g. pre-eclampsia

Nephrotic syndrome

Complications
- Venous thrombosis
- Sepsis
- Acute kidney infection
- Chronic kidney disease
- Hyperlipidaemia
- Hypertension

Management

Lifestyle
- Fluid and salt restriction
- Smoking cessation
- Exercise and balanced diet with adequate calorific intake and sufficient protein content (1–2g/kg daily)
- Monitor weight regularly to help determine fluid status

Treat underlying cause
- Immunotherapy regimen e.g. prednisolone and cyclophosphamide
- Stop offending drugs
- Treat underlying cancer

Treat complications
- Treat fluid overload: diuretics
- Treat proteinuria: ACE inhibitors/ angiotensin 2 receptor blockers
- Treat hyperlipidaemia: statins
- Patients with severely low albumin levels may require admission to receive IV albumin therapy
- Infection prophylaxis: influenza and pneumococcal vaccinations
- Thrombosis risk: avoid prolonged bed rest, consider prophylactic anticoagulation
- Treat hypertension

Investigations
- **Urine** Dipstick analysis, Bence Jones protein, albumin : creatinine ratio – to quantify proteinuria
- **Bloods** FBC, coagulation screen, U&Es, ESR/ CRP, fasting glucose, immunoglobulins, serum electrophoresis, autoimmune screen, hepatitis B and C and HIV serology, lipids
- **CXR** To check for pulmonary oedema/pleural effusion
- **US abdomen/kidneys** To check for ascites, the presence of two kidneys, the size and shape of the kidneys and for any urinary tract obstruction
- **Renal biopsy** Under ultrasound to guide diagnosis

Symptoms

- Oedema
- Tiredness
- Frothiness of urine
- Breathlessness (related to pleural effusion)

Signs

- Oedema: periorbital oedema (see *Fig. 1*) (commonly in children), lower limb oedema, oedema of genitals, ascites
- Leuconychia (see *Fig. 2*)
- Signs of fluid overload e.g. oedema, raised JVP
- Signs of pleural effusion e.g. dyspnoea, stony dull percussion of chest, reduced breath sounds at bases
- Signs of dyslipidaemia: eruptive xanthomata, xanthelasma (see *Fig. 3*)

Clinical features

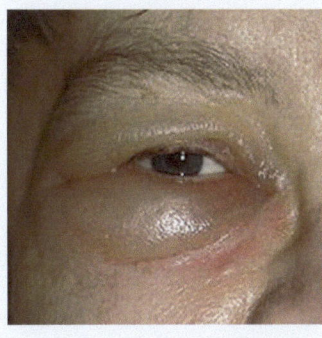

Fig. 1 Periorbital oedema

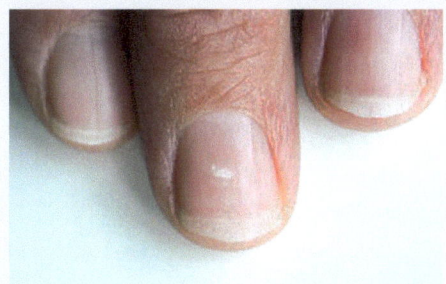

Fig. 2 Leuconychia, which can be caused by hypoalbuminaemia

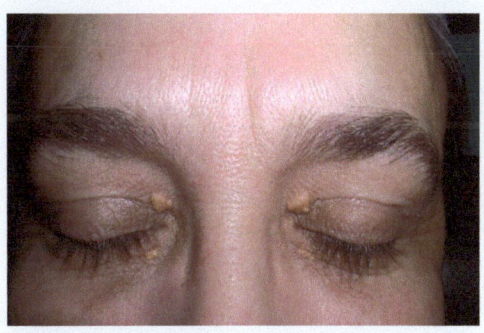

Fig. 3 Xanthelasma: yellow fat deposits underneath the skin, usually on or around the eyelids

Notes

Urinary tract infection (UTI) is presence of characteristic symptoms and significant bacteriuria from kidneys to bladder.

Classification

- **Lower UTI** Generally considered infection of the bladder (cystitis)
- **Upper UTI** Includes pyelitis (infection of the proximal part of the ureters) and pyelonephritis (infection of the kidneys and the proximal part of the ureters)
- **Recurrent UTI** May be due to relapse (recurrent UTI with the same strain of organism) or re-infection (recurrent UTI with a different strain or species of organism)
- **Uncomplicated UTI** Infection of the urinary tract by a usual pathogen in a person with a normal urinary tract and with normal kidney function
- **Complicated UTI** Where anatomical, functional or pharmacological factors predispose the person to persistent infection, recurrent infection or treatment failure e.g. abnormal urinary tract
- **Urethral syndrome or painful bladder syndrome** Symptoms of cystitis in the absence of UTI; this syndrome is also called interstitial cystitis, bladder pain syndrome and trigonitis

Definition

Complications

- Pyelonephritis
- Perinephric and intrarenal abscess
- Hydronephrosis or pyonephrosis
- Acute kidney injury
- Sepsis

Urinary tract infection

Management

Conservative

- Education about the condition and avoidance of certain risk factors e.g. spermicide use
- Vaginal oestrogen therapy in post-menopausal women should be considered as a preventative measure
- There is no significant evidence that drinking cranberry juice, increasing fluid intake or personal hygiene measures makes a difference
- D-mannose can be used to prevent UTIs

Pharmacological

- Empirical treatment: trimethoprim or nitrofurantoin for 3 days – the drugs of choice for the empirical treatment of uncomplicated lower UTI
- Oral ciprofloxacin for 7–10 days or co-amoxiclav or cefalexin are choices for upper UTI
- Pregnant women with symptomatic bacteriuria should be treated with an antibiotic for 7 days; a urine culture should be sent
- Men, patients with 'complicated UTI' and catheterised patients should be treated for 7 days
- Prophylactic antibiotics with low-dose trimethoprim or nitrofurantoin can be used for recurrent cystitis
- Paracetamol and/or NSAIDs can be used for symptomatic treatment

Investigations

- **Urine dipstick** Often positive for nitrite and/or leucocytes, may show microscopic haematuria
- **Urine microscopy, culture and sensitivity** Shows high WCC, causative organism and sensitivities to antibiotics
- **US/CT KUB** Should be considered to rule out urinary obstruction/collection in acute uncomplicated pyelonephritis or to rule out structural causes for recurrent UTIs or complicated UTIs

- Female (due to shorter urethra and proximity to anus)
- Increasing age
- Recent instrumentation of the renal tract
- Abnormality of the renal tract
- Incomplete bladder emptying
- Sexual activity
- New sexual partner
- Use of spermicide
- Diabetes
- Catheterisation
- Institutionalisation
- Pregnancy
- Immunocompromised/ immunosuppressed

- *E. coli* (80%)
- *P. mirabilis*
- *Klebsiella* spp.
- Enterococci
- *Enterobacter* spp.
- *Staphylococcus saprophyticus*: the 2nd leading cause in sexually active females
- *Pseudomonas aeruginosa*
- *Candida albicans* (rare)

- Entry of bacteria into the urinary tract may be:
  - Retrograde, with ascension through urethra into bladder most commonly from faecal origin
  - Via the bloodstream; is more likely in people who are immunosuppressed
  - Direct, e.g. insertion of a catheter into the bladder, instrumentation or surgery
- The urinary system has defences to prevent UTI such as micturition, secreted factors and mucosal defences but when these defences are overcome by bacterial virulence factors then the patient is prone to developing a UTI
- Virulence factors include fimbriae which allow binding, and a bacterial capsule that resists phagocytosis (uropathogenic *Escherichia coli*); *Proteus mirabilis* produces urease and increases the pH of urine

Risk factors

Causes

Pathophysiology

Notes

Urinary tract infection

Clinical features

- Urinary frequency
- Dysuria
- Haematuria
- Foul-smelling ± cloudy urine
- Urgency
- Urinary incontinence
- Suprapubic pain and tenderness
- Loin/flank pain and tenderness (suggest upper UTI)
- Rigors
- Pyrexia
- Nausea ± vomiting
- Acute confusional state (delirium): particularly elderly patient

Chapter 5

Endocrinology

Acromegaly is a rare disorder caused by excessive secretion of **growth hormone (GH)** and it is almost always due to a **benign pituitary adenoma**. It is very rarely caused by ectopic production of GH or unregulated GH-releasing hormone (GHRH) secretion. It results in an overgrowth of all organ systems, bones, joints and soft tissues.

Definition

- Under the influence of **GHRH** and **somatostatin** (SST), both produced by the hypothalamus, GH is secreted in a pulsatile manner
- Hypoglycaemia stimulates GH secretion while hyperglycaemia has the opposite effect
- GHRH stimulates GH production by the somatotrophs of the anterior pituitary gland, and somatostatin-14 inhibits both GH and thyroid-stimulating hormone (TSH) secretion
- Ghrelin hormone produced by the GI tract acts on the hypothalamus to stimulate GHRH and also acts on the anterior pituitary gland directly to promote GH secretion
- GH acts on adipose tissue (to promote lipolysis), on the liver (to promote gluconeogenesis and stimulate the release of **insulin-like growth factor 1**, **IGF-1**) and on muscle (to promote protein synthesis)
- IGF-1 itself ↑somatic cell growth, chondrocyte function and bone modelling/remodelling
- The negative feedback effects on the control of GH secretion are via IGF-1 and by feedback of GH on the hypothalamus (see *Fig. 1*)

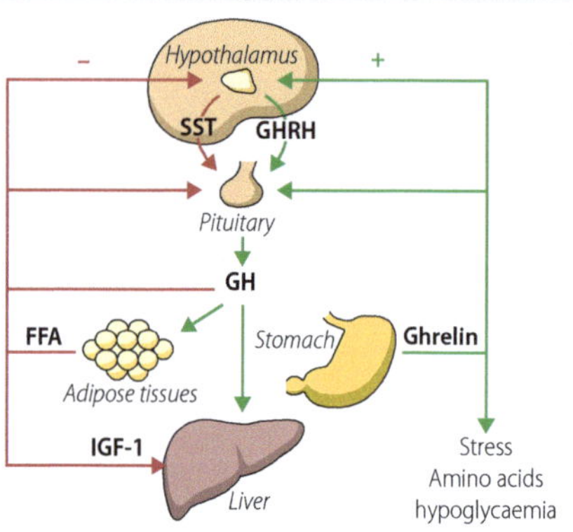

Fig. 1 Control of GH secretion; FFA, free fatty acids

Growth hormone physiology

Acromegaly

Complications

- Impaired glucose tolerance or diabetes
- Cardiovascular disease: hypertension, ischaemic heart disease, cardiomyopathy, heart failure
- Colonic polyps and adenocarcinoma of the colon
- Obstructive sleep apnoea
- Hyperprolactinaemia, ↓glucocorticoids, sex steroids and thyroid hormone
- Hypopituitarism (post-surgery or radiotherapy)

Management

Pharmacological

- **SST analogues** 1st-choice medical treatment, e.g. octreotide
- **Dopamine agonists** Effective (e.g. cabergoline) but less so than SST analogues
- **GH receptor antagonists** e.g. Pegvisomant is licensed for the treatment of acromegaly in patients with inadequate response to surgery, radiotherapy or somatostatin analogues

Surgical

- **Trans-sphenoidal surgery** Treatment of choice in most cases

Radiotherapy

- Used for refractory disease, as an adjuvant for large invasive tumours and when surgery is contraindicated

Investigations

- Blood: glucose, serum phosphate, urinary calcium and serum triglycerides (may all be raised)
- **IGF-1:** used for initial screening as it is highly sensitive (normal level usually excludes acromegaly)
- **Oral glucose tolerance test:** if the glucose load fails to suppress GH it is diagnostic of acromegaly
- Prolactin, adrenal, thyroid and gonadal hormones (tumour may cause hypopituitarism)
- Visual field assessment: the most common defect is a bitemporal hemianopia due to compression of the optic chiasm
- MRI of the pituitary gland and hypothalamus to confirm the pituitary tumour
- Cardiac assessment: ECG, ECHO (to rule out cardiovascular complications)

- **Headache** Common and often unrelated to size of adenoma
- **Facial changes** (*see Figs. 2 and 3*)
- **Skin changes** Include excess sweating and skin tags
- **Sexual dysfunction** Subfertility, amenorrhoea, loss of libido
- **Hands and feet** These grow (*see Fig. 4*) leading to difficulty in wearing rings and increase in shoe size
- **Visual field defects** (*see Fig. 5*)
- **Joint pain** Common, mainly load-bearing joints and kyphoscoliosis
- **Fatigue**
- **Carpal tunnel syndrome**
- **Galactorrhoea**

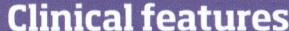

Clinical features

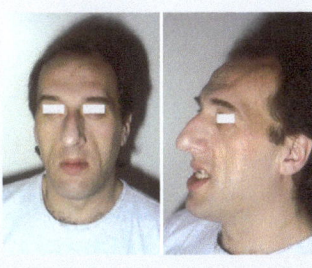

Fig. 2 Characteristic facial features of acromegaly including coarsening of the general appearance, widening of the nose, thicker lips, development of frontal bossing and prognathism

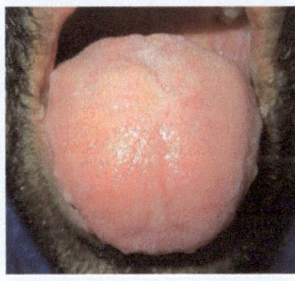

Fig. 3 Macroglossia seen in a patient with acromegaly

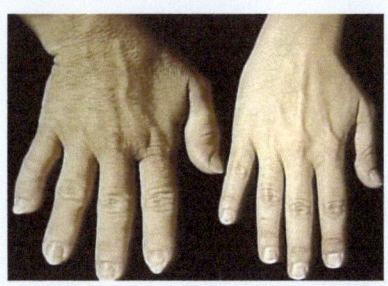

Fig. 4 The hand of a patient with acromegaly: 'spade like' (left) compared with someone with normal-sized hands

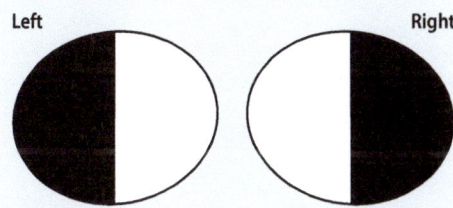

Fig. 5 The most common defect is a **bitemporal hemianopia** caused by compression of the optic chiasm by the pituitary adenoma

Causes

- **Pituitary adenoma** (95% of cases)
- **Ectopic GH** from non-endocrine tumours (rare) e.g. lung cancer, pancreatic cancer, ovarian cancer
- **Familial:** as part of MEN-1, familial acromegaly, Carney's complex or McCune–Albright syndrome

Notes

Acromegaly

Definition

Adrenal insufficiency is a group of disorders in which there is a failure to produce adequate amounts of adrenal hormones, i.e. **glucocorticoids (cortisol)** and/or **mineralocorticoids (aldosterone)**.

Pathophysiology

- **Adrenal insufficiency** May be primary, secondary or tertiary
- **Primary adrenal insufficiency** The adrenal gland cortex is destroyed therefore it has impaired ability to secrete hormones (but hypothalamus and pituitary gland function remain intact); this leads to loss of both cortisol and aldosterone secretion
- **Addison's disease** Most common cause of primary adrenal insufficiency in the West; there is progressive destruction of the adrenal glands via autoimmune mechanisms and antibodies against steroid 21-hydroxylase can be found in about 85% of patients
- **Addison's disease** Associated with other autoimmune conditions e.g. autoimmune thyroid disease, type 1 diabetes and pernicious anaemia
- **Tuberculosis** The leading cause of primary adrenal insufficiency worldwide and is often in combination with HIV infection
- **Secondary adrenal insufficiency** Results from disruption of adrenocorticotropic hormone (ACTH) secretion by the pituitary gland (hypopituitarism) and **tertiary adrenal insufficiency** results from loss of CRH secretion due to hypothalamic damage or long-term glucocorticoid treatment
- **Secondary and tertiary causes** Result in glucocorticoid but not aldosterone deficiency as aldosterone is not under the control of ACTH

Adrenal insufficiency

Notes

Adrenal insufficiency

Management

Acute (Addisonian crisis)

- Aggressive fluid resuscitation with IV normal saline
- Immediate administration of hydrocortisone e.g. 100mg IV or IM
- Continuous cardiac and electrolyte monitoring
- Treatment of the underlying precipitating disorder, e.g. treat infection with antibiotics

Long-term

- **Hormone replacement** Hydrocortisone and fludrocortisone
- **Patient education**:
  - Information about the condition
  - Medical emergency identification bracelet and steroid card
  - Importance of not missing steroids/stopping them abruptly
  - Intercurrent illness: if tolerating oral medication then double dose, and if unable to take orally seek urgent medical help
  - Advice for travel: carry extra medication and an emergency self-injection kit

Causes

Primary adrenal insufficiency

- **Autoimmunity (Addison's disease):** accounts for approx. 85% of cases of primary adrenal insufficiency in the developed world
- Infections: TB (most common cause of primary adrenal insufficiency world-wide), HIV, histoplasmosis, cryptococcosis, syphilis
- Trauma
- Post adrenalectomy
- Invasion: e.g. neoplastic, sarcoidosis, amyloidosis, haemochromatosis

Secondary adrenal insufficiency

- Pituitary disorders: e.g. tumours, irradiation, infiltration, Sheehan syndrome
- Isolated ACTH deficiency
- Chronic opiate usage

Tertiary adrenal insufficiency

- Long-term glucocorticoid treatment (accounts for approx. 99% of cases of adrenal insufficiency)
- Directly following cure of Cushing syndrome
- Hypothalamic impairment: infiltrative disease e.g. sarcoidosis, tumours, irradiation

Clinical features

Acute (may present as a 'crisis')

- Hypotension
- Hypovolaemic shock
- Acute abdominal pain
- Low-grade fever and vomiting
- Collapse

Chronic ('develops insidiously and may be mild')

▶**Symptoms:**

- Lethargy
- Weakness
- Anorexia
- Nausea and vomiting
- Abdominal pain
- Weight loss
- 'Salt-craving'
- Confusion/personality change
- Diarrhoea
- Constipation
- Syncope or dizziness
- Irritability

▶**Signs:**

- Hyperpigmentation (primary adrenal insufficiency only, see *Fig. 1*): often at buccal mucosa, lips, palmar creases, new scars (not present in secondary adrenal insufficiency)
- Hypotension
- Postural hypotension

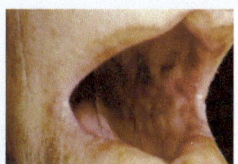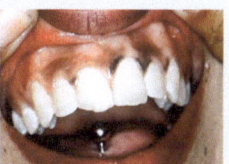

Fig. 1 Hyperpigmentation in buccal mucosa in patients with primary adrenal insufficiency

Investigations

Screening tests

- **Bloods** FBC (possibly anaemia, mild eosinophilia and lymphocytosis), U&Es ($\downarrow Na^+$, $\uparrow K^+$), LFTs (possible raised ALT), glucose ($\downarrow$), Ca^{2+} (possibly $\uparrow$), adrenal autoantibodies e.g. anti-21-hydroxylase for Addison's
- **ABG** As above and may show metabolic acidosis
- **Imaging** CXR (rule out lung cancer), CT or MRI of adrenal gland (investigate primary causes) or hypothalamic pituitary region (investigate secondary causes)

Diagnostic tests

- **ACTH** ($\uparrow$ in 1° adrenal insufficiency and $\downarrow$ in 2° adrenal insufficiency)
- **Cortisol levels** (0900h) Low; ≥500nmol/L makes Addison's very unlikely
- **Insulin tolerance test** Hypoglycaemia is induced by an insulin infusion and the cortisol response is monitored; confirms 2° adrenal insufficiency
- **ACTH stimulation (Synacthen®) test** ACTH is administered IV or IM, and cortisol levels measured 30min later; the normal response is $\uparrow$ in cortisol; in 1° adrenal insufficiency this does not occur
- **CRH test** Used to differentiate between 2° and 3° adrenal insufficiency; after administration of CRH, ACTH response is measured. Patients with 2° adrenal insufficiency, i.e. pituitary disease, do not respond whereas those with hypothalamic disease, i.e. 3° adrenal insufficiency, do respond

Cushing syndrome is the term used to describe a range of signs and symptoms which occur as a result of prolonged exposure to **glucocorticoids**.

Definition

- Glucocorticoids, most importantly cortisol, are produced by the adrenal cortex
- The release of cortisol is under the control of **corticotropin-releasing hormone (CRH)** by the hypothalamus and **adrenocorticotropic hormone (ACTH)** by the anterior pituitary gland (see *Fig. 1*)
- The cause of Cushing syndrome can be either **exogenous** (most common) or **endogenous**
- Endogenous causes result from the adrenal gland itself producing excessive cortisol (**ACTH independent**) or in response to excessive stimulation from ACTH (**ACTH dependent**) produced by the anterior pituitary gland or from elsewhere

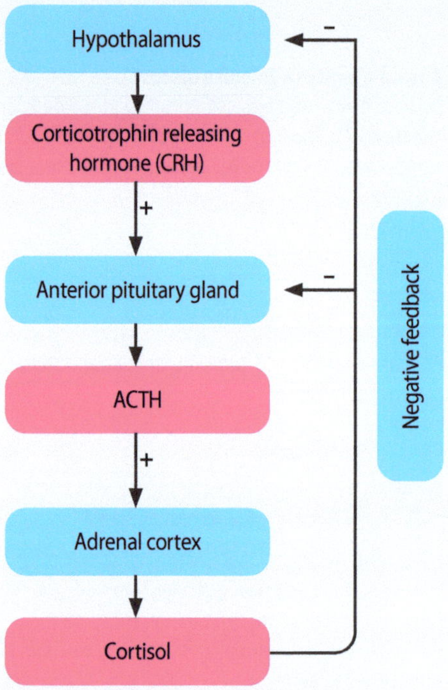

Fig. 1 The hypothalamus–pituitary–adrenal axis

Pathophysiology

Cushing syndrome

Complications

- 'Steroid diabetes'
- Osteoporosis
- Hypertension
- Coagulopathy
- Metabolic syndrome
- Immunosuppression
- Nelson syndrome: ACTH-secreting tumour develops following therapeutic total bilateral adrenalectomy (TBA) for Cushing syndrome
- Cataracts

Management

- Stop/reduce dose of offending drug for exogenous Cushing syndrome
- Consider steroid-sparing agents such as azathioprine for exogenous Cushing syndrome
- Trans-sphenoidal microsurgery or radiotherapy-adjunct for pituitary tumours (Cushing disease)
- Adrenalectomy: 'cures' adenomas but rarely cures cancer
- Treat underlying cancer in ectopic cortisol secretion
- Metyrapone, ketoconazole, and mitotane can all be used to lower cortisol by directly inhibiting synthesis and secretion in the adrenal gland

1. Confirm raised cortisol

- **Urinary free cortisol** Simple and non-invasive; very sensitive but not specific
- **Overnight dexamethasone suppression test** Give dexamethasone 1mg PO at midnight and measure serum cortisol at 0800h; in Cushing syndrome, there is no cortisol suppression
- **Low-dose dexamethasone suppression test** Patient is given dexamethasone 0.5mg/6h orally for 2 days; measure cortisol at 0 and 48h; in Cushing syndrome, there is failure to suppress cortisol
- **Midnight salivary cortisol** Reflects free plasma cortisol since there is no cortisol-binding globulin in saliva; has good sensitivity and specificity

Causes

ACTH dependent

- Cushing disease: excess ACTH from the pituitary (80%)
- Ectopic ACTH-producing tumour: e.g. small cell lung cancer (5–10%)
- Excess exogenous ACTH administration

ACTH independent

- Excess exogenous glucocorticoid administration (most common)
- Adrenal adenoma
- Adrenal carcinoma (rare)
- Familial Cushing syndrome and other rare causes such as MEN-1, McCune–Albright syndrome, adrenal macronodular hyperplasia and food-induced Cushing syndrome

Clinical features

Signs

- 'Moon-shaped' face (see Fig. 2)
- Striae (see Fig. 3)
- Proximal muscle weakness
- Plethoric facies
- Easy bruising
- Weight gain with poor linear growth (in children and adolescents)
- Buffalo hump (fat pad sign)
- Central obesity
- Thin skin and poor healing
- Hirsutism with crown hair loss
- Acne
- Virilisation, short stature, advanced or delayed puberty in children
- ↑Pigmentation (ACTH-dependent Cushing syndrome only)

Symptoms

- Depression
- Difficulty with weight management
- Fatigue
- Psychotic features
- Decreased libido
- Menstrual abnormalities
- Back pain

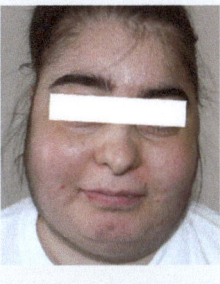

Fig. 2 'Moon-shaped' face

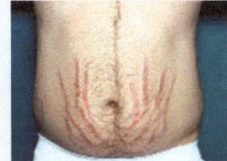

Fig. 3 Abdominal striae

Investigations

Diagnosis of Cushing syndrome involves a 2 step process: first, confirming raised cortisol levels, followed by investigating the underlying cause (provided an obvious cause such as exogenous corticosteroids is not present)

2. Establish cause for ↑cortisol

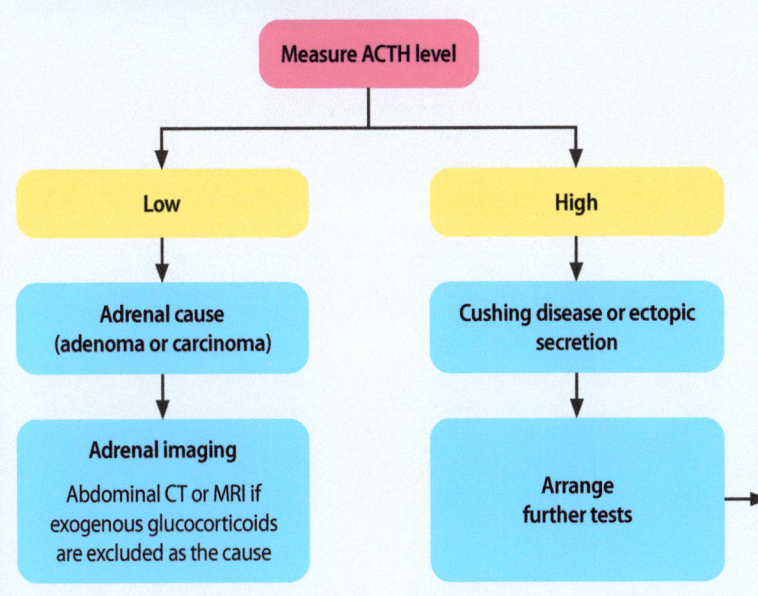

Measure ACTH level

Low → **Adrenal cause (adenoma or carcinoma)** → **Adrenal imaging** — Abdominal CT or MRI if exogenous glucocorticoids are excluded as the cause

High → **Cushing disease or ectopic secretion** → **Arrange further tests**

- **High-dose dexamethasone suppression test** >90% reduction in basal urinary free cortisol levels supports pituitary adenoma diagnosis
- **Blood gas** Hypokalaemia alkalosis >95% in ectopic tumour secretion, <10% in Cushing disease
- **Inferior petrosal sinus (IPS) sampling** Performed with CRH stimulation; a higher IPS to peripheral ACTH ratio suggests pituitary adenoma rather than ectopic secretion
- **MRI pituitary** To determine pituitary adenoma
- **Full body CT scan** To look for underlying malignancy
- **Plasma CRH** Ectopic CRH production is a very rare cause of Cushing disease

Diabetes insipidus (DI) is a condition caused by hyposecretion of, or insensitivity to the effects of, **antidiuretic hormone (ADH)**, also known as **arginine vasopressin (AVP)**. Its deficiency or failure to act causes an inability to concentrate urine in the distal renal tubules, leading to the passage of copious volumes of dilute urine.

- Increased plasma osmolality is detected by osmoreceptors in the anterior hypothalamus which stimulates the posterior pituitary gland to secrete ADH
- ADH acts on the distal convoluted tubule and collecting duct resulting in ↑water reabsorption thus restoring plasma osmolality (see *Fig. 1*)
- ADH secretion is suppressed when plasma osmolality is below 280mOsm/kg, allowing maximal water diuresis

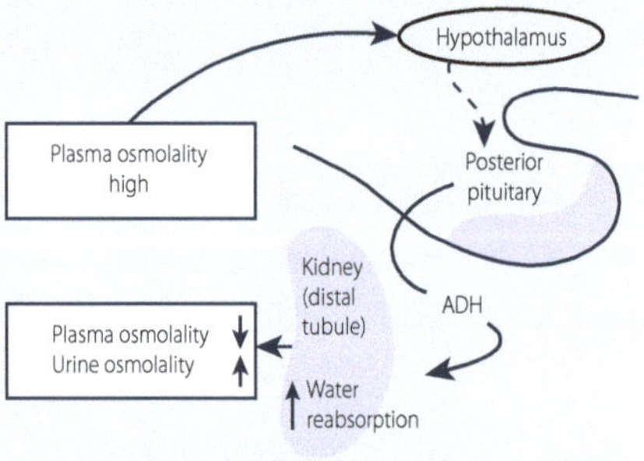

Fig. 1 ADH release

- There are two major forms of DI:
  - **Cranial DI** Decreased secretion of ADH resulting in reduced ability to concentrate urine
  - **Nephrogenic DI** Reduced ability to concentrate urine because of resistance to ADH in the kidney
- DI must be distinguished from **primary polydipsia**, which is a psychiatric disturbance characterised by excessive intake of water, and other causes of polyuria and polydipsia e.g. hyperglycaemia

Definition

ADH physiology

Pathophysiology

Diabetes insipidus

Investigations

- **Urine** 24-h urine collection (>3L/24h), osmolality (↓osmolality, <300mOsm/kg)
- **Water deprivation test** The patient is deprived of fluids for up to 8h or until 5% loss of body weight, following which desmopressin 2µg IM is given (see *Table 1*)
- **Bloods** Glucose/HbA1c (exclude diabetes), U&Es, plasma osmolality (↑)
- **MRI** Pituitary, hypothalamus and surrounding tissues
- **US KUB** May be used to assess for obstructive complications caused by the high urinary back-pressure

Table 1 Water deprivation test interpretation

Urine osmolality after fluid deprivation (mOsm/kg)	Urine osmolality after desmopressin (mOsm/kg)	Likely diagnosis
>600	>600	Normal
<300	>800	Cranial DI
<300	<300	Nephrogenic DI
>800	>800	Primary/psychogenic polydipsia (PP)
300–800	<800	Partial cranial DI or nephrogenic DI or PP or diuretic abuse

Management

Cranial DI

- **Desmopressin** (a synthetic replacement for vasopressin) to increase water reabsorption
- Treat any underlying infections
- Surgical excision of tumours

Nephrogenic DI

- Have access to drinking water and to drink enough to satiate thirst
- Correct any metabolic abnormality
- Stop any drugs that may be causing the problem
- High-dose desmopressin may be used with success in mild-to-moderate cases of nephrogenic DI
- Thiazide diuretic and NSAIDs

Cranial

- Idiopathic
- Tumours e.g. craniopharyngioma, germinoma, hypothalamic metastases
- Head injury
- Granulomatous conditions e.g. sarcoidosis, TB, Wegener's granulomatosis
- Infections e.g. encephalitis, meningitis, cerebral abscess
- Post radiotherapy
- Vascular e.g. haemorrhage/thrombosis, aneurysms, Sheehan syndrome
- Congenital defects in the ADH gene: DIDMOAD

Nephrogenic

- Inherited (mutations in the ADH receptor)
- Metabolic: hypercalcaemia and hypokalaemia
- Chronic kidney disease
- Drugs e.g. lithium, meclocycline

Causes

- Polyuria
- Polydipsia
- Nocturia
- Urinary incontinence (may result if there is damage to the bladder through chronic overdistension)
- Signs of dehydration
- Palpable bladder
- In infants may present with irritability, failure to thrive, protracted crying, fever, anorexia and fatigability or feeding problems

Clinical features

Notes

Diabetes insipidus

Diabetes mellitus is a group of metabolic disorders in which persistent hyperglycaemia is caused by deficient insulin secretion, resistance to the action of insulin, or both:
- **Type 1 diabetes mellitus (T1DM):** an absolute insulin deficiency which causes persistent hyperglycaemia
- **Type 2 diabetes mellitus (T2DM):** insulin resistance and a relative insulin deficiency resulting in persistent hyperglycaemia

- Diabetes is one of the most common chronic diseases in the UK, and its prevalence is increasing
- NICE estimates that by 2025, more than 5 million people in the UK will be diagnosed with diabetes
- T1DM can occur at any age but it most commonly presents in children and young people
- Approx. 90% of those with diabetes have T2DM; they are usually older at presentation (>30 years) but it is increasingly being diagnosed in children and adolescents due to increasing obesity

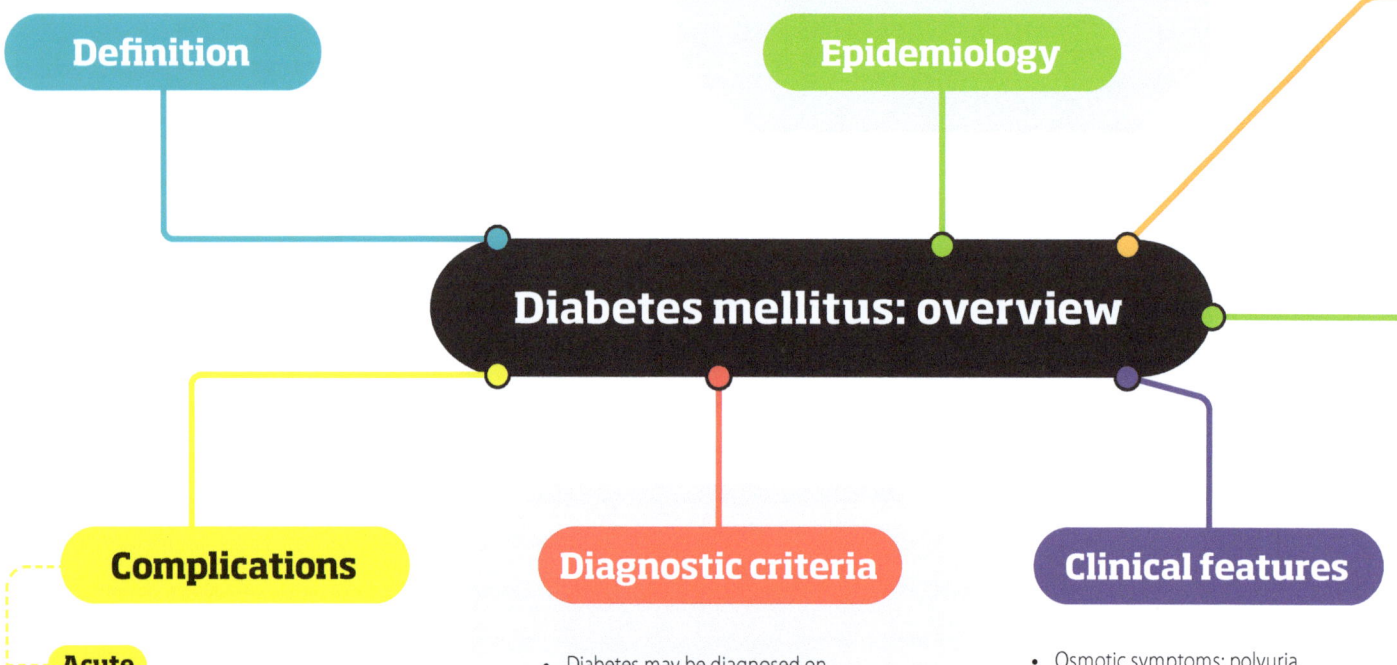

Definition

Epidemiology

Diabetes mellitus: overview

Complications

Acute

- Hypoglycaemia
- Diabetic ketoacidosis
- Hyperglycaemic hyperosmolar state (HHS)

Long-term

Microvascular complications:
- Nephropathy
- Retinopathy
- Peripheral neuropathy
- Autonomic neuropathy

Macrovascular complications:
- Cardiovascular disease e.g. myocardial infarction
- Cerebrovascular disease e.g. stroke, TIA
- Peripheral arterial disease e.g. intermittent claudication

Diagnostic criteria

- Diabetes may be diagnosed on the basis of **1 abnormal plasma glucose + diabetic symptoms** or **2 abnormal tests** in an **asymptomatic individual:**
  - **Fasting plasma glucose ≥7.0mmol/L**
  - **Random plasma glucose ≥11.1mmol/L**
  - **Oral glucose tolerance test (OGTT)** Plasma glucose concentration ≥11.1mmol/L 2h after 75g anhydrous glucose
  - **HbA1c** ≥48mmol/mol (6.5%)
- Increased risk of diabetes:
  - **Impaired glucose tolerance (IGT)** Fasting plasma venous glucose **<7mmol/L** and 2 OGTT plasma venous glucose **7.8–11.0mmol/L**
  - **Impaired fasting glucose** Plasma venous glucose of **6.1–6.9mmol/L**
  - **Pre-diabetes** HbA1c **42–47mmol/mol (6–6.4%)**

Clinical features

- Osmotic symptoms: polyuria, polydipsia
- Lethargy
- Boils, pruritus vulvae or with frequent, recurrent or prolonged infections
- Patients with T1DM may present acutely with weight loss, dehydration, ketonuria and hyperventilation
- Presentation in patients with T2DM tends to be subacute with a longer duration of symptoms or with complications e.g. retinopathy picked up on routine optician appointment or asymptomatic and picked up on routine bloods

T1DM

▶Genetics:

- Family history: about 15% of people with T1DM have a 1st-degree relative with the condition
- The class II gene products HLA-DR3 and -DR4 have been associated with increased risk of T1DM

▶Environmental:

Genetically susceptible people, unknown infectious agents or components of early childhood diet can trigger the development of autoimmunity to the beta cells in the pancreatic islets of Langerhans

T2DM

- Obesity (especially central adiposity)
- Sedentary lifestyle
- Ethnicity: South Asian, African–Caribbean, Middle Eastern at greater risk of T2DM compared with White population
- History of gestational diabetes
- Impaired glucose tolerance/impaired fasting glucose
- Drug therapy e.g. combined use of a thiazide diuretic with a beta blocker, statins
- Low-fibre, high-glycaemic index diet
- Metabolic syndrome
- Polycystic ovary syndrome
- Family history (2.4-fold increased risk)
- Adults who had low birth weight for gestational age

Risk factors

Pathophysiology

T1DM

- The development of T1DM is based on a combination of a genetic predisposition and an autoimmune process that results in gradual destruction of the beta cells of the pancreas, leading to absolute insulin deficiency
- There is usually a pre-diabetic phase where autoimmunity has already developed, with insulin autoantibodies being detected in genetically predisposed individuals as early as 6–12 months of age
- These include islet cell antibodies against cytoplasmic proteins in the beta cells, antibodies to glutamic acid decarboxylase (GAD-65) and insulin autoantibodies to protein tyrosine phosphatase
- Possible triggers for the process may include viruses, dietary factors, environmental toxins and emotional or physical stress

T2DM

- T2DM is characterised by a combination of peripheral insulin resistance and inadequate insulin secretion by pancreatic beta cells
- Insulin resistance is strongly linked to obesity and physical inactivity in genetically susceptible individuals
- In patients with T2DM, there has been found to be elevated levels of free fatty acids and pro-inflammatory cytokines in the plasma which lead to decreased glucose transport into muscle cells, elevated hepatic glucose production and increased breakdown of fat
- The beta cell mass is reduced by about a half at the time of diagnosis

Notes

Diabetes mellitus: overview

Education and information

All adults with type 1 diabetes mellitus (T1DM) should be referred to a structured education programme of proven benefit e.g. the DAFNE (dose adjustment for normal eating) programme.

Dietary advice

- A low glycaemic index diet for blood glucose control should not be advised
- Patients should be offered carbohydrate-counting training as part of the structured education programme for self-management
- Advise adults with T1DM on the importance of a healthy, balanced diet in reducing the risk of cardiovascular disease; the diet should be low in fat, sugar and salt, and contain at least 5 portions of fruit and vegetables a day
- Dietitian support may be required to help optimise body weight and blood glucose control

Exercise

- Adults with T1DM should be advised to regularly exercise (30min 5 times/week) as this lowers blood glucose levels and reduces their increased cardiovascular risk long term
- They should also be advised on the effect of activity on blood glucose levels when insulin levels are adequate i.e. risk of hypoglycaemia
- The recommendations of exercise are the same as those of T2DM (see *Ch5: Diabetes mellitus: type 2 management*)

Insulin and other pharmacological agents

Insulin

- All patients with T1DM will require insulin treatment
- Almost all insulin preparations are synthetic (recombinant) human insulin
- Insulin is injected into the subcutaneous tissue of the abdomen, thighs or upper arm
- Choice of insulin regimen depends on several factors, e.g. age, duration of diabetes, family lifestyle, school support and socioeconomic factors
- Multiple daily injection (MDI) basal-bolus insulin is the regimen of choice
- **Long-acting insulin** e.g. Twice-daily insulin detemir as basal insulin therapy for adults with T1DM
- **Rapid-acting insulin** Offer rapid-acting insulin analogues injected before meals e.g. insulin aspart for mealtime insulin replacement
- **Mixed insulin** Consider a twice-daily human mixed insulin regimen for adults with T1DM if an MDI basal-bolus insulin regimen is not possible
- Common complications of insulin therapy include hypoglycaemia, lipohypertrophy (at injection site), insulin resistance and weight gain
- **Continuous subcutaneous insulin infusion (or 'insulin pump') therapy** is recommended as a treatment option if attempts to achieve target HbA1c levels with multiple daily injections result in the person experiencing disabling hypoglycaemia, or if HbA1c remains high despite being on MDI therapy

Metformin

NICE recommend considering adding metformin if BMI ≥25kg/m²

Modification of other risk factors

Blood pressure

- If there is no albuminuria or features of the metabolic syndrome, the threshold for starting antihypertensive treatment in an adult is a BP ≥135/85mmHg
- If there is albuminuria, or 2 or more features of the metabolic syndrome, the threshold for starting antihypertensive treatment is a BP ≥130/80mmHg
- ACE inhibitors or angiotensin-II receptor antagonists are 1st-line treatment for treating hypertension

Lipids

- Statin treatment should be offered with atorvastatin 20mg for the primary prevention of CVD if the person:
  - Is older than 40 years, *or*
  - Has had diabetes for more than 10 years, *or*
  - Has established nephropathy, *or*
  - Has other CVD risk factors (such as obesity and hypertension)
- Statin treatment with atorvastatin 80mg for the secondary prevention of CVD

Smoking

Patients with T1DM who smoke should be given advice on smoking cessation and appropriately referred to smoking cessation services.

Alcohol

- Patients with diabetes should drink alcohol within the safe limits (14 units/week)
- Alcohol can exacerbate or prolong hypoglycaemia, or cause signs of hypoglycaemia to be less clear or delayed, and therefore patients should avoid drinking on an empty stomach, avoid binging and wear some form of diabetes identification (as the reduced awareness of hypoglycaemia may be confused with alcohol intoxication) e.g. medic alert bracelet

Screening and managing complications

(see *Ch5: Diabetes mellitus: type 2 management*)

Monitoring and targets

HbA1c

- Should be monitored every 3–6 months
- Adults should have a target HbA1c level of 48mmol/mol (6.5%) or lower
- Individual factors such as the person's daily activities, aspirations, likelihood of complications, comorbidities, occupation and history of hypoglycaemia should be strongly taken into account

Self-monitoring of blood glucose

- Recommend testing at least 4 times a day, including before each meal and before bed
- More frequent monitoring is recommended if frequency of hypoglycaemic episodes increases; during periods of illness; before, during and after sport; when planning pregnancy, during pregnancy and while breastfeeding
- Recommended blood glucose levels:
  - 5–7mmol/L on waking *and*
  - 4–7mmol/L before meals at other times of the day

DVLA and diabetes mellitus

(see *Ch5: Diabetes mellitus: type 2 management*)

Sick day rules

During a period of illness (that does not warrant admission), the patient should adhere to the following 'sick day rules':
- Not stop their insulin therapy
- The dose of insulin may need to be altered during periods of illness; they should seek advice from their diabetes team if unsure of how to adjust insulin doses
- Monitor blood glucose levels more frequently; this should be done at least every 3–4h including through the night, and sometimes every 1–2h
- Consider ketone monitoring (blood or urine); if the urine ketone level is greater than 2+, or blood ketone levels are greater than 3mmol/L, the person should contact the GP or diabetes care team immediately
- Maintain normal meal pattern (where possible) if appetite is reduced; normal meals could be replaced with carbohydrate-containing drinks (such as milk, milk shakes, fruit juices and sugary drinks)
- Aim to drink at least 3L (5 pints)/day to prevent dehydration; if vomiting or diarrhoea is persistent, they should seek immediate medical advice as IV fluids may be required
- Seek urgent medical advice if they are violently sick, drowsy or unable to keep fluids down

Diabetes mellitus: type 2 management

Patient education

Patients with type 2 diabetes mellitus (T2DM) or at risk of T2DM should be offered referral to a structured education programme such as the DESMOND (Diabetes Education for Self-Management for Ongoing and Newly Diagnosed) programme.

Dietary advice

- High-fibre diet low glycaemic index sources of carbohydrates
- Low-fat dairy products and oily fish
- Reduce the intake of foods containing saturated fats and trans fatty acids
- Initial target weight loss in an overweight person is 5–10%
- Discourage the use of foods marketed specifically for people with diabetes
- Consider referral to dietitian

Exercise

Regular exercise may lower blood glucose levels; exercise recommendations include:
- At least 150min/week of moderate intensity physical activity e.g. brisk walking or cycling in bouts of ≥10min, or
- 75min vigorous intensity activity (such as running or playing football) spread across the week or combinations of moderate and vigorous intensity activity
- All adults should also undertake physical activity to improve muscle strength on at least 2 days per week
- Time spent being sedentary should be minimised
- Older adults (≥65 years) who are at risk of falls should incorporate physical activity to improve balance and coordination on at least 2 days per week

Antidiabetic medication
(see *Fig. 1* and *Table 1* on *Notes* page overleaf)

Modification of other risk factors

Blood pressure

- If <80y target clinical BP <140/90mmHg and if ≥80y target clinical BP <150/90mmHg
- ACE inhibitors or angiotensin-II receptor antagonists are 1st line in patients with diabetes

Lipids

Patients with a 10-year cardiovascular risk >10% (using QRISK2) should be offered a statin; 1st-line statin of choice is atorvastatin 20mg ON for primary prevention and atorvastatin 80mg ON for secondary prevention

Smoking

Patients with T2DM who smoke should be given advice on smoking cessation and appropriately referred to smoking cessation services.

Alcohol

- Patients with diabetes should drink alcohol within the safe limits (14units/week)
- Alcohol can exacerbate or prolong hypoglycaemia, or cause signs of hypoglycaemia to be less clear or delayed; therefore patients should avoid drinking on an empty stomach, avoid binging and wear some form of diabetes identification (as the reduced awareness of hypoglycaemia may be confused with alcohol intoxication) e.g. medic alert bracelet

Screening and managing complications

Ensure the person is screened for the following at diagnosis and then at least annually:

- **Retinopathy** Patients should receive retinal examination as part of the NHS retinopathy screening programme
- **Diabetic foot problems** Check for neuropathy (including use of a 10g monofilament), ulcers, callus formation, infection, deformity, gangrene and Charcot arthropathy; foot care advice should be given including appropriate footwear and for patients to regularly check their own feet; they may require referral to podiatry
- **Nephropathy** Check serum U&Es and urine albumin: creatinine ratio (ACR); patients with nephropathy should be put on ACE inhibitor or ARB provided there are no contraindications
- **Cardiovascular risk factors** Check smoking status, blood pressure, BMI and cholesterol and manage these accordingly (see above)
- Peripheral and autonomic neuropathy, erectile dysfunction and gastroparesis: ask specifically in the history and manage accordingly

Monitoring and targets

HbA1c

- Individual targets should be agreed with patients to encourage motivation; HbA1c targets are dependent on treatment:
  - **Managed by lifestyle only 48mmol/mol (6.5%)** target
  - **Managed by lifestyle and metformin 48mmol/mol (6.5%)** target
  - **Management includes any drug which may cause hypoglycaemia 53mmol/mol (7.0%)** target
  - **Already on one drug, but HbA1c has risen to 58mmol/mol (7.5%) 53mmol/mol (7.0%)** target
- HbA1c should be checked every 3–6 months until stable, then 6-monthly
- A more conservative approach should be taken for people who are older or frail due to risk of hypoglycaemia

Self-monitoring

Patients with T2DM do not need to routinely monitor their glucose unless:
- The person is on insulin, *or*
- There is evidence of hypoglycaemic episodes, *or*
- The person is on oral medication that may increase their risk of hypoglycaemia while driving or operating machinery, *or*
- The person is pregnant or is planning to become pregnant
- Starting treatment with corticosteroids or to confirm suspected hypoglycaemia
- There is acute intercurrent illness at risk of worsening hyperglycaemia; review treatment as necessary

DVLA and diabetes mellitus

Group 1 driving entitlement

- If diet-controlled alone then no requirement to inform Driver and Vehicle Licensing Agency (DVLA)
- If on tablets (that do not cause hypoglycaemia) or glucagon-like peptide-1 (GLP-1) analogue there is no need to notify DVLA
- Do not need to inform DVLA if on tablets that may induce hypoglycaemia (e.g. sulfonylureas) unless there has been more than one episode of severe hypoglycaemia (requiring the assistance of another person) within the preceding 12 months
- If on insulin they need to inform the DVLA; the patient can drive a car as long as they have hypoglycaemic awareness, not more than one episode of severe hypoglycaemia within the preceding 12 months and no relevant visual impairment

Group 2 driving entitlement

The following standards need to be met for patients on insulin or other hypoglycaemic drugs, e.g. sulfonylureas:
- There has not been any severe hypoglycaemic event in the previous 12 months
- The driver has full hypoglycaemic awareness
- The driver must show adequate control of the condition by regular blood glucose monitoring, at least twice daily and at times relevant to driving
- The driver must demonstrate an understanding of the risks of hypoglycaemia

Sick day rules

During a period of illness (that does not warrant admission), the patient should adhere to 'sick day rules' (see *Ch5: Diabetes mellitus: type 1 management*).

Bariatric surgery

- Bariatric surgery may be indicated for people with a BMI of 35 or over
- Bariatric surgery has been shown to induce remission of diabetes or reduce the need for medications with long-term results in morbidly obese patients
- The two common types of surgery are gastric banding and gastric bypass surgery

Diabetes mellitus: type 2 management notes

T2DM pharmacological management algorithm

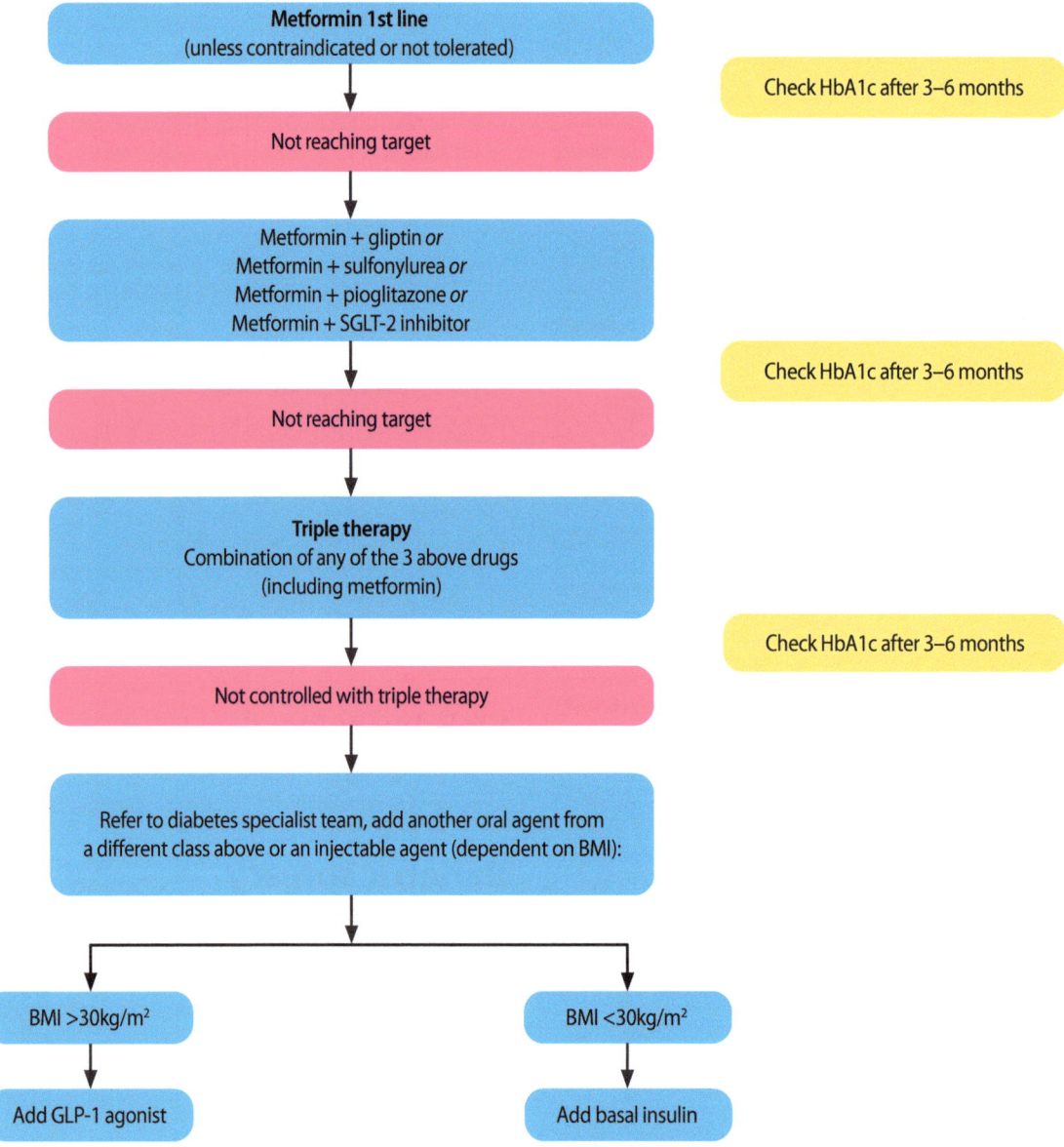

Fig. 1 Algorithm of the pharmacological management of T2DM; medication should be continued at each stage if either individualised HbA1c target reached or HbA1c falls >0.5% (5.5mmol/mol in 3–6 months); medication should be discontinued if ineffective or not tolerated; reinforce advice on diet, lifestyle and adherence to antidiabetic drug treatment at each review; GLP-1, glucagon-like peptide-1; SGLT-2, sodium-glucose co-transporter 2

Table 1 T2DM medication

Drug	Notes
Metformin	• **Methods of action** ↓Hepatic gluconeogenesis, ↑tissue sensitivity to insulin, ↑peripheral glucose uptake and use, ↓intestinal absorption of glucose • **Dosage** Initially 500mg OD, maximum daily dose of 2g to be given in 2–3 divided doses • **Efficacy** Moderate • **Advantages** Weight reduction, cardiovascular (CV) benefit and hypoglycaemic risk is low • **Disadvantages and common side effects** GI side effects are common; a rare but important side effect is lactic acidosis • **Cautions** Avoid if eGFR is <30ml/min/1.73m^2
Sulfonylureas	• **Examples** Gliclazide, glibenclamide, tolbutamide • **Dosage example** Gliclazide initially 40–80mg OD, increased if necessary up to 160mg OD, maximum 320mg in 2–3 divided doses per day • **Method of action** Stimulate beta cells of the pancreas to release insulin • **Advantages** High efficacy • **Disadvantages and common side effects** No CV benefit, side effects of weight gain and hypoglycaemia • **Cautions** Obesity, elderly, G6PD deficiency
Thiazolidinediones	• **Examples** Pioglitazone is the only licensed medication from this class • **Dosage** Initially 15–30mg OD, adjusted according to response • **Method of action** Binds to and activates PPAR-gamma which is a nuclear receptor that regulates a large number of genes including lipid metabolism and insulin action by reducing hepatic glucose production and enhancing peripheral glucose uptake • **Advantages** High efficacy • **Disadvantages and common side effects** Causes weight gain, oedema and increased risk of fractures, bladder cancer and heart failure
SGLT-2 inhibitors	• **Examples** Canagliflozin, dapagliflozin, empagliflozin • **Dosage example** Canagliflozin 100mg OD; increased if tolerated to 300mg OD if required • **Method of action** Reduces renal tubular glucose reabsorption, producing a reduction in blood glucose without stimulating insulin release • **Advantages** CV benefit, causes weight loss and low risk of hypoglycaemia • **Disadvantages and common side effects** Genital thrush is common. Can cause diabetic ketoacidosis. • **Cautions** Avoid initiation if eGFR <60ml/min/1.73m^2
DDP-4 inhibitors (gliptins)	• **Examples** Sitagliptin, linagliptin • **Dosage example** Sitagliptin 100mg OD • **Methods of action** In normal physiology an oral glucose load results in a greater release of insulin than if the same load is given intravenously – known as the incretin effect; this effect is largely mediated by GLP-1 and is known to be decreased in T2DM; increasing GLP-1 levels either by the administration of an analogue (GLP-1 mimetic, e.g. exenatide) or inhibiting its breakdown (DPP4 inhibitors – the gliptins) is therefore the target of two recent classes of drug • **Advantages** Weight neutral; well tolerated with few side effects • **Disadvantages and common side effects** Low/moderate effect; no CV benefit • **Cautions** Reduce dose in CKD stage 3
GLP-1 analogues	• **Examples** Exenatide, dulaglitide, liraglutide • **Dosage example** Exenatide initially 5μg BD for at least 1 month, then increased if necessary up to 10μg BD by SC injection • **Method of action** As above, GLP-1 stimulates the release of insulin • **Advantages** High efficacy; has CV benefits; hypoglycaemic risk is low and causes weight loss; dose unchanged in CKD • **Disadvantages and common side effects** Main side effect is pancreatitis

DKA is a medical emergency characterised by the triad of marked **hyperglycaemia, acidosis and ketonaemia**. It may be a complication of existing T1DM or be the first presentation. DKA may also rarely occur in T2DM. It results from the absolute or relative deficiency of insulin in the presence of an increase in the counter-regulatory hormones (glucagon, cortisol, growth hormone and adrenaline). Rarely, under conditions of extreme stress, patients with T2DM may also develop DKA.

- Glucose >11mmol/L or known diabetes mellitus
- pH <7.3 or bicarbonate <15mmol/L
- Ketones >3mmol/L or urine ketones ++ on dipstick

Diagnostic criteria

Definition

Diabetic ketoacidosis

Management

IV fluids

- Wide-bore cannula and bolus resuscitation as required with 0.9% saline
- Followed by maintenance fluids (see *Fig. 1*)
- Maintain K⁺ between 4.0 and 5.5mmol/L (see *Table 1*)

Insulin

Fixed rate IV insulin infusion (FRIII) should be administered: 50 units human soluble insulin (Actrapid, Humulin S) made up to 50ml with 0.9% NaCl; infuse at a fixed rate of 0.1U/kg/h. If the patient normally takes long-acting insulin SC, continue this at the usual dose and usual time.

Monitoring

- Measure blood ketones and capillary glucose hourly
- Check the rates of ketone fall, glucose fall and bicarbonate rise
- Measure venous blood gas (VBG) for pH, HCO_3^- and K⁺ at 60 min, 2h and 2h thereafter
- Continue the FRIII until the ketone measurement is <0.6mmol/L, venous pH >7.3 and/or venous HCO_3^- >18mmol/L
- If the glucose falls <14.0mmol/L, commence 10% glucose given at 125ml/h alongside the 0.9% NaCl

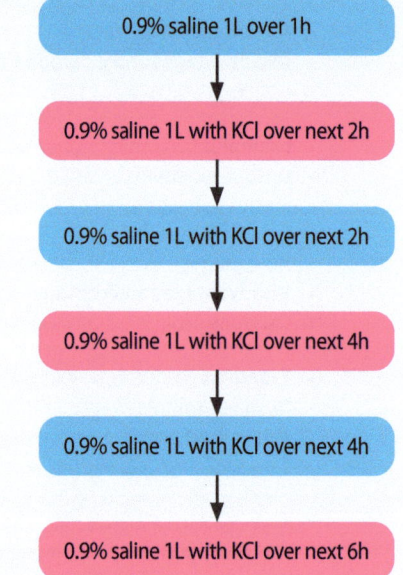

Fig. 1 Example of IV fluid maintenance regime in DKA

Table 1 Potassium replacement in DKA

K⁺ level in first 24h (mmol/L)	K⁺ replacement in infusion solution
>5.5	Nil
3.5–5.5	40mmol/L
<3.5	Senior review as additional potassium required (via central line in HDU)

- Infection
- Cessation of insulin (unintentional or deliberate)
- Inadequate insulin
- Cardiovascular disease e.g. stroke or myocardial infarction
- Drugs e.g. steroids, thiazides or sodium-glucose co-transporter 2 (SGLT-2) inhibitors

Note: No obvious precipitant may be present

- Polyuria
- Polydipsia
- Vomiting
- Dehydration
- Altered mental state
- Coma
- Weight loss
- Weakness
- Lethargy
- Kussmaul respiration
- Acetone breath smell

- Gastric stasis
- Thromboembolism
- Arrhythmias 2° to hyperkalaemia/ iatrogenic hypokalaemia
- Iatrogenic cerebral oedema
- Hypokalaemia
- Hypoglycaemia
- Acute respiratory distress syndrome
- Acute kidney injury

Causes

Clinical features

Complications

Investigations

Severity

≥1 of the following may indicate severe DKA:
- Blood ketones >6mmol/L
- HCO_3^- level <5mmol/L
- Venous/arterial pH <7.0
- Hypokalaemia on admission
- Glasgow Coma Scale (GCS) score <12
- O_2 saturation <92%
- Systolic BP <90mmHg
- HR >100 or <60
- Anion gap >16

Bedside tests

- Capillary blood glucose and ketone: significantly elevated
- Urine dipstick: ketone and glucose positive, may show underlying infection
- 12-lead ECG: rule out MI and arrhythmias

Blood tests

- **Plasma glucose** Elevated
- **FBC** ↑WCC in sepsis
- **CRP** ↑ In sepsis
- **U&Es** Na⁺ may be high (dehydration) or low due to interference of glucose/ ketones, or normal; K⁺ may be ↑ due to acidosis, normal or occasionally low; urea and creatinine may be raised
- **Plasma osmolality** >290mOsm/kg in cases of DKA; if new presentation and osmolality >320mOsm/kg and there is not significant ketonaemia/ketonuria then hyperosmolar hyperglycaemic state (HHS) may be the diagnosis
- **Cardiac enzymes (e.g. troponin)** If MI suspected, creatine kinase is raised if rhabdomyolysis co-exists
- **Amylase** If pancreatitis suspected
- **Blood cultures** If sepsis suspected

Venous blood gas

- Shows metabolic acidosis with low pH and low HCO_3^- and hyperglycaemia
- Useful for working out anion gap:
  - Anion gap = $(Na^+ + K^+) - (Cl^- + HCO_3^-)$
  - Usually >13 in DKA
- Regular VBGs vital for monitoring

Imaging

- **CXR** Look for source of infection
- **AXR** If indicated by history/examination
- **CT/MRI** If there is impairment of consciousness or focal neurology

Hyperosmolar hyperglycaemic state

Definition

Hyperosmolar hyperglycaemic state (HHS), formerly known as **hyperosmolar hyperglycaemic non-ketotic coma (HONK)** is a potentially life-threatening illness that occurs in T2DM. It is characterised by severe hyperglycaemia, hypovolaemia and raised plasma osmolality. Ketosis does not occur due to the presence of basal insulin secretion sufficient to prevent ketogenesis. A mixed picture of HHS and DKA may however occur.

Precipitating factors

Intercurrent or co-existing illness

- MI
- Infection (most common): e.g. UTI, pneumonia, cellulitis, systemic sepsis
- Stroke/TIA/intracranial haemorrhage
- Hyperthermia or hypothermia
- Endocrine: hyperthyroidism, Cushing syndrome or ACTH-secreting tumour
- Intestinal ischaemia/infarction
- AKI or decompensated CKD
- Pancreatitis
- PE
- Burns

Drugs

- Calcium channel blockers
- Beta blockers
- Chemotherapeutic agents
- Glucocorticoids
- Loop diuretics
- Alcohol and illicit drugs including cocaine, amphetamines and MDMA (Ecstasy)

Diabetes related

- First presentation of diabetes mellitus: unsuspected, undiagnosed
- Poor diabetic control/non-compliance: intentional, accidental, neglect

Clinical features

The patient is often elderly and may be presenting for the first time:
- Hyperglycaemia
- Dehydration with marked thirst
- Marked drowsiness
- Convulsions, coma and focal CNS signs

Diagnostic features

- **Hypovolaemia**
- **Marked hyperglycaemia** (≥30mmol/L) without significant hyperketonaemia (7.3, HCO_3^- >15mmol/L)
- **Raised plasma osmolality** usually ≥320mOsm/kg

Investigations

Same as for DKA

Management

- **Fluid replacement** IV 0.9% NaCl with K^+ added as required as with DKA; fluid replacement will reduce blood glucose; a rapid fall should be avoided (aim for a reduction of 4–6mmol/h)
- **Insulin** Fixed rate intravenous insulin infusion (FRIII) (0.05U/kg/h) is recommended, ideally reducing blood glucose by up to 5mmol/L/h; reassess fluid intake and renal function once blood glucose has ceased to decline during initial fluid replacement
- **Treatment in HDU** in severe cases (see *below*)
- **Regular monitoring** VBGs as with DKA
- **Antibiotics** Give antibiotics when there is clinical, imaging or laboratory evidence of infection
- **Anticoagulation** Patients in HHS are at increased thrombotic risk and should receive prophylactic treatment for this (LMWH) throughout admission, unless contraindicated

Care in HDU/ITU should be considered if ≥1 of following:

- Osmolality >350mOsm/kg
- Na^+ >160mmol/L
- Venous/arterial pH <7.1
- Hypokalaemia (<3.5mmol/L) or hyperkalaemia (>6mmol/L) on admission
- GCS <12 or abnormal AVPU (alert, voice, pain, unresponsive) scale
- Oxygen saturation <92% on air (assuming normal baseline respiratory function)
- SBP <90mmHg
- Pulse >100 or <60bpm
- Urine output <0.5ml/kg/h
- Serum creatinine >200µmol/L
- Hypothermia
- Macrovascular event (e.g. myocardial infarction or stroke)
- Other serious comorbidity

Complications

- Ischaemia or infarction affecting any organ, particularly MI and cerebrovascular event
- Thromboembolic disease, including DVT and PE
- Renal failure and multi-organ failure
- Acute respiratory distress syndrome
- Disseminated intravascular coagulation
- Rhabdomyolysis
- Cerebral oedema
- Central pontine myelinolysis
- Iatrogenic complications: hypoglycaemia due to over-administration of insulin; fluid overload leading to cardiac failure

Definition

Hyperaldosteronism can be defined as excessive levels of aldosterone which may be independent of the renin–angiotensin axis (**primary hyperaldosteronism**) or due to elevated renin levels (**secondary hyperaldosteronism**).

Physiology

- Aldosterone is a steroid hormone and is the main mineralocorticoid secreted by the zona glomerulosa of the adrenal cortex
- The control of aldosterone synthesis and release is through the **renin–angiotensin–aldosterone system (RAAS)**
- The most important physiological effect of aldosterone is stimulation of Na^+ reabsorption and K^+ excretion in the late distal tubule and collecting duct, thereby indirectly influencing water retention or loss, blood pressure and blood volume
- Hyperaldosteronism therefore causes high plasma Na^+, hypertension and low K^+
- This may be independent of the RAAS (primary hyperaldosteronism) or due to elevated renin levels (secondary hyperaldosteronism)

Hyperaldosteronism

Management

- **Conn syndrome** Laparoscopic adrenalectomy; medical management with spironolactone is used in the period prior to surgery
- **Hyperplasia** Managed with spironolactone, amiloride or eplerenone
- **GRA** Dexamethasone for 4 weeks
- **Adrenal carcinoma** Surgically treated

Investigations

- **U&Es** May show hypokalaemia and hypernatraemia
- **Plasma aldosterone : renin ratio** Raised
- **Blood gas** Hypokalaemia, alkalosis
- **ECG** May show arrhythmias from electrolyte imbalance
- **CT/MRI adrenal glands** To locate an adrenal adenoma, hyperplasia or carcinoma
- **Selective adrenal villous sampling** Gold standard for localising the cause of primary hyperaldosteronism
- **Genetic testing** Available for GRA

Clinical features

- **Hypertension** Usually asymptomatic
- **Hypokalaemia** Weakness, cramps, paraesthesia, polyuria, polydipsia
- **Metabolic alkalosis**
- Sodium may be raised

Primary hyperaldosteronism

- **Adrenal adenoma (Conn syndrome)** Accounts for >80% of all cases of hyperaldosteronism; usually unilateral and solitary
- **Adrenal hyperplasia** Accounts for approx. 15% of all cases of hyperaldosteronism; majority of cases are bilateral
- **Familial hyperaldosteronism** There are 2 forms: type 1 is glucocorticoid-remediable aldosteronism (GRA) and type 2 is characterised by inherited aldosterone-producing adenoma or inherited bilateral adrenal hyperplasia
- **Adrenal carcinoma** A rare cause of primary hyperaldosteronism

Secondary hyperaldosteronism

Caused by ↑renin due to ↓renal perfusion:
- Renal artery stenosis
- Diuretics
- CCF
- Hepatic failure
- Nephrotic syndrome
- Malignant hypertension

Causes

Notes

Hyperaldosteronism

Calcium physiology

- Serum calcium levels are regulated by PTH and vitamin D on the kidneys, bone and GI tract (see *Fig. 1*)
- PTH increases calcium levels by increasing reabsorption of calcium and activation of vitamin D in the kidneys and stimulating calcium release from bone
- The active form of vitamin D (**1,25-dihydroxyvitamin D**) increases intestinal calcium absorption
- The normal range of calcium is 2.2–2.6mmol/L

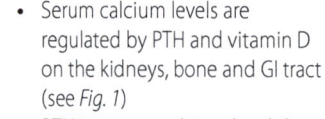

Sunlight

Skin
7-dehydrocholesterol

Food → Vitamin D

Liver

(25-hydroxylase)

25(OH)D

Kidney

PTH activates

(1-hydroxylase)

1,25(OH)$_2$D

Fig. 1 Calcium homeostasis

Definition

Hypocalcaemia is a low plasma calcium i.e. <2.2mmol/L. Hypocalcaemia is nearly always due to deficiency or resistance to PTH or vitamin D deficiency.

Hypocalcaemia

Management

Acute treatment

- Treat where symptomatic or severe hypocalcaemia i.e. <1.90mmol/L
- Treat with calcium bolus i.e. **10**ml of **10**% calcium gluconate over **10**min (repeat as necessary) or calcium infusion
- Oral calcium may be needed in addition
- Monitor serum calcium concentrations regularly (ITU monitoring may be required)
- Correct magnesium if low

Long-term treatment/prevention

- Oral calcium replacement e.g. with calcium carbonate
- Oral vitamin D replacement: cholecalciferol
- Ensure adequate dietary intake: foods rich in calcium or supplements
- Monitor those at risk

Investigations

- **Calcium** (adjusted) <2.2mmol/L
- **Phosphate** ↑ In CKD and hypoparathyroidism and ↓ in vitamin D deficiency
- **ALP** ↑ In CKD and vitamin D deficiency
- **Vitamin D** To exclude vitamin D deficiency
- **U&Es** To exclude CKD
- **PTH** To evaluate likely cause
- **CK** To exclude rhabdomyolysis
- **Amylase** To exclude pancreatitis
- **ECG** To exclude dysrhythmias and prolonged QT interval
- **X-ray hand** Shorter 4th and 5th metacarpals in pseudohypoparathyroidism
- **ECHO** Cardiac structural defects in DiGeorge syndrome

↓PTH

- **Parathyroid destruction:** surgery (thyroidectomy, parathyroidectomy, radical neck dissection), radiotherapy, infiltration by metastases or systemic disease (e.g. sarcoidosis, amyloidosis, HIV, syphilis)
- **Parathyroid agenesis**
- **Reduced parathyroid secretion:** due to gene defects e.g. DiGeorge syndrome, hypomagnesaemia, hungry bone disease (after parathyroidectomy), mutation in calcium-sensing receptor (CASR)
- **Isolated autoimmune hypoparathyroidism**

↑PTH

- **Vitamin D deficiency:** due to nutritional lack, malabsorption, liver disease, receptor defects
- **Vitamin D resistance:** renal tubular dysfunction (Fanconi syndrome) or receptor defect
- **PTH resistance:** pseudohypoparathyroidism, hypomagnesaemia

Other causes

- Hyperventilation
- Drugs: calcium chelators, bone resorption inhibitors (bisphosphonates, calcitonin), phenytoin, ketoconazole, foscarnet
- Acute pancreatitis
- Acute rhabdomyolysis
- Malignancy: tumour lysis syndrome, osteoblastic metastases
- Toxic shock syndrome

Causes

Notes

Hypocalcaemia

Clinical features

Symptoms

- Usually asymptomatic
- Paraesthesia (usually fingers, toes and around mouth)
- Tetany
- Carpopedal spasm (wrist flexion and fingers drawn together)
- Muscle cramps

Signs

- Chvostek's sign (see *Fig. 2a*)
- Trousseau's sign (see *Fig. 2b*)
- Seizures
- Ventricular fibrillation (VF) or heart block
- Laryngospasm/bronchospasm
- With prolonged hypocalcaemia: subcapsular infarct, papilloedema, abnormal teeth, confusion

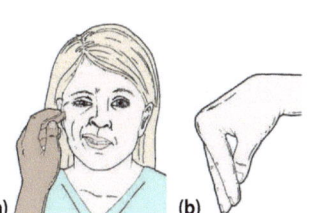

Fig. 2 (a) Chvostek's sign (muscular spasm provoked by tapping of the facial nerve below the zygomatic arch); **(b)** Trousseau's sign (carpopedal spasm provoked by inflating a blood pressure cuff for several minutes)

Hypercalcaemia is elevated calcium levels, commonly caused by an excessive release of PTH or it may be independent of PTH.

- **Mild hypercalcaemia** 2.65–3.00mmol/L
- **Moderate hypercalcaemia** 3.01–3.40mmol/L
- **Severe hypercalcaemia** >3.40mmol/L

- Serum calcium levels are regulated by PTH and vitamin D on the kidneys, bone and gastrointestinal (GI) tract
- PTH causes increased calcium levels by increasing reabsorption of calcium and activation of vitamin D in the kidneys and increased calcium release from bone; the active form of vitamin D (1,25-dihydroxyvitamin D, calcitriol) promotes intestinal calcium absorption
- Normal calcium range is 2.2–2.6mmol/L

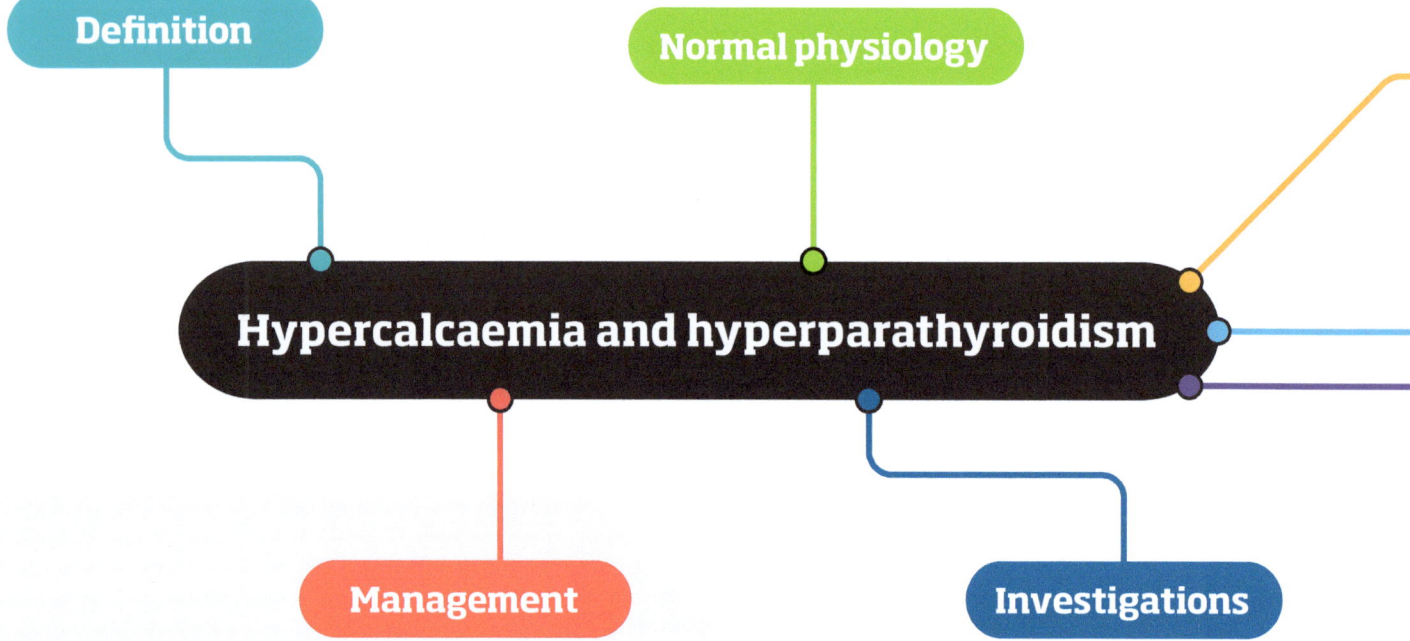

Definition

Normal physiology

Hypercalcaemia and hyperparathyroidism

Management

Investigations

- Stop offending drugs
- **IV fluids** 0.9% saline helps to increase the urinary output of calcium and should be used 1st line in patients with moderate and severe hypercalcaemia
- **Bisphosphonates** After rehydration, bisphosphonates may be administered; IV pamidronate and zoledronic acid are commonly used
- **Loop diuretics** e.g. Furosemide is occasionally used
- **Treat underlying cause** e.g. Malignancy
- **Calcitonin** Has fewer side effects than bisphosphonates but is less effective in reducing calcium levels
- **Glucocorticoids** Useful for hypercalcaemia due to vitamin D

toxicity, sarcoidosis and lymphoma
- **Cinacalcet hydrochloride** A calcimimetic agent that effectively reduces PTH levels in patients with secondary hyperparathyroidism
- **Paricalcitol** Licensed for the prevention and treatment of secondary hyperparathyroidism associated with CKD
- **Denosumab** Useful for patients with persistent or relapsed hypercalcaemia of malignancy
- **Haemodialysis** Should be considered for patients with advanced underlying kidney disease and refractory severe hypercalcaemia

- **PTH** Raised in primary, secondary and tertiary hyperparathyroidism and decreased in vitamin D excess/ milk alkali syndrome, granulomatous disease, adrenal insufficiency and thyrotoxicosis
- **Serum phosphate** Usually low in primary hyperparathyroidism and raised in secondary and tertiary hyperparathyroidism
- **Serum ALP** Raised in malignancy (not haematological malignancy)
- **Vitamin D** Raised in vitamin D intoxication
- **Urine calcium** Low in familial hypocalciuric hypercalcaemia
- **CXR** To rule out lung malignancy, sarcoidosis, TB
- **U&Es** To assess renal function and dehydration
- **FBC** May show iron deficiency anaemia or anaemia of chronic disease
- **Serum electrophoresis** To rule out myeloma
- **Plain X-ray** May show features indicative of bone abnormalities e.g. demineralisation, bone cysts, pathological fractures or bony metastases
- **ECG** Severe hypercalcaemia can cause cardiac arrhythmias and shortened QT interval
- **US technetium scan** Of parathyroid glands if hyperparathyroidism is suspected

PTH mediated

- **Primary hyperparathyroidism** Most common cause of hypercalcaemia
- **Familial** MEN-1 and MEN-2A, familial hypocalciuric hypercalcaemia
- **Tertiary hyperparathyroidism** Secondary to acute renal failure

Non PTH mediated

- **Malignancy** Common; mechanism is through parathyroid-related peptide or bone metastases
- **Medications** Thiazide diuretics, lithium, teriparatide, excess vitamin D, excess vitamin A, theophylline toxicity
- **Chronic granulomatous conditions** Sarcoidosis, TB
- **Endocrine conditions** Hyperthyroidism, acromegaly, phaeochromocytoma, adrenal insufficiency
- **Miscellaneous** Immobilisation, milk alkali syndromes

Causes

Primary hyperparathyroidism

- Most common cause of hypercalcaemia
- Causes: adenoma (80–85%), multiple gland hyperplasia (10–15%), parathyroid cancer (<1%)
- Diagnosis: ↑serum Ca^{2+} and ↑PTH; ultrasound or technetium scan of the parathyroid glands

Secondary hyperparathyroidism

- Not a cause of hypercalcaemia but an appropriate increase in PTH in response to low Ca^{2+}
- Causes: most commonly chronic renal failure or vitamin D deficiency
- Calcium will be low or normal in presence of raised PTH; vitamin D is usually low and phosphate high

Tertiary hyperparathyroidism

- Progression of secondary hyperparathyroidism to an autonomous overproduction of PTH resulting in hypercalcaemia
- Differs from primary hyperparathyroidism as phosphate often remains elevated

Hyperparathyroidism

Clinical features

'Bones, stones, abdominal groans and psychic moans'
- **GI** Anorexia, nausea, vomiting, constipation, pancreatitis, peptic ulcer disease
- **Musculoskeletal** Muscle weakness, bone pain, osteopenia/osteoporosis
- **Renal** Polyuria, polydipsia, kidney stones, distal renal tubular acidosis, nephrogenic diabetes insipidus
- **Neurological** Decreased concentration, confusion, fatigue, stupor, coma
- **Cardiovascular** Cardiac arrhythmias, shortened QT interval

Notes

Hypercalcaemia and hyperparathyroidism

Hyperprolactinaemia is defined as a raised level of prolactin in the blood. Hyperprolactinaemia can be physiological, e.g. during pregnancy and stress, or pathological.

- Prolactin is primarily synthesised and released by the lactotrophs of the anterior pituitary gland although extrapituitary prolactin synthesis is also recognised in immune, mammary, epithelial and fat cells
- The control of prolactin secretion is highlighted in *Fig. 1*
- In humans, the only clearly defined physiological role of prolactin is stimulation of lactation during pregnancy when prolactin levels are raised

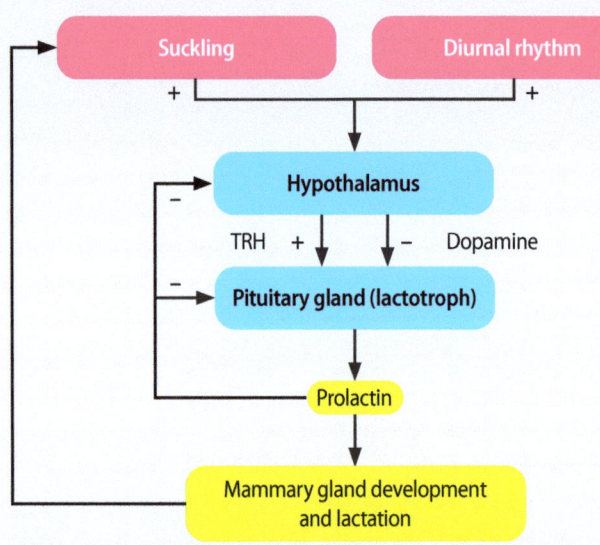

Fig. 1 Control of prolactin secretion

Definition

Normal physiology

Hyperprolactinaemia

Complications

Related to hypogonadism

- Osteoporosis
- ↓Fertility
- Erectile dysfunction

Related to tumour size

- Visual loss
- Headache
- Pituitary apoplexy
- CSF rhinorrhoea

Management

Conservative

- Observation
- Microadenomas in asymptomatic patients may not need observation
- Stop offending drugs (if possible)
- Treat underlying reversible causes e.g. hypothyroidism

Medical

- Dopamine agonists e.g. cabergoline, bromocriptine
- Exclude cardiac valve fibrosis and pulmonary fibrosis before starting treatment
- After 1 month of therapy, the patient should be evaluated for side effects and serum prolactin should be measured

Surgical

- Recommended on basis of tumour size and symptoms, inadequate response or intolerant to dopamine agonists
- Often using a trans-sphenoidal route to remove a tumour
- Combined with postoperative radiotherapy for large tumours, often restores normoprolactinaemia
- Unfortunately there is a high risk of recurrence

- Unlike other hormones of the anterior pituitary gland, prolactin secretion is mainly under inhibitory control (predominantly by **dopamine**) rather than secretion from a hypothalamic-releasing hormone
- Hyperprolactinaemia can be caused by a number of stimuli of prolactin release e.g. prolactinomas or loss of dopamine inhibition
- The loss of dopamine inhibition may be due to a true dopamine deficiency (e.g. tumours of the hypothalamus), a defect in transport of dopamine from hypothalamus to the pituitary gland (e.g. a pituitary or stalk tumour), antagonism of dopamine by certain drugs (e.g. antipsychotics) or unregulated stimulation of lactotrophs e.g. chest wall injury resulting in mimicking of 'suckling' reflex

- **Physiological causes** Stress (physical or psychological), pregnancy, breastfeeding
- **Hypothalamus disease** Trauma, radiotherapy, infiltration (sarcoidosis, histiocytosis), tumours e.g. craniopharyngioma, metastatic disease
- **Pituitary disease** Prolactinomas (micro- or macro-), mixed lactotroph/mammotroph adenoma, stalk compression (from any pituitary/sellar pathology)
- **Endocrine** Hypothyroidism (due to ↑ synthesis of thyrotropin-releasing hormone, TRH), Cushing syndrome, PCOS, acromegaly
- **Drugs** Oestrogens, anti-emetics (domperidone, metoclopramide), antipsychotics e.g. haloperidol, antidepressants (SSRIs), opioids
- **Impairment of metabolism/excretion** Chronic renal failure or severe liver disease
- **Chest wall trauma or surgery**

Pathophysiology

Causes

Investigations

- **TFTs** To exclude hypothyroidism as a cause of ↑prolactin
- **Beta HCG** (urine or serum) To exclude pregnancy
- **Basal serum prolactin** (non-stressful venepuncture) If mildly elevated, it should be repeated, a prolactin level >5000mU/L usually indicates a true prolactinoma
- **Visual field assessment** Often bitemporal hemianopia
- **MRI pituitary** To identify a pituitary tumour

Clinical features

Related to tumour size (usually macroadenomas)

- Headache
- Visual disturbances (typically bitemporal hemianopia or upper temporal quadrantanopia)
- Cranial nerve palsies
- Symptoms/signs of hypopituitarism

Related to hypogonadism

Males

- Reduced libido
- Reduced beard growth
- Erectile dysfunction
- Galactorrhoea

Females

- Amenorrhoea/oligomenorrhoea
- Galactorrhoea
- Subfertility
- Hirsutism
- Reduced libido

- The thyroid gland is a bi-lobed structure which is found in the anterior neck (see *Fig. 1*)
- The hypothalamus secretes thyrotropin-releasing hormone (TRH) which stimulates the anterior pituitary to secrete thyroid-stimulating hormone (TSH); this then acts on the thyroid gland increasing the production of thyroxine (T_4) and tri-iodothyronine (T_3), the two main thyroid hormones (see *Fig. 2*)
- These then act on a wide variety of tissues, helping to regulate the use of energy sources, protein synthesis, and control the body's sensitivity to other hormones

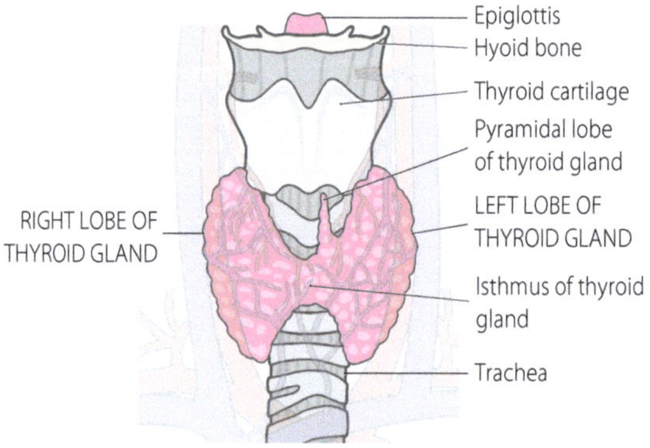

Hypothyroidism is the clinical result of impaired production of the thyroid hormones, thyroxine (T_4) and tri-iodothyronine (T_3), which are essential for normal growth, development and metabolism.

Fig. 1 Location of the thyroid gland and neighbouring structures

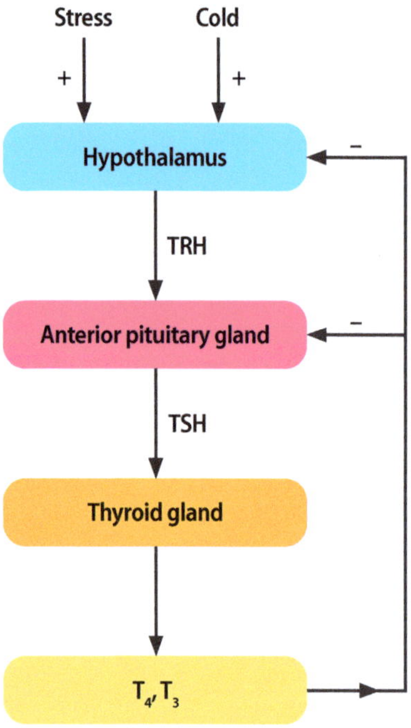

Fig. 2 The hypothalamus–pituitary–thyroid axis

Definition

Thyroid physiology

Hypothyroidism

- Impaired quality of life
- Cardiovascular complications: dyslipidaemia, coronary artery disease, heart failure
- Hyperthyroidism (from overtreatment of hypothyroidism)
- Reproductive complications: impaired fertility, obstetric complications e.g. pre-eclampsia
- Myxoedema coma

Complications

Management

Thyroxine replacement

- Lifelong replacement with **levothyroxine** is the mainstay of treatment
- For adults aged over 18 years, the initial dose of levothyroxine is 50–100µg once daily
- There are certain patients for whom the recommended initial dose of levothyroxine is 25µg, including:
  - Patients with cardiac disease
  - Patients with severe hypothyroidism
  - Patients aged over 50 years
- Once TFTs are stabilised, TSH should be checked annually

Investigations

- **Thyroid function tests (TFTs)**:
  - 1° hypothyroidism: ↑TSH, ↓T_3, T_4
  - 2° hypothyroidism: ↓TSH, ↓T_3, T_4
  - Subclinical hypothyroidism: ↑TSH, →T_3, T_4
- **Autoantibodies** Antithyroid peroxidase (anti-TPO) antibodies or antithyroglobulin antibodies are found in 90–95% of patients with autoimmune thyroiditis; TSH receptor antibodies may also be found
- **FBC, lipid profile, CK** Untreated hypothyroidism can cause ↑CK, ↑cholesterol and triglycerides and anaemia (normocytic or macrocytic)
- **Imaging** E.g. ultrasonography, to rule out neoplastic lesions if the patient has an asymmetrical goitre

Pathophysiology

- **Iodine deficiency** is the most common cause of primary hypothyroidism worldwide
- **Hashimoto's thyroiditis** is the most common cause of primary goitrous hypothyroidism in non-iodine deficient areas:
  - There is autoimmune destruction of thyroid cells by cell- and antibody-mediated immune processes
  - The major environmental triggers of autoimmune thyroid disease include iodine, medications, infection, smoking and possibly stress
  - Most patients have serum antibodies to thyroglobulin, thyroid peroxidase enzyme and antibodies that block TSH to its receptor
  - The result is inadequate thyroid hormone secretion, although, initially both preformed T_4 and T_3 may 'leak' into the circulation from damaged cells causing transient hyperthyroidism
  - It is associated with HLA-DR5; monozygotic twin studies indicate that there is about 70% genetic contribution to autoimmune thyroid disease
  - It is 5–10 × more common in women than men
  - It is associated with other autoimmune disorders e.g. IDDM, Addison's and pernicious anaemia
- **Secondary hypothyroidism** is rare and produces disruption in the feedback loop because of problems at the level of the pituitary gland

Causes

Primary

- **Hashimoto's thyroiditis**
- **De Quervain's thyroiditis:** associated with a painful goitre and raised ESR
- **Riedel thyroiditis:** fibrous tissue replacing the normal thyroid parenchyma; it causes a painless goitre
- **Post-partum thyroiditis**
- **Drugs:** amiodarone, contrast media, iodides, lithium and antithyroid medication
- **Iodine deficiency**
- **Infiltration of thyroid:** e.g. amyloidosis, sarcoidosis and haemochromatosis
- **Post thyroidectomy/radioactive iodine therapy**
- **Congenital hypothyroidism:** due to a problem with thyroid dysgenesis or thyroid dyshormonogenesis

Secondary

- **Isolated TSH deficiency**
- **Hypopituitarism:** neoplasm, infiltrative, infection e.g. TB, Sheehan syndrome, radiotherapy
- **Hypothalamic disorders:** neoplasms and trauma

Clinical features

Symptoms

- Tiredness, lethargy
- Intolerance to cold
- Dry skin and hair loss
- Slowing of intellectual activity
- Constipation
- Decreased appetite with weight gain
- Deep hoarse voice
- Menorrhagia and later oligomenorrhoea or amenorrhoea
- Impaired hearing due to fluid in middle ear
- Reduced libido

Signs (see *Fig. 3*)

- Dry coarse skin
- Hair loss (typically scalp and lateral third of eyebrow)
- Cold peripheries
- Puffy face, hands and feet (myxoedema)
- Bradycardia
- Delayed tendon reflex relaxation
- Carpal tunnel syndrome
- Serous cavity effusions: e.g. pericarditis or pleural effusions

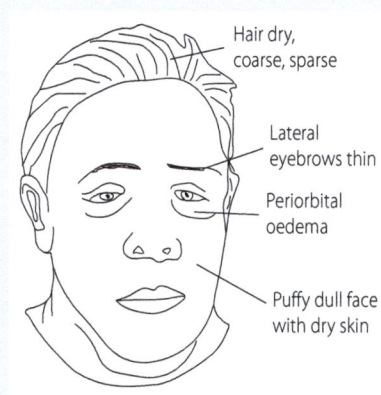

Hair dry, coarse, sparse

Lateral eyebrows thin

Periorbital oedema

Puffy dull face with dry skin

Fig. 3 Facial signs of hypothyroidism

Interpreting thyroid function tests

Diagnosis	TSH	Free T$_4$
Thyrotoxicosis	↓	↑
Primary hypothyroidism	↑	↓
Secondary hypothyroidism	↓	↓
Sick euthyroid syndrome*	↓	↓
Subclinical hypothyroidism**	↑	→
Poor compliance with thyroxine***	↑	→

*Common in hospital inpatients; changes are reversible upon recovery from the systemic illness and no treatment is usually needed

**Common finding and represents patients who are likely to go on and develop hypothyroidism but still have normal thyroxine levels

***Patients who are poorly compliant may only take their thyroxine in the days before a routine blood test; the thyroxine levels are hence normal but the TSH 'lags' and reflects longer-term low thyroxine levels

Myxoedema coma

- Myxoedema coma is a medical emergency seen mostly in elderly patients and is associated with a high mortality rate
- Patients may be on treatment for hypothyroidism or be previously undiagnosed
- Infections and discontinuation of thyroid supplements are the major precipitating factors

Clinical features

- A reduced level of consciousness
- Seizures
- Hypothermia
- Features of hypothyroidism

Management

- IV levothyroxine is the mainstay of therapy
- T$_3$ therapy may also be used but this can cause arrhythmias
- Supportive therapy, e.g. IV fluids, correction of metabolic disturbances, hypothermia correction
- Intubation and ventilation if respiratory impairment is severe
- IV hydrocortisone as impaired adrenal function is present in profound hypothyroidism

Subclinical hypothyroidism

- Subclinical hypothyroidism occurs when a patient has a TSH level above the upper limit of the reference range and free T$_4$ levels are within the normal reference range
- There is some controversy over whether to treat these patients; symptoms may improve on T$_4$ but there are concerns over risk of reduced bone mineral density and atrial fibrillation
- The following patients should be considered for treatment with levothyroxine:
  - Those with TSH level >10mU/L
  - Those who are symptomatic
  - Those with a history of radio-iodine treatment or positive thyroid antibody test (as this subgroup almost always progress to overt hypothyroidism)
  - If there has been previous treatment of Graves' disease or other organ-specific autoimmune disease
- If none of the above is present, then TSH should be monitored every 6–12 months

Hypothyroidism in pregnancy

- Women of childbearing age should be encouraged to wait until they are euthyroid prior to trying to conceive
- It is important to maintain a euthyroid state throughout pregnancy, especially during the first trimester
- TFTs should be measured during the 1st, 2nd and 3rd trimesters for all pregnant women with hypothyroidism (TSH is a sensitive marker of thyroid dysfunction during pregnancy)
- Treating clinical and subclinical hypothyroidism can reduce adverse obstetric outcomes
- Levothyroxine dose may need to be increased by more than 50% during pregnancy; the dose can usually be reduced postpartum

Hyperthyroidism occurs when an excess of circulating thyroid hormones (**thyrotoxicosis**) is produced by an overactive thyroid gland.

Definition

- Primary hyperthyroidism is the term used when the pathology is within the thyroid gland
- Secondary hyperthyroidism is rare and occurs when the thyroid gland is stimulated by excessive thyroid-stimulating hormone (TSH) in the circulation due to pathology of the pituitary gland
- **Graves' disease** is the most common cause of primary hyperthyroidism and is the result of IgG antibodies binding to the TSH receptor and stimulating excess thyroid hormone production
- TSH receptor stimulating antibodies and **antithyroid peroxidase** antibodies are present in most patients with Graves' disease
- Graves' disease is associated with other autoimmune disorders e.g. pernicious anaemia and myasthenia gravis

Pathophysiology

Hyperthyroidism

Complications

- Atrial fibrillation
- High-output cardiac failure
- Osteoporosis
- Cardiomyopathy
- Thyroid storm

Management

Conservative

- Education
- Smoking cessation

Pharmacological

- **Symptomatic control** Propranolol for tremor and palpitations
- **Antithyroid drugs (carbimazole or propylthiouracil):**
  - Act very quickly and inhibit the production of thyroid hormones
  - Two potential methods of treating hyperthyroid patients: 'block and replace' (antithyroid drugs are given with thyroxine replacement), and 'dose titration' (only antithyroid drugs are used and doses are adjusted to achieve normalisation of TFTs); both methods are equally effective
  - **Carbimazole** is usually used 1st line; agranulocytosis is an important adverse effect and patients should be warned to seek urgent medical help if they develop a fever, sore throat etc; it is teratogenic and therefore women of childbearing potential should use effective contraception during treatment
  - **Propylthiouracil** Known to cause severe liver failure, particularly in children, and therefore reserved for use in pregnancy and thyroid storm

Radioiodine

- Usually the treatment of choice in relapsed Graves' disease and in those patients with toxic nodular hyperthyroidism
- Radioactive iodine is given to the patient as a drink and is taken up by the thyroid gland, causing destruction of the gland; it can take up to 3–4 months to take effect
- It is contraindicated in pregnancy and breastfeeding, and women must be advised not to get pregnant for at least 6 months
- Hypothyroidism is a potential and common complication

Surgical

- **Subtotal** or near **total thyroidectomy** achieves a 98% cure rate; it is indicated if there is suboptimal response to antithyroid medication or radioiodine (particularly in patients who are pregnant or who have Graves' orbitopathy)
- Patients should be returned to the euthyroid state with antithyroid drugs before surgery to avoid thyroid storm
- Complications are rare but include haemorrhage, hypoparathyroidism and vocal cord paralysis

- **Graves' disease:** the most common cause of thyrotoxicosis; as well as typical features of thyrotoxicosis other features may be seen including thyroid eye disease
- **Toxic multinodular goitre:** autonomously functioning thyroid nodules that secrete excess thyroid hormones
- **Solitary thyroid nodule:** palpable, toxic adenoma
- **De Quervain's thyroiditis:** a transient form of hyperthyroidism that probably results from a viral infection; often accompanied by pyrexia and a painful goitre (see *Fig. 1*)
- **Other forms of thyroiditis:** subacute thyroiditis, silent thyroiditis and postpartum thyroiditis
- **Drugs:** e.g. amiodarone, lithium, exogenous iodine and thyroid hormone
- **Follicular carcinoma of the thyroid gland:** associated with metastatic disease
- **TSH-secreting pituitary adenoma**

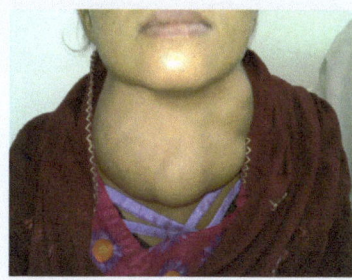

Fig. 1 Thyroid goitre

Causes

Clinical features

Symbols

Symptoms

- Weight loss or gain
- Increased or decreased appetite
- Irritability
- Weakness and fatigue
- Diarrhoea ± steatorrhoea
- Sweating
- Tremor
- Mental illness: anxiety, depression, psychosis
- Heat intolerance
- Loss of libido
- Oligomenorrhoea or amenorrhoea

Signs

- Palmar erythema
- Sweaty and warm palms
- Fine tremor
- Tachycardia: may present as atrial fibrillation and/or heart failure (common in the elderly)
- Hair thinning or diffuse alopecia
- Pretibial myxoedema (see *Fig. 2*)
- Thyroid acropachy
- Urticaria, pruritus
- Brisk reflexes
- Goitre
- Anxiety
- Proximal myopathy (muscle weakness ± wasting)
- Gynaecomastia
- Lid lag (may be present in any cause of hyperthyroidism)
- Thyroid eye disease (see *Notes*) including exophthalmos (see *Fig. 3*) and ophthalmoplegia

Investigations

- **Thyroid function tests (TFTs)** (see *Notes*)
- **Autoantibodies** Antimicrosomal antibodies against thyroid peroxidase, antithyroglobulin antibodies and TSH-receptor antibodies are all positive in most patients with Graves' disease
- **Imaging:**
  - US scan of nodules
  - Isotope scan to locate hot (overactivity) and cold (no activity) spots
- **Inflammatory markers** CRP and ESR are often raised in patients with subacute thyroiditis
- **Fine-needle aspiration** Aspirate nodules to rule out malignancy

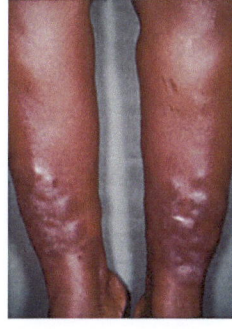

Fig. 2 Pretibial myxoedema

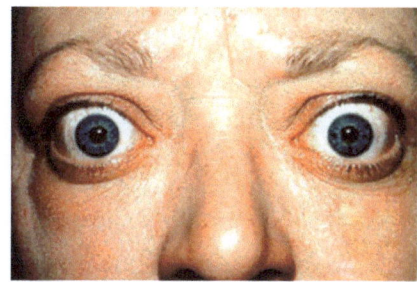

Fig. 3 Exophthalmos

Thyroid eye disease

Thyroid eye disease affects between 25 and 50% of patients with Graves' disease and patients may be eu-, hypo- or hyperthyroid at the time of presentation.

Pathophysiology

- It is thought to be caused by an autoimmune response against an autoantigen, possibly the TSH receptor causing retro-orbital inflammation
- Smoking is the most important modifiable risk factor for the development of thyroid eye disease
- Radioiodine treatment may increase the inflammatory symptoms seen in thyroid eye disease

Clinical features

- Exophthalmos
- Conjunctival oedema
- Optic disc swelling
- Ophthalmoplegia
- Increased risk of exposure keratopathy

Management

- Smoking cessation
- Topical lubricants to help prevent corneal inflammation caused by exposure
- High-dose systemic steroids e.g. prednisolone to reduce inflammation
- Radiotherapy
- Surgery

Subclinical hyperthyroidism

- Subclinical hyperthyroidism is defined as: normal serum free T_4 and T_3 levels with a TSH below normal range (usually <1mIU/L)
- Common causes include multinodular goitre and excessive thyroxine treatment
- The importance in recognising subclinical hyperthyroidism lies in the potential effect on the cardiovascular system (can precipitate atrial fibrillation) and bone metabolism (increase likelihood of osteoporosis); it may also impact on quality of life and increase the likelihood of dementia
- TSH levels often revert to normal; therefore levels must be persistently low to warrant intervention and often only monitoring is required; a reasonable treatment option is a therapeutic trial of low-dose antithyroid agents for approximately 6 months in an effort to induce a remission

Thyroid storm

Hyperthyroid crisis, or thyrotoxic storm, is an extreme manifestation of thyrotoxicosis due to overproduction of thyroid hormones; it classically occurs in patients with underlying Graves' disease or toxic multinodular goitre.

Presentation

Often, there is sudden onset of severe hyperthyroidism with:
- Hyperpyrexia (>41°C), dehydration
- Heart rate >140bpm (with or without AF/other arrhythmias), hypotension, congestive heart failure
- Nausea, jaundice, vomiting, diarrhoea, abdominal pain
- Confusion, agitation, delirium, psychosis, seizures or coma

Common precipitants

- Infection or other acute illness
- Withdrawal of or non-compliance with antithyroid medication
- Recent trauma, surgical stress, recent thyroid surgery
- MI, stroke, pulmonary embolism
- Diabetic ketoacidosis, hyperosmolar coma or hypoglycaemia
- Following childbirth
- Drugs: radioiodine, amiodarone, radiographic contrast media
- Overdose of thyroid hormone tablets
- Vigorous palpation of the thyroid gland in hyperthyroid patients

Management

- Treatment of the precipitating cause, e.g. any suspected infection
- Resuscitation: oxygen, IV fluids and nasogastric tube if there is vomiting
- Antithyroid treatment: carbimazole or propylthiouracil orally
- Lugol's solution (aqueous iodine oral solution)
- Beta blockers (initially IV propranolol 5mg, then orally) unless contra-indicated; diltiazem can be used if propranolol is contraindicated
- Hydrocortisone administration is also recommended
- For severe agitation, sedate with chlorpromazine
- Keep cool with tepid sponging and paracetamol (avoid aspirin which can increase T_4 levels)
- Patients who fail medical therapy should be treated with therapeutic plasma exchange or thyroidectomy

Definition

Hypoglycaemia is a lower than normal level of blood glucose. It can be defined as 'mild' if the episode is self-treated and 'severe' if assistance by a third party is required. Although definitions of hypoglycaemia vary greatly, any blood glucose **<4.0mmol/L** should be treated.

Causes (EXPLAINS)

- **Ex**ogenous e.g. insulin and oral hypoglycaemics (most common), alcohol excess, ACE inhibitors, salicylate poisoning
- **P**ituitary insufficiency
- **L**iver causes including severe liver failure, glycogen storage disease, galactosaemia
- **A**drenal insufficiency, congenital **A**drenal hyperplasia, **A**fter bariatric surgery ('Dumping syndrome')
- **I**nsulinoma, **I**mmune hypoglycaemia (e.g. anti-insulin receptor antibodies in Hodgkin's disease), **I**nfection e.g. malaria
- **N**on-pancreatic neoplasms (e.g. fibroma, sarcoma, hepatoma), **N**esidioblastosis
- **S**tarvation

Hypoglycaemia

Management

Acute

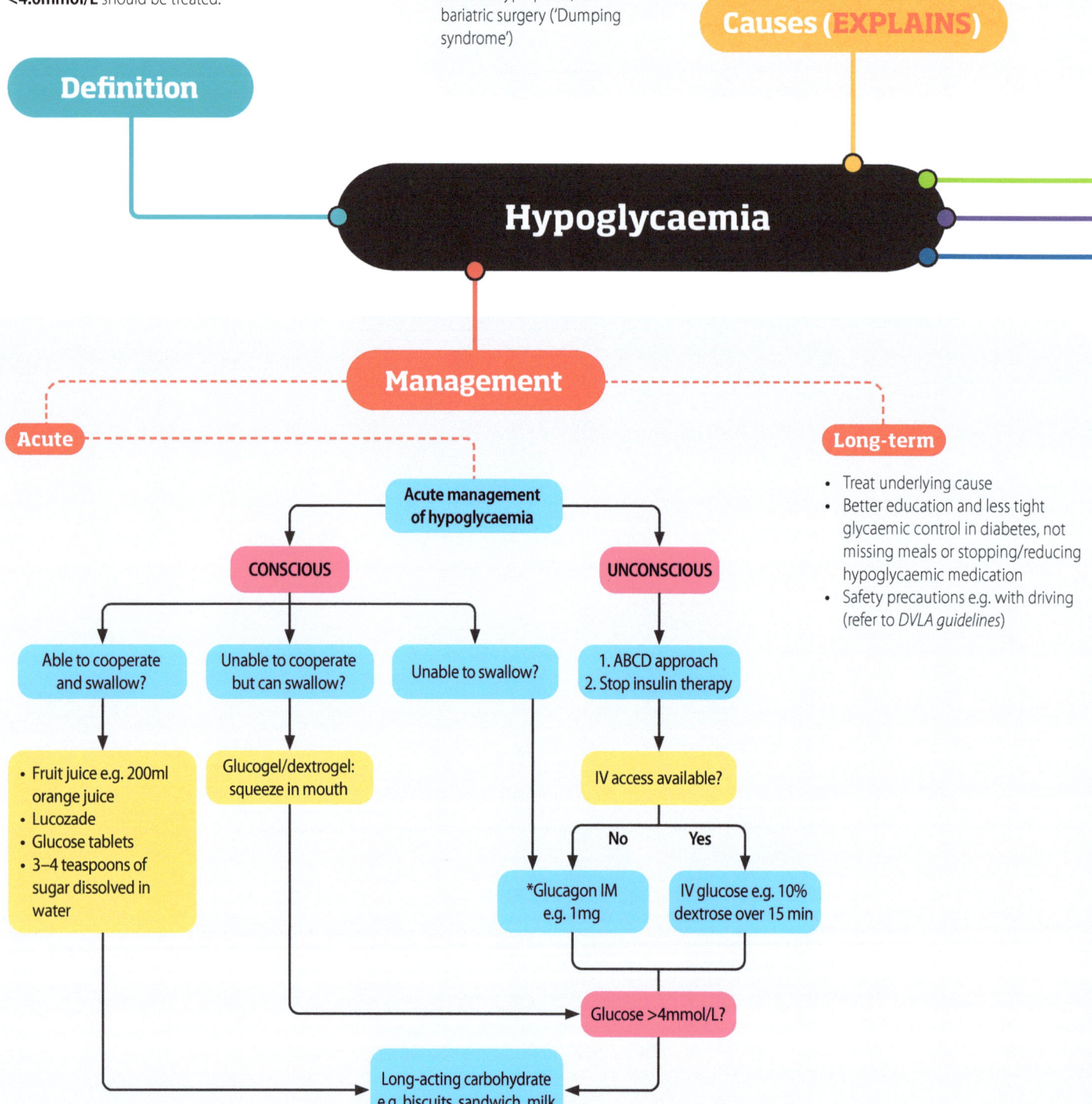

Acute management of hypoglycaemia

CONSCIOUS

- Able to cooperate and swallow?
  - Fruit juice e.g. 200ml orange juice
  - Lucozade
  - Glucose tablets
  - 3–4 teaspoons of sugar dissolved in water

- Unable to cooperate but can swallow?
  - Glucogel/dextrogel: squeeze in mouth

- Unable to swallow?

UNCONSCIOUS

1. ABCD approach
2. Stop insulin therapy

- IV access available?
  - **No** → *Glucagon IM e.g. 1mg
  - **Yes** → IV glucose e.g. 10% dextrose over 15 min

Glucose >4mmol/L?

Long-acting carbohydrate e.g. biscuits, sandwich, milk

Long-term

- Treat underlying cause
- Better education and less tight glycaemic control in diabetes, not missing meals or stopping/reducing hypoglycaemic medication
- Safety precautions e.g. with driving (refer to *DVLA guidelines*)

*Note: IM glucagon has a relatively slow onset of action and relies on glycogen stores; therefore it may not be suitable for those in starved states, liver disease and in young children (IV glucose should be given instead)

- Although rare, insulinomas are the most common cause of endogenous hyperinsulinaemia in adults
- Around 5–7% are malignant and around 7–10% occur in association with MEN-1
- Diagnosis: low glucose (<2.2mmol/L) at the same time as inappropriately high insulin and C-peptide; this is usually diagnosed with an overnight fast but in less clear-cut cases a prolonged fast of up to 72h may be carried out under observation in hospital
- Insulinomas may be too small to be seen on CT scans and further investigation with endoscopic ultrasound should be considered
- Surgical removal is the mainstay of treatment

Insulinoma

Autonomic symptoms

- Sweating
- Anxiety
- Hunger
- Tremor
- Palpitations
- Dizziness

Neuroglycopenic symptoms

- Confusion, change in behaviour
- Fatigue, drowsiness
- Blurred vision
- Weakness
- Dizziness
- Slurred speech
- Seizures
- Coma

General malaise

- Headache
- Nausea

Clinical features

Diagnosis/investigations

Confirming diagnosis (see *Fig. 1*)

- Capillary glucose *or*
- Plasma glucose <4mmol/L

Exploring underlying cause

(usually not required if taking hypoglycaemic agents)
- HbA1c, LFTs, TFTs, U&Es, 0900h cortisol ± short Synacthen test (if suspected adrenal insufficiency)
- Blood and urine assays for sulfonylureas: to detect factitious hypoglycaemia caused by these drugs
- Plasma insulin, glucose and C-peptide: hypoglycaemic insulinaemia is present with insulinoma, sulfonylureas and exogenous insulin administration, but C-peptide is only raised with endogenous insulin i.e. with insulinoma

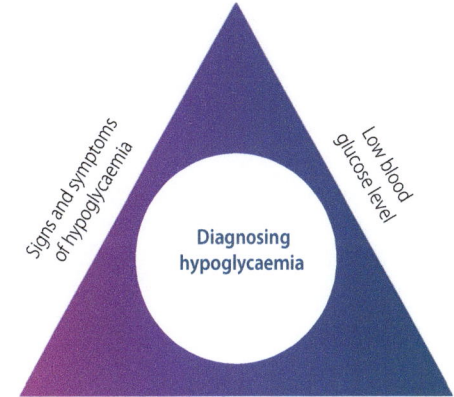

Signs and symptoms of hypoglycaemia

Low blood glucose level

Diagnosing hypoglycaemia

Relief of symptoms with increased blood glucose

Fig. 1 According to Whipple's triad, the diagnosis of hypoglycaemia rests on the 3 criteria shown

Definition

Hyponatraemia refers to a low concentration of sodium in the blood and is defined as a serum sodium <136mmol/L.

Causes

This depends on plasma osmolality and fluid status (see *Fig. 1*)

Classification

By severity

- **Mild hyponatraemia** Serum Na+ 130–135mmol/L
- **Moderate hyponatraemia** Serum Na+ 125–129mmol/L
- **Severe hyponatraemia** Serum Na+ <125mmol/L

By rate of onset

- **Acute hyponatraemia** Duration <48h
- **Chronic hyponatraemia** Duration ≥48h

Hyponatraemia

Complications

- Cerebral oedema
- Cerebral herniation
- Death
- Central pontine myelinolysis: if hyponatraemia corrected too fast

Management

The management of hyponatraemia depends on the fluid status and underlying cause; hyponatraemia should be corrected slowly as if corrected too fast it can result in central pontine myelinolysis.

Hypovolaemia

- Stop underlying cause e.g. diuretics
- Treat with IV normal saline

Euvolaemia

- Fluids restriction: 500–1000ml/day
- Demeclocycline: licensed to treat hyponatraemia associated with SIADH secondary to malignant disease where fluid restriction is ineffective and patient does not have cirrhosis

- Hypertonic saline can be used in severe hyponatraemia in ITU/HDU setting
- Vasopressin receptor antagonist, e.g. tolvaptan, may be useful for SIADH; however, can induce thirst and can increase Na+ levels too rapidly

Hypervolaemia

- Fluid restrict
- Treat underlying cause, e.g. heart failure, with loop diuretics

Symptoms

- Usually asymptomatic
- Anorexia
- Nausea
- Headache
- Lethargy
- Personality change
- Muscle cramps
- Weakness
- Confusion
- Ataxia
- Drowsiness

Signs

- Decreased level of consciousness
- Cognitive impairment (e.g. short-term memory loss, disorientation, confusion, depression)
- Focal or generalised seizures
- Signs of hypovolaemia e.g. dry mucous membranes, tachycardia, prolonged capillary refill time
- Signs of hypervolaemia e.g. raised JVP, pulmonary and peripheral oedema

Clinical features

Investigations

Blood tests

- **U&Es** To confirm hyponatraemia
- **TFTs** Severe hypothyroidism can cause hyponatraemia
- **Plasma osmolality** (paired with urine osmolality) (see *Fig. 1*)
- **Glucose** Hyperglycaemia can cause hyponatraemia
- **Cortisol (0900h)** Adrenocortical deficiency can cause hyponatraemia
- **Lipids and albumin** Raised levels can result in pseudohyponatraemia

Urine

- **Urine osmolality** (paired with plasma osmolality)
- **Urinary sodium** (see *Fig. 1*)

Imaging

- **CXR** (rule out infection/lung malignancy in SIADH)
- **CT chest, abdomen, pelvis** (rule out malignancy in SIADH)

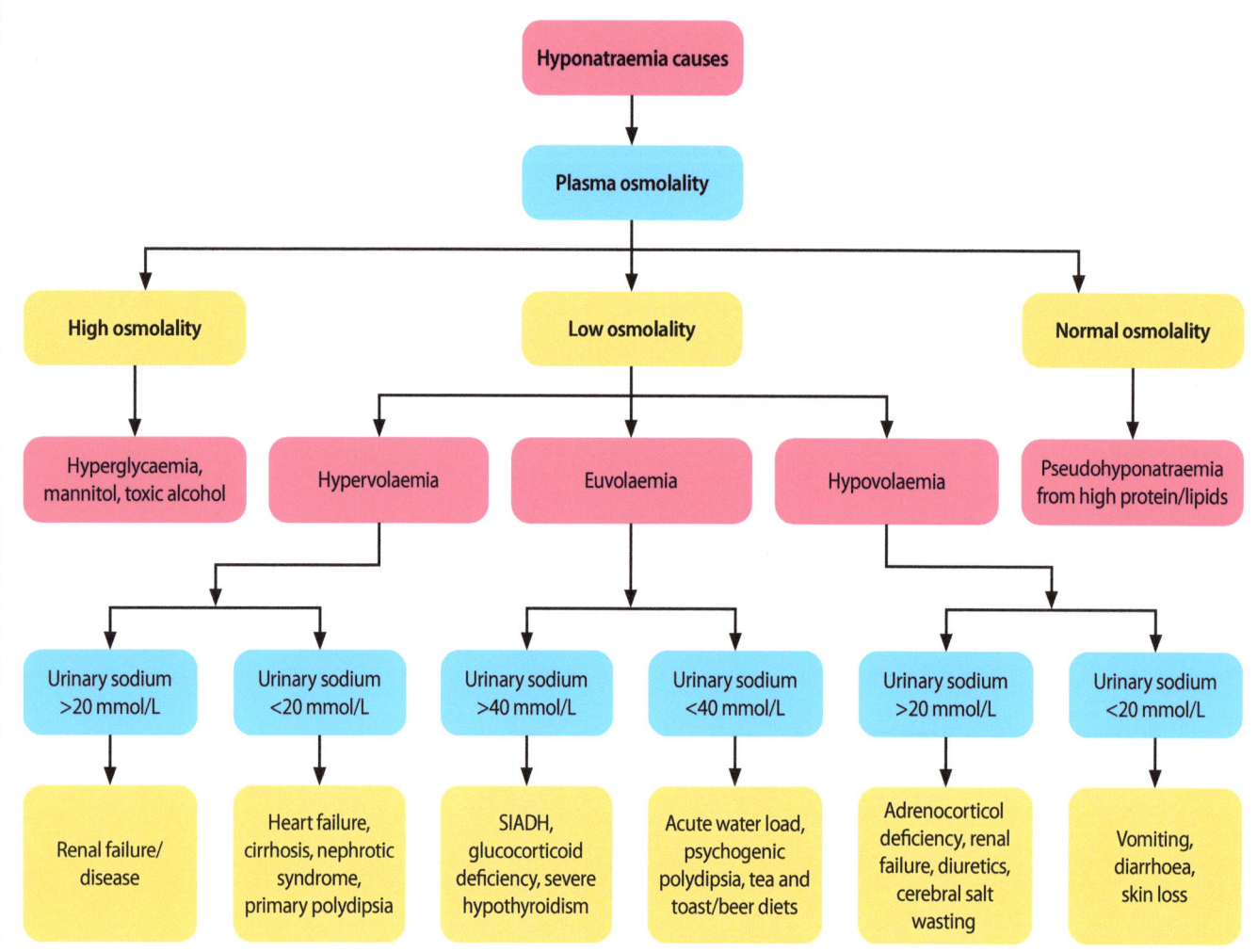

Fig. 1 Causes of hyponatraemia according to plasma osmolality, fluid status and urinary sodium

Syndrome of inappropriate ADH secretion (SIADH)

Definition

SIADH is inappropriate ADH secretion from the posterior pituitary gland or from an ectopic source despite low serum osmolality.

Causes

- **Neurological** Tumour, meningoencephalitis, head trauma, infection, Guillain–Barré syndrome, multiple sclerosis, SLE, subarachnoid or subdural haemorrhage, sinus thrombosis, AIDS, porphyria
- **Pulmonary** Lung small cell carcinoma, mesothelioma, pneumonia, cystic fibrosis
- **Malignancies** Lung small cell carcinoma, pancreas, prostate, thymus, lymphoma
- **Drugs** e.g. SSRIs, opiates, thiazide diuretics, carbamazepine, tricyclic antidepressants, vincristine, cyclophosphamide, phenothiazines, oxytocin

Diagnostic features

- Hyponatraemia
- Plasma hypo-osmolality proportional to hyponatraemia
- Inappropriately elevated urine osmolality
- Persistent urine Na^+ >30mmol/L with normal salt intake
- Euvolaemia
- Normal thyroid and adrenal function

Management

- Fluid restriction
- Treat underlying cause e.g. malignancy, infection
- Hypertonic saline in acute severe case
- As above; demeclocycline and vasopressin receptor antagonists e.g. tolvaptan can also be used

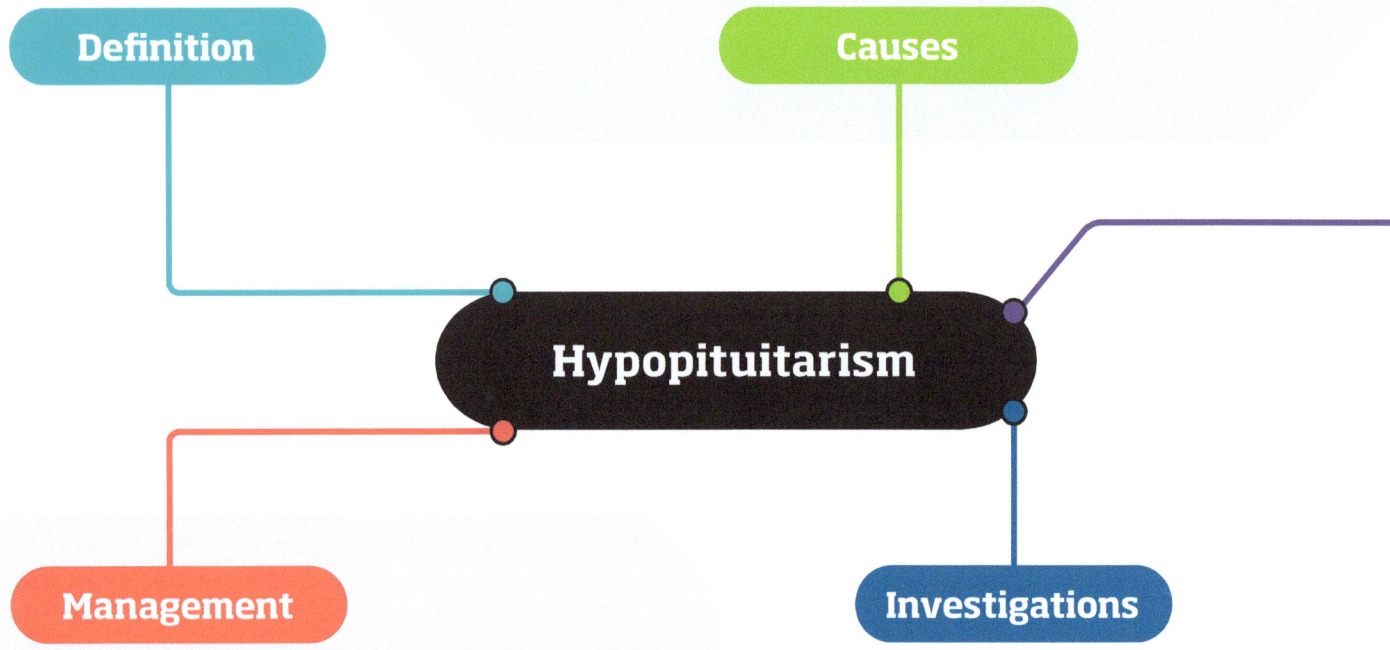

Hypopituitarism is the inability of the pituitary gland to provide sufficient hormones usually due to pituitary disease or hypothalamic abnormalities associated with reduced stimuli to hormonal secretion.

Definition

Causes

- **Pituitary tumours** For example, adenomas
- **Non-pituitary tumours** Craniopharyngiomas, meningiomas, gliomas, chordomas, ependymomas, metastases
- **Infiltrative processes:** Sarcoidosis, histiocytosis X, haemochromatosis, lymphocytic hypophysitis
- **Infections** Cerebral abscess, meningitis, encephalitis, tuberculosis, syphilis
- **Ischaemia and infarction** Subarachnoid haemorrhage, ischaemic stroke, Sheehan syndrome (postpartum haemorrhage with anterior pituitary infarction), pituitary apoplexy (caused by an acute infarction of a pituitary adenoma)
- **Empty sella syndrome** Radiological diagnosis of absence of normal pituitary within the sella turcica; usually benign and asymptomatic but may develop headaches and hypopituitarism
- **Iatrogenic** Irradiation, neurosurgery, withholding previous chronic glucocorticoid replacement
- **Traumatic head injury**
- **Congenital** Kallmann syndrome (congenital hypogonadotropic hypogonadism with anosmia)
- **Pituitary hypoplasia/aplasia**
- **Genetic cause** e.g. HEXS1, LHX3, PIT1, PROP1 gene mutations, septo-optic dysplasia
- **Idiopathic**

Hypopituitarism

Management

- Acute pituitary failure may require resuscitation, including IV fluids
- Surgical or medical removal of lesion if tumour is the underlying cause; removal of macroadenomas that do not respond to medical therapy
- In pituitary apoplexy, prompt surgical decompression may be life-saving
- Hormone replacement as appropriate and treatment of the underlying cause:
  - **Glucocorticoids** (usually hydrocortisone but occasionally prednisolone or dexamethasone) is required if the ACTH–adrenal axis is impaired, especially in acute presentations; increased doses of glucocorticoids are required following any form of emotional or physical stress (e.g. during an infection) to prevent acute decompensation
  - Secondary hypothyroidism: **thyroid hormone** replacement; in panhypopituitarism is important to restore cortisol levels before thyroxine
  - Gonadotropin deficiency: **testosterone** replacement in men and **oestrogens** (with or without progesterone) for women (combined oral contraceptive pill for premenopausal women); gonadotropins or pulse gonadotropin-releasing hormone if fertility is required and the defect is hypothalamic (with intact pituitary)
  - **Growth hormone** replacement for growth hormone deficiency
  - **Vasopressin** replacement for diabetes insipidus

Investigations

- **Blood glucose, U&Es** Disturbances of renal function, glucose and electrolytes are common
- **Hormone assays** TFTs, prolactin, gonadotropins, testosterone and cortisol
- **Measure gonadotropins, TSH, growth hormone, glucose** and **cortisol** Following triple stimulation with gonadotropin-releasing hormone (GnRH), thyrotropin-releasing hormone (TRH) and insulin-induced hypoglycaemia
- **Pituitary function tests:**
  - For growth hormone deficiency: IGF-1 (low levels suggest growth hormone deficiency), insulin-stress test (measures growth hormone response to IV insulin)
  - For ACTH deficiency: Synacthen test (measures the adrenal response to ACTH), insulin-stress test (measuring ACTH response to insulin-induced hypoglycaemia)
  - For TSH deficiency: TRH stimulation test (TSH response to IV-administered TRH)
- **Cranial MRI** To exclude tumours and other lesions of the sellar and parasellar region after hypopituitarism has been confirmed

Presentation varies from asymptomatic to acute pituitary failure with acute collapse and coma, depending on the aetiology, rapidity of onset, and predominant hormones involved.

- **ACTH deficiency** Fatigue, pallor, anorexia, weight loss, weakness, dizziness, nausea, vomiting, circulatory collapse, shock
- **TSH deficiency:**
  - **Adults** Tiredness, cold intolerance, constipation, hair loss, dry skin, hoarseness, weight gain, bradycardia and hypotension
  - **Children** Delayed development, growth restriction and intellectual impairment
- **Gonadotropin deficiency:**
  - **Women** Oligomenorrhoea, loss of libido, dyspareunia, breast atrophy, infertility, osteoporosis
  - **Men** Loss of libido, impotence, mood impairment, loss of facial, scrotal and body hair; decreased muscle mass, osteoporosis
  - **Children** Delayed puberty
- **Growth hormone deficiency** Short stature, decreased muscle mass and strength, visceral obesity, fatigue, decreased quality of life, impairment of attention and memory, dyslipidaemia, premature atherosclerosis, growth restriction (children)
- **Antidiuretic hormone deficiency** Polyuria and polydipsia

Clinical features

Notes

Hypopituitarism

Phaeochromocytoma is a rare tumour that secretes **catecholamines**. It is derived from chromaffin cells, usually in the adrenal medulla; however, occasionally (18%) there are extra-adrenal phaeochromocytomas (called **paragangliomas**).

Definition

Adrenaline physiology

- The **adrenal medulla** is the location of the majority of the body's chromaffin cells which produce catecholamines
- It plays an important role in the fight-or-flight response:
  - **Cardiovascular:** ↑heart rate, ↑force of heart contraction, mainly vasoconstriction and vasodilatation in the cardiac and skeletal muscle
  - **Metabolic and endocrine actions:** ↑glycogenolysis, ↑lipolysis, ↑glucagon secretion, ↓insulin secretion, ↑renin secretion
  - **Miscellaneous:** dilation of pupils, contraction of spleen, ejaculation, inhibition of micturition

Pathophysiology

- 10–15% are malignant in nature
- The clinical manifestations of a phaeochromocytoma arise from excessive catecholamine secretion by the tumour
- Catecholamines typically secreted are **noradrenaline** and **adrenaline**; but some tumours produce dopamine
- Excessive and uncontrolled catecholamine results in increased stimulation of alpha- and beta-adrenergic receptors in various parts of the body

Phaeochromocytoma

Prognosis

- For non-malignant phaeochromocytoma the 5-year survival rate is >95%
- For malignant phaeochromocytoma the 5-year survival rate is <50%

Management

- Associated MEN conditions must be searched for and, if found, managed accordingly, including genetic counselling
- Surgical resection of the tumour is the treatment of choice:
  - Preoperative treatment with alpha blockers (phenoxybenzamine is started at least 7–10 days before operation) and beta blockers (e.g. propranolol) is required to control BP and prevent intraoperative hypertensive crises
  - A 24-h urine collection for total catecholamines, metanephrines and VMA must be checked 2 weeks after operation
- Lifelong annual biochemical testing is recommended to detect recurrent or metastatic disease

Investigations

Biochemistry

- **Urine** 24-h collection of total catecholamines, vanillylmandelic acid (VMA) and metanephrines
- **Bloods** ↑Plasma catecholamines and plasma metanephrines; calcium and glucose may be raised

Imaging

To localise the tumour:

- CT abdomen and pelvis ± mediastinum and neck
- MRI abdomen and pelvis ± mediastinum and neck
- Meta-iodobenzylguanidine (MIBG) scan
- PET scan

- Approx. 70% are **sporadic**
- Up to 30% are inherited as part of:
  - **Multiple endocrine neoplasia (MEN) syndrome 2:** occurs bilaterally in 70% of MEN syndromes
  - **Neurofibromatosis type 1:** incidence of phaeochromocytoma is approx. 1%
  - **von Hippel–Lindau (VHL) disease:** 15–20% develop phaeochromocytoma and approx. 50% are bilateral

Causes

Symptoms
- Headache
- Sweating
- Palpitations
- Tremor
- Nausea
- Weight loss
- Weakness
- Anxiety
- Sense of doom
- Epigastric/flank pain

Signs
- Hypertension
- Postural hypotension
- Tremor
- Tachycardia
- Hyperglycaemia
- Hypertensive retinopathy
- Pallor
- Fever

Clinical features

Hypertensive crisis

Any of the following may precipitate a hypertensive crisis:
- Induction of anaesthesia
- Opiates
- Dopamine antagonists
- Decongestants such as pseudoephedrine
- Drugs that inhibit the reuptake of catecholamines, including tricyclic antidepressants and cocaine
- X-ray contrast media
- Childbirth

Notes

Phaeochromocytoma

Polycystic ovary syndrome (PCOS) is a complex endocrine disorder thought to affect 5–20% of women of reproductive age, with clinical features that include hirsutism and acne (due to **excess androgens**), **oligomenorrhoea** or **amenorrhoea**, and **multiple cysts** in the ovary.

Note: Polycystic ovaries on US are very common and can be seen in up to 33% of women of reproductive age; however, the majority of women with polycystic ovaries do not have features of PCOS and do not require treatment.

- The pathophysiology of PCOS is not completely understood but it is thought to be centred on **hyperandrogenism**
- **Insulin resistance** is an important part of the syndrome that leads to hyperinsulinaemia causing insulin to stimulate LH receptors in the theca cells to further increase androgen secretion
- This is compounded by central adiposity which contributes to reduced sex hormone binding globulin (SHBG) thus increasing the free circulating androgen index
- Hyperandrogenism results in an increased number of growing follicles which subsequently produce **anti-Müllerian hormone** resulting in a lack of dominant follicle selection and **anovulation** thus contributing to menstrual disturbance and subfertility

- Menstrual disturbance: oligomenorrhoea or amenorrhoea
- Infertility or subfertility
- Acne
- Hirsutism (see *Fig. 1*)
- Alopecia
- Obesity or difficulty losing weight
- Psychological symptoms: mood swings, depression, anxiety, poor self-esteem
- Sleep apnoea
- Acanthosis nigricans (brown to black, poorly defined, velvety hyperpigmentation of the skin); it is associated with insulin resistance

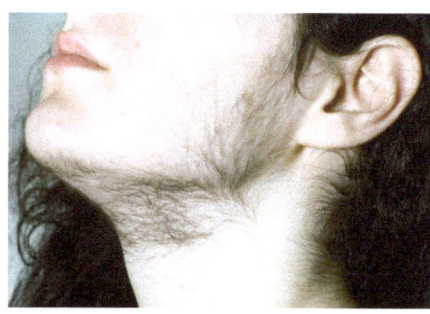

Fig. 1 Hirsutism

Definition

Pathophysiology

Clinical features

Polycystic ovary syndrome

- Impaired glucose tolerance and T2DM
- Cardiovascular disease
- Dyslipidaemia
- Infertility
- Pregnancy complications
- Sleep apnoea
- Endometrial cancer

Complications

Management

General measures

- **Weight loss and exercise** have been shown to improve fertility, psychological symptoms and metabolic features
- **COCP:** to control menstrual irregularity in women that require contraception

Hirsutism and acne management

- Local therapy: physical methods (waxing, shaving, bleaching, plucking, depilation and electrolysis), laser treatment, eflornithine cream
- A **COCP** may be used to help manage hirsutism
- **Co-cyprindiol** (ethinylestradiol and cyproterone): licensed for treating hirsutism and acne
- **Spironolactone**, **flutamide** and **finasteride** may be used under specialist supervision

Metabolic management

- **Weight loss** and **exercise**
- **Metformin** for impaired glucose tolerance
- Orlistat can help with weight loss in obese women with PCOS and may improve insulin sensitivity

Subfertility management

- **Clomiphene** induces ovulation and has been proven to improve pregnancy rates
- **Metformin** may be used instead of or together with clomiphene to improve pregnancy rates
- **Gonadotropins** are 2nd-line treatment for inducing ovulation in those resistant to clomiphene
- **Laparoscopic ovarian drilling** is 2nd-line treatment for inducing ovulation

- **Sex hormones** ↑Total testosterone or normal (because SHBG is suppressed in PCOS), ↑free testosterone; biochemical evidence requires ↑free androgen index (serum total testosterone/SHBG)
- **FSH, LH** ↑LH with ↑LH:FSH ratio (>2)
- **Prolactin** May be ↑ but done mainly to exclude hyperprolactinaemia as a cause for symptoms
- **TSH** Exclude thyroid dysfunction
- **OGTT/HbA1c** ↑Risk of impaired glucose tolerance and diabetes in PCOS
- **Lipids** ↑Risk of dyslipidaemia in PCOS
- **Pelvic US** The average volume is three times that of normal ovaries; however, the syndrome can exist without the presence of polycystic ovaries

Investigations

The Rotterdam criteria

1. **Menstrual disturbance:**
   Amenorrhoea (absent periods) or oligomenorrhoea (infrequent periods)
2. **Hyperandrogenism:**
   Clinical hyperandrogenism (Ferriman–Gallwey score >8) or biochemical hyperandrogenism (elevated total/free testosterone)
3. **Polycystic ovaries:**
   Polycystic ovaries on US (≥12 antral follicles in one ovary or ovarian volume ≥10cm³) (see *Fig. 2*)

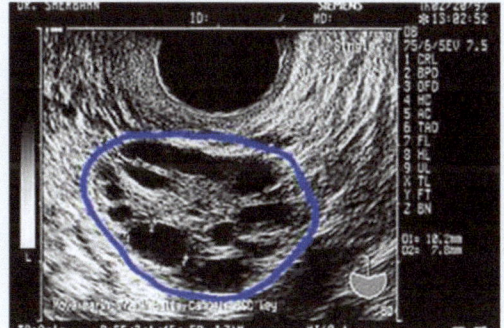

Fig. 2 Polycystic ovary

Diagnostic criteria

Notes

Polycystic ovary syndrome

Chapter 6

Neurology

Definition

An acute, unilateral, partial or complete paralysis of the face due to idiopathic unilateral **lower motor neurone facial nerve palsy**. It is the most common cause of facial nerve palsy but it is often a diagnosis of exclusion as other important diagnoses such as stroke, infections, parotid tumours, middle ear disease should be excluded first.

Pathophysiology

- Likely cause is ischaemic compression of the facial nerve within the facial canal due to inflammation
- Inflammation is most likely caused by a viral infection (with herpes simplex virus and varicella zoster virus being the likely culprits) although the exact pathogenesis remains unclear
- There may be a familial component in recurrent cases, possibly due to anatomical abnormality of the facial canal

Epidemiology/risk factors

- Overall, it is relatively uncommon with an incidence of approx. 20–30 people per 100 000 each year
- Most commonly seen at age 15–60 years
- It is more common in people who are diabetic, immunocompromised, obese, hypertensive or have upper respiratory conditions, or in pregnant women

Bell's palsy

Prognosis

- Most people with Bell's palsy begin to recover, even without treatment, within 2–3 weeks (approx. 85%); complete recovery usually occurs within 3–4 months
- If untreated, around 15% of patients have permanent moderate to severe weakness
- Poor prognostic features include:
  - Complete palsy or severe degeneration (on electrophysiology)
  - No signs of recovery by 3 weeks
  - Age >60 years
  - Severe pain
  - Ramsay Hunt syndrome
  - Associated with hypertension, diabetes or pregnancy

Management

Eye care

- ↓Tear production and difficulty closing the eye puts people at risk of corneal dryness, ulceration and even blindness; appropriate eye care is vital
- Prescription of artificial tears and eye lubricants should be considered
- Taping the eyelids shut at night is recommended
- If the cornea remains exposed after attempting to close the eyelid, urgent referral to ophthalmology should be considered

Steroids

- Should be prescribed for patients within 72h of onset of Bell's palsy
- Prednisolone 1mg/kg or 60mg OD for 5 days then reducing by 10mg each day for a further 5 days (10 days in total)

- Antivirals such as aciclovir are NO LONGER recommended

Physiotherapy

'Facial re-training' to improve facial motor function may help but evidence of its effectiveness is lacking.

Botulinum

Botulinum toxin can augment facial symmetry.

Surgery

- Facial nerve decompression is an option for patients with facial palsy not responding to medical treatment
- If residual paralysis after 6–9 months, referral to plastic surgery should be considered for surgical nerve grafting

Rapid onset (<72h):
- Unilateral sagging of the mouth
- One-sided facial paralysis (see *Fig. 1*)
- Drooling of saliva
- Speech difficulty
- Hyperacusis
- Altered taste (loss of taste sensation in the anterior two-thirds of tongue)
- Failure of eye closure: may cause watery or dry eyes

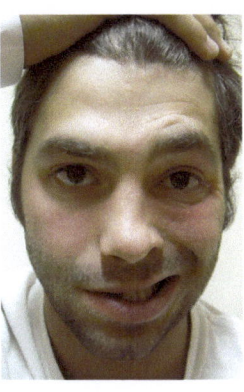

Fig. 1 Bell's palsy showing right facial paralysis when the patient was asked to smile

Clinical features

Idiopathic
- Bell's palsy (most common) (see *Fig. 1*)

Infectious
- Ramsay Hunt syndrome
- Lyme disease
- Meningitis
- TB
- Other viruses: HIV, EBV, CMV

Intracranial lesions
- Stroke
- Brain tumours
- Multiple sclerosis (MS)

Systemic disease
- Diabetes mellitus
- Sarcoidosis
- Guillain–Barré syndrome (usually bilateral facial nerve palsy)
- Rheumatoid arthritis and Sjögren syndrome
- Vasculitides

ENT
- Acoustic neuroma
- Otitis media
- Parotid tumours
- Cholesteatoma

Trauma
- Basal skull fracture
- Forceps delivery
- Post acupuncture haematoma
- Diving (barotrauma)

Causes of facial nerve palsy

Investigations

The diagnosis of Bell's palsy is clinical and investigations are not usually required but may be done to rule out other causes or determine the severity of palsy:
- **Serology** Raised borrelia antibodies (in Lyme disease) or varicella zoster virus antibodies (in Ramsay Hunt syndrome)
- **MRI brain** To rule out stroke, space-occupying lesion or MS
- **Nerve conduction studies** Predict delayed recovery by showing axonal degeneration
- **Schirmer's tear test** Shows reduced flow of tears on the side of the palsy
- **Stapedial reflex** (audiological test) Absent if stapedius muscle is affected

Notes

Bell's palsy

Neuroanatomy of the facial nerve (7th cranial nerve)

- The facial nerve is largely motor in function, supplying the muscles of facial expression
- In addition it has two major branches which arise during its intracranial course through the facial canal of the petrous temporal bone:
  - The chorda tympani, which carries taste from the anterior two-thirds of the tongue
  - Nerve to stapedius muscle, which has a damping effect to protect the ear from loud noise
- Therefore damage to the facial nerve in the temporal bone (e.g. in Bell's palsy) causes hyperacusis and taste disturbance to the anterior two-thirds of the tongue
- Within the parotid gland, the nerve terminates by splitting into five extracranial branches which can be remembered by the mnemonic 'Two Zebras Bit My Coccyx': Temporal, Zygomatic, Buccal, Mandibular and Cervical

Clinically distinguishing upper vs lower motor neurone lesions that cause facial weakness

- It is vital to be able to distinguish clinically facial weakness caused by an upper (central) vs a lower (peripheral) motor neurone lesion as this will significantly alter the management plan
- Upper motor neurone lesions, such as a **stroke**, cause contralateral face weakness **sparing** the **forehead**, while lower motor neurone lesions, such as a facial nerve injury, typically cause weakness involving the whole ipsilateral face (see *Fig. 2*)

Ramsay Hunt syndrome

Definition

Ramsay Hunt syndrome (herpes zoster oticus) is caused by the reactivation of the varicella zoster virus in the geniculate ganglion of the 7th cranial nerve.

Epidemiology

It most commonly occurs in elderly people (over 60 years) although it can affect all ages.

Clinical features

- Auricular pain (often first feature)
- Facial nerve palsy on affected side (as above)
- Vesicular rash around the ear (see *Fig. 3*)
- Vertigo and tinnitus

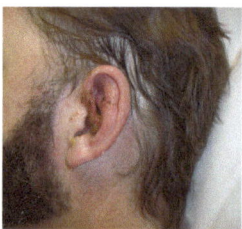

Fig. 3 Vesicular rash in Ramsay Hunt syndrome

Management

- Oral corticosteroids: prednisolone regime as above
- Oral antivirals e.g. aciclovir
- Analgesia: paracetamol (± codeine) and NSAIDs are 1st line; tricyclic antidepressants, gabapentin, pregabalin, and opioids are other options
- Eye care as above

Prognosis

- Recovery of facial nerve function is less likely than in Bell's palsy
- The prognosis is excellent for younger and otherwise healthy patients
- Elderly people have increased risk of post-herpetic neuralgia, bacterial infections and scarring

Peripheral facial palsy

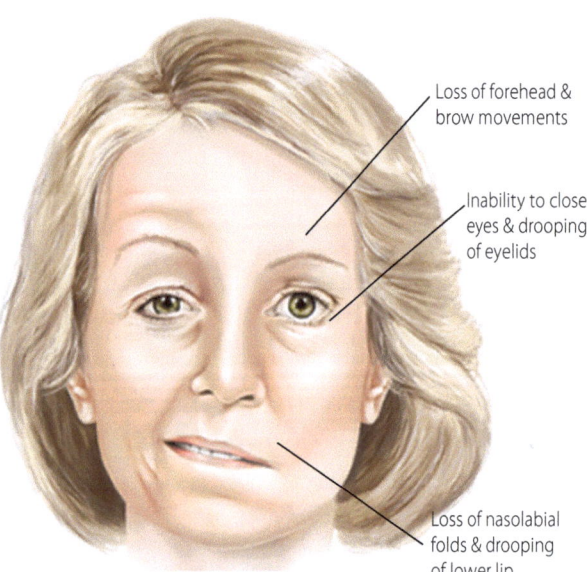

Loss of forehead & brow movements

Inability to close eyes & drooping of eyelids

Loss of nasolabial folds & drooping of lower lip

Central facial palsy

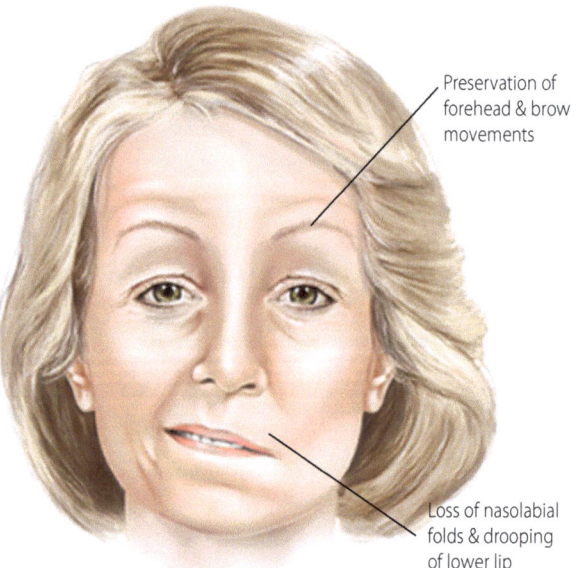

Preservation of forehead & brow movements

Loss of nasolabial folds & drooping of lower lip

Fig. 2 The innervation to the muscles of the upper face originates on both sides of the brain, whereas the innervation to the muscles of the lower face is from the contralateral side of the brain only; when the cortex is injured, e.g. in a stroke, there is weakness in the contralateral lower face only, therefore 'forehead sparing'; when the facial nerve is injured, there is weakness in the ipsilateral upper and lower face

Delirium

Definition

An acute, transient, global organic disorder of CNS functioning resulting in impaired consciousness and attention. There are different types of delirium: hypoactive, hyperactive and mixed.

Classification

- **Hypoactive** (40%) Characterised by people who become withdrawn, quiet and sleepy; most common type of delirium but often goes unrecognised
- **Hyperactive** (25%) Characterised by people who have heightened arousal and can be restless, agitated or aggressive
- **Mixed** (35%) Demonstrate both hyperactive and hypoactive features

Risk factors

- Older age ≥65 years
- Dementia
- Renal impairment
- Sensory impairment
- Recent surgery
- Multiple comorbidities
- Physical frailty
- Male sex
- Previous episodes
- Severe illness

Management

Treat underlying cause:

- Treat any infections
- Correct any electrolyte disturbances
- Stop any offending drugs
- Laxatives for faecal impaction
- Temporary catheterisation for urinary retention
- Give analgesia if pain suspected

Reassurance and reorientation

- Reassure patient to reduce anxiety and disorientation; patient should be reminded of time, place, day and date regularly

Provide appropriate environment

- Quiet, well-lit side room; consistency in care and staff; reassuring nursing staff; encourage family and friends to attend; optimise sensory acuity e.g. glasses, well-lit room, orientation aids

Manage disturbed, violent or distressing behaviour

- Oral low-dose haloperidol (0.5–4mg) or olanzapine (2.5–10mg)

Investigations

Routine investigations

- **Urine dipstick ± culture** To exclude UTI
- **Bloods** FBC (infection), U&Es (electrolyte disturbance), LFTs (alcoholism, liver disease), calcium (hypercalcaemia), glucose (hypo/hyperglycaemia), CRP (infection/inflammation), TFTs (hyperthyroidism), vitamin B_{12}, folate, ferritin (nutritional deficiencies), blood culture (sepsis)
- **ECG** (cardiac abnormalities, acute coronary syndrome)
- **CXR** (pneumonia/heart failure)

Investigations based on history/examination

- **Arterial blood gas** (hypoxia)
- **CT head** (head injury, intracranial bleed, CVA)
- **Lumbar puncture** (meningitis, encephalitis)
- **EEG** (epilepsy)

- **H**ypoxia Respiratory failure, MI, cardiac failure, PE
- **E**ndocrine Hyperthyroidism, hypothyroidism, hyperglycaemia, hypoglycaemia, Cushing syndrome
- **I**nfection Pneumonia, UTI, encephalitis, meningitis
- **S**troke And other intracranial events
- **N**utritional Thiamine deficiency, vitamin B_{12}, nicotinic acid, folate
- **T**heatre (post-op) Anaesthetic, opioid analgesics + other complications
- **M**etabolic Hypoxia, electrolyte disturbance, hypoglycaemia, hepatic impairment, renal impairment
- **A**bdominal Faecal impaction, malnutrition, urinary retention, bladder catheterisation
- **A**lcohol Intoxication or withdrawal
- **D**rugs Benzodiazepines, opioids, anticholinergics, anti-parkinsonian medications, steroids

Causes (HE ISN'T MAD)

Acute and fluctuating course (often worse at night) DELIRIUM:
- **D**isordered thinking: slowed irrational, incoherent thoughts
- **E**uphoric, fearful, depressed or angry
- **L**anguage impaired: rambling speech, repetitive and disruptive
- **I**llusions, delusions: transient persecutory or delusions of misidentification
- **R**eversal of sleep–wake pattern: may be tired during the day and hypervigilant at night
- **I**nattention
- **U**naware/disoriented: disoriented to time, place and person
- **M**emory deficits

Clinical features

Diagnostic criteria

Several screening tools can be used to help diagnosis delirium (see *Notes*):
- **Abbreviated mental test score (AMTS)**
- **Confusion assessment method (CAM)**
- **4 As test (4AT)**

Notes

Delirium

Delirium vs dementia

	Delirium	Dementia
Sleep–wake cycle	Disrupted	Usually normal
Attention	Markedly reduced	Normal/reduced
Arousal	Increased/decreased	Usually normal
Autonomic features	Abnormal	Normal
Duration	Hours to weeks	Months to years
Delusions	Fleeting	Complex
Course	Fluctuating	Stable/slow/progressive
Conscious level	Impaired	Not impaired
Hallucinations	Common	Less common
Onset	Acute/subacute	Chronic
Psychomotor activity	Usually abnormal	Usually normal

Confusion assessment method (CAM)

The confusion assessment method (CAM) involves assessing a patient for 4 features; diagnosis involves the presence of 1 and 2 + either 3 or 4:

1. Acute onset and fluctuating course
2. Inattention
3. Disorganised thinking
4. Altered consciousness

Abbreviated mental test score (AMTS)

1. Age? (1)
2. Time to the nearest hour? (1)
3. Recall address at end: '42 West Street' (1)
4. 'What year it is?' (1)
5. 'Where are you right now?' (1)
6. Identify two people (e.g. doctor, nurse) (1)
7. 'What is your date of birth?' (1)
8. 'When did the Second World War end?' (1)
9. 'Who is the current monarch?' (1)
10. Count backwards from 20 to 1 (1)

(**<8 correct** Cognitive impairment likely)

4AT

1. Alertness *This includes patients who may be markedly drowsy (e.g. difficult to rouse and/or obviously sleepy during assessment) or agitated/hyperactive. Observe the patient. If asleep, attempt to wake with speech or gentle touch on shoulder. Ask the patient to state their name and address to assist rating.*	
Normal (fully alert, but not agitated, throughout assessment)	0
Mild sleepiness for <10sec after waking, then normal	0
Clearly abnormal	4
2. AMT4 *Age, date of birth, place (name of the hospital or building), current year*	
No mistakes	0
1 mistake	1
2 or more mistakes/untestable	2
3. Attention *Months of the year backwards*	
Achieves 7 months or more correctly	0
Starts but scores <7 months/refuses to start	1
Untestable (cannot start because unwell, drowsy, inattentive)	2
4. Acute change or fluctuating course *Evidence of significant change or fluctuation in: alertness, cognition, other mental function (e.g. paranoia, hallucinations) arising over the last 2 weeks and still evident in last 24h*	
No	0
Yes	4

4 or above Possible delirium ± cognitive impairment
1–3 Possible cognitive impairment
0 Delirium or cognitive impairment unlikely

Epilepsy is a neurological condition characterised by recurrent seizures unprovoked by any immediately identifiable cause. An epileptic seizure is the sudden transient attack of symptoms and signs due to abnormal electrical activity in the brain, leading to a disturbance of consciousness, behaviour, emotion, motor function or sensation.

Definition

Classification

Focal seizures

- Previously termed partial seizures
- These start in a specific area, on one side of the brain
- The level of awareness can be used to further classify focal seizures: **focal aware** (previously termed 'simple partial'), **focal impaired awareness** (previously termed 'complex partial') and **awareness unknown**
- Focal seizures can also be classified as being motor, non-motor (e.g. déjà vu, jamais vu) or having other features such as aura

Generalised seizures

- These involve both sides of the brain at the onset
- Consciousness is lost immediately
- Can be further subdivided into **motor** (e.g. tonic–clonic) and **non-motor** (e.g. absence)
- Specific types include **tonic–clonic** (grand mal), **tonic**, **clonic**, **absence** (petit mal) and **atonic**

Epilepsy

Management

General advice

- Take precautions e.g. avoid swimming alone, avoid dangerous sports, e.g. rock climbing, leave door open when having a bath
- Driving:
  - All patients must not drive and must inform the DVLA
  - For first unprovoked seizure: 6 months off if there are no relevant structural abnormalities on brain imaging and no definite epileptiform activity on EEG (if not met then this is increased to 12 months)
  - For patients with established epilepsy or those with multiple unprovoked seizures: may qualify for a driving licence if they have been free from any seizure for 12 months

Neurosurgical treatment

- Neurosurgical treatment has particular benefit for selected people with refractory focal epilepsy
- Some neurosurgical procedures involve resection of part of the brain and the aim is to obtain complete seizure freedom
- For the most commonly performed procedures, involving anterior and medial temporal lobe resection, about 70% of patients will become seizure-free

Anti-epileptics (see *Table 1*)

Anti-epileptics are usually started following a second epileptic seizure; NICE guidelines suggest starting anti-epileptics after the first seizure if any of the following are present:
- the patient has a neurological deficit
- brain imaging shows a structural abnormality
- the EEG shows unequivocal epileptic activity
- the patient or their family or carers consider the risk of having a further seizure unacceptable

- Idiopathic (most common)
- Cerebrovascular disease: cerebral infarction, cerebral haemorrhage and venous thrombosis
- Head injury
- Post cranial surgery
- CNS infections: meningitis or encephalitis
- Neurodegenerative diseases: Alzheimer's and multi-infarct dementia are risk factors for epilepsy
- Autoimmune disease: e.g. anti-NMDA receptor encephalitis and anti-LG11 encephalitis
- Brain neoplasm
- Genetic diseases: e.g. Dravet syndrome
- Drugs: e.g. phenothiazines, isoniazid, tricyclic antidepressants, benzodiazepines, binge alcohol drinking or alcohol withdrawal
- Metabolic medical disorders: uraemia, hypoglycaemia, hyponatraemia, hypernatraemia, hypercalcaemia and hypocalcaemia

Causes

- A seizure results when a sudden imbalance occurs between the excitatory and inhibitory forces within the network of cortical neurones in favour of a sudden-onset net excitation
- This imbalance can result from an alteration at many levels of brain function, from genes and subcellular signalling cascades to widespread neuronal circuits
- If the affected cortical network is in the visual cortex, the clinical manifestations are visual phenomena; other affected areas of primary cortex give rise to sensory, gustatory or motor manifestations; the psychic phenomenon of déjà vu occurs when the temporal lobe is involved

Pathophysiology

- Injuries sustained during seizures
- Social stigmatisation and occupational issues
- Anxiety/depression
- Status epilepticus
- Sudden unexplained death in epilepsy (SUDEP)
- Increased mortality rate from SUDEP, deaths due to accidents during seizures, deaths due to status epilepticus

Complications

Investigations

- **Bloods** e.g. Glucose, Ca^{2+}, LFTs to identify potential causes
- **EEG** Supports the diagnosis of epilepsy and may be used to help to determine seizure type and epilepsy syndrome; it is however often normal in between attacks (therefore normal EEG does not rule out epilepsy) but during a seizure it almost always shows an abnormal pattern (typically showing a cortical spike or generalised spike activity); long-term video or ambulatory EEG may be used if diagnostic uncertainty remains after clinical assessment and standard EEG
- **ECG** In all those with altered consciousness, particularly those in older age groups, when disorders of cardiac rhythm may simulate epilepsy; 24-h ambulatory ECG and other cardiovascular tests e.g. implantable loop devices may also be helpful
- **Neuroimaging** (used to identify structural abnormalities):
  - **MRI brain** Imaging investigation of choice and particularly important in those with a focal onset on history (unless examination or EEG suggests evidence of benign focal epilepsy), and in those who do not respond to 1st-line medication
  - **CT brain** To identify gross pathology if MRI is not available or is contraindicated
- **Polysomnography** May be used to confirm a diagnosis of sleep-related epilepsy
- **Handheld video recordings** Asking family members or friends to video record events should be considered in patients with uncertain diagnosis (after consent from patient)

Clinical features

- **Aura** Subjective symptoms at the start of the seizure (the patient is aware of this) – suggestive of focal epilepsy e.g. strange feeling in the gut, déjà vu, strange smells or flashing lights
- **Potential triggers** Sleep deprivation, stress, light sensitivity or alcohol use
- Specific features of the seizure:
  - **Tonic** Short-lived, abrupt, generalised muscle stiffening (may cause a fall) with rapid recovery – suggestive of tonic seizure
  - **Generalised tonic–clonic** Generalised stiffening and subsequent rhythmic jerking of the limbs, urinary incontinence and tongue biting
  - **Absence seizure** Brief pauses, e.g. suddenly stop talking full sentence then carrying on where left off (presents in childhood)
  - **Atonic seizure** Sudden onset of loss of muscle tone causing falls
  - **Myoclonic seizure** Brief, 'shock-like' involuntary single or multiple jerks
- **Post-ictal phenomena** (residual symptoms after the attack) e.g. Drowsiness, headaches, amnesia or confusion (usually occur only after generalised tonic and/or clonic seizures).

Epilepsy notes

Anti-epileptics

Table 1 Anti-epileptics

Sodium valproate	• **Indication** 1st-line treatment for patients with generalised seizures including generalised tonic–clonic, absence and myoclonic seizures • **Mechanism of action** Blockage of voltage-gated Na$^+$ channels and increased brain levels of gamma-aminobutyric acid (GABA) • **Side effects** Include nausea/vomiting, weight gain, hair loss, confusion, drowsiness, hepatotoxicity, thrombocytopenia, teratogenicity, encephalopathy, oedema, SIADH • **Cautions/contraindications** Pregnancy, acute porphyrias, known or suspected mitochondrial disorders, liver failure, urea cycle disorders
Carbamazepine	• **Indications** 1st-line treatment for focal seizures • **Mechanism of action** Preferentially binds to voltage-gated Na$^+$ channels in their inactive form • **Side effects** Rash, vomiting, drowsiness, hyponatraemia, leucopenia, thrombocytopenia, vision disturbance, movement disorders • **Cautions/contraindications** Pregnancy, acute porphyrias, AV conduction abnormalities, bone marrow depression
Lamotrigine	• **Indications** 1st-line treatment for focal seizures and 2nd-line for generalised tonic–clonic seizures • **Mechanism of action** Blocks Na$^+$ channels and suppresses the release of glutamate and aspartate • **Side effects** Aggression, agitation, diarrhoea, dizziness, drowsiness, sleep disorders, tremor, vomiting, aplastic anaemia • **Cautions/contraindications** Myoclonic seizures (may be exacerbated), Parkinson's disease (may be exacerbated), caution in hepatic and renal impairment
Levetiracetam	• **Indications** 2nd-line treatment for patients with focal seizures • **Mechanism of action** Exact mechanism unclear but binding to synaptic vesicle protein 2A (SV2A) appears to be the key driver • **Side effects** Depression/anxiety, diarrhoea/vomiting, dyspepsia, insomnia, vertigo, blood dyscrasias • **Cautions/contraindications** Caution in severe hepatic impairment and dose adjustment in renal impairment
Ethosuximide	• **Indications** 1st-line treatment for people with absent seizures • **Mechanism of action** Binds to T-type voltage-sensitive calcium channels • **Side effects** Aggression, agranulocytosis, reduced appetite, concentration impaired, generalised tonic–clonic seizure, headache, bone marrow disorders • **Cautions/contraindications** Acute porphyrias, pregnancy, caution in hepatic failure and renal failure
Phenytoin	• **Indications** Used for generalised, focal seizures and status epilepticus but not used 1st line in generalised and focal seizures due to side effects and narrow therapeutic index • **Mechanism of action** Blocks voltage-dependent Na$^+$ channels • **Side effects** Gingival hyperplasia, hirsutism, coarsening of facial features, drowsiness, megaloblastic anaemia, peripheral neuropathy, lymphadenopathy, dyskinesia, teratogenicity; toxicity causes dizziness, diplopia, nystagmus, slurred speech, ataxia, confusion, seizures • **Monitoring** Phenytoin levels do not need to be monitored routinely but trough levels, immediately before dose, should be checked if: adjustment of phenytoin dose, suspected toxicity or detection of non-adherence to the prescribed medication • **Contraindications** Pregnancy, second- and third-degree heart block, sino-atrial block, sinus bradycardia, Stokes–Adams syndrome; caution in hepatic impairment
Phenobarbital	• **Indications** All seizures (including status epilepticus) except absent seizures • **Mechanism of action** Acts on GABA$_A$ receptors enhancing synaptic inhibition • **Side effects** Rash, sedation, bone disorders, depression, ataxia • **Cautions/contraindications** Pregnancy, history of porphyria, severe hepatic impairment, caution in renal impairment

Status epilepticus (*Fig. 1*)

Convulsive status epilepticus is defined as a convulsive seizure which continues for a prolonged period (e.g. longer than 5 min), or when convulsive seizures occur one after the other with no recovery between. Convulsive status epilepticus is an emergency and requires immediate medical attention

Management

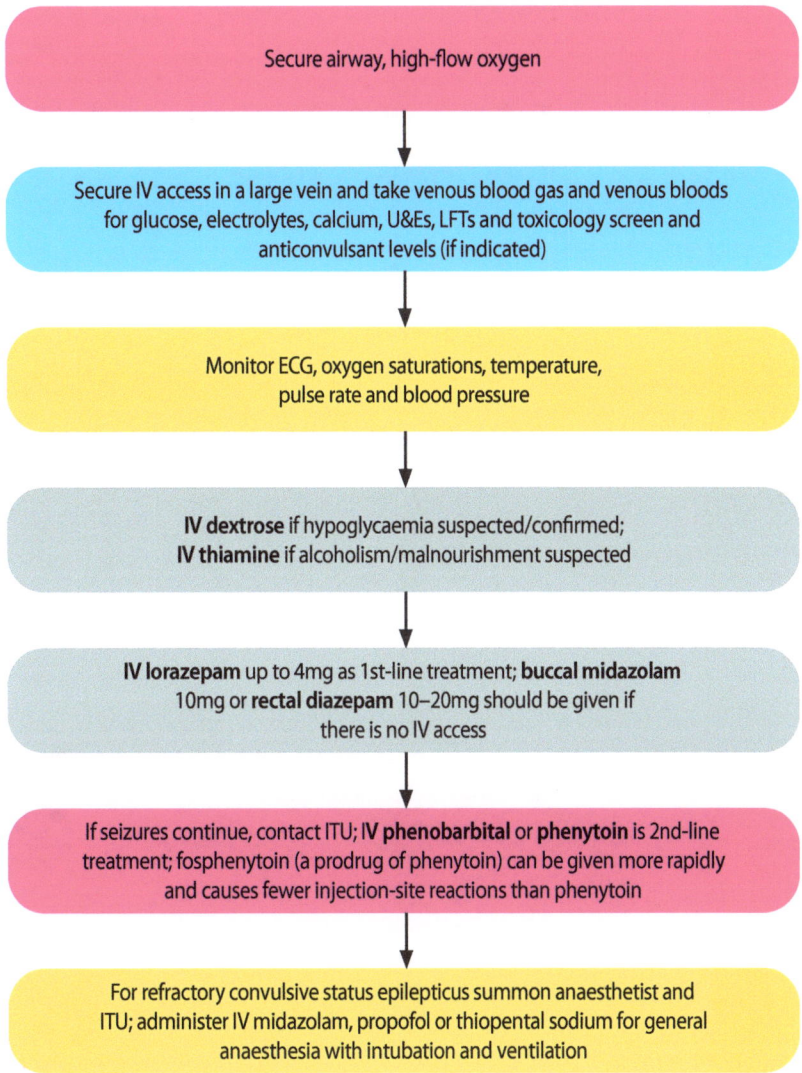

Secure airway, high-flow oxygen

Secure IV access in a large vein and take venous blood gas and venous bloods for glucose, electrolytes, calcium, U&Es, LFTs and toxicology screen and anticonvulsant levels (if indicated)

Monitor ECG, oxygen saturations, temperature, pulse rate and blood pressure

IV dextrose if hypoglycaemia suspected/confirmed; **IV thiamine** if alcoholism/malnourishment suspected

IV lorazepam up to 4mg as 1st-line treatment; **buccal midazolam** 10mg or **rectal diazepam** 10–20mg should be given if there is no IV access

If seizures continue, contact ITU; **IV phenobarbital** or **phenytoin** is 2nd-line treatment; fosphenytoin (a prodrug of phenytoin) can be given more rapidly and causes fewer injection-site reactions than phenytoin

For refractory convulsive status epilepticus summon anaesthetist and ITU; administer IV midazolam, propofol or thiopental sodium for general anaesthesia with intubation and ventilation

Fig. 1 Management of status epilepticus

Extradural haematoma is the collection of blood between the dura and the bone (usually skull but may be spinal column) (see *Fig. 1*). It is immediately life-threatening.

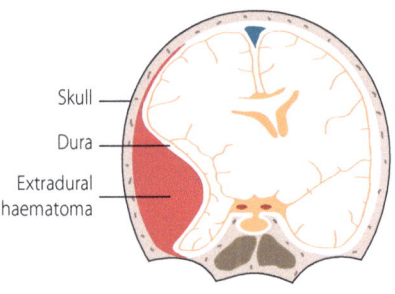

Fig. 1 Diagram of an extradural haematoma

- Skull
- Dura
- Extradural haematoma

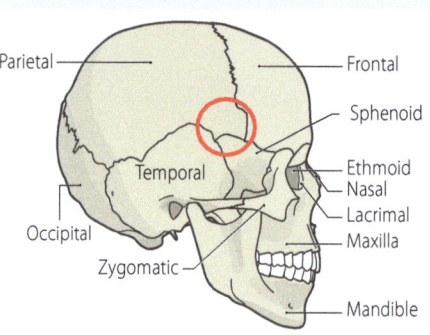

- Parietal
- Frontal
- Sphenoid
- Ethmoid
- Nasal
- Lacrimal
- Maxilla
- Temporal
- Occipital
- Zygomatic
- Mandible

Fig. 2 The pterion, the weakest part of the skull; a traumatic blow to the pterion may rupture the middle meningeal artery causing an epidural haematoma

- Most commonly caused by a fractured temporal or parietal bone which causes damage to the **middle meningeal artery** or vein
- Typically caused by trauma to the **pterion**, the region where the frontal, parietal, temporal and sphenoid bones join together (see *Fig. 2*).
- Young people are more commonly affected, not only because of the prevalent demographics of patients with a head injury, but it also relates to the changes that occur in the dura in older patients, as the dura is much more adherent to the inner surface of the skull
- Children are less likely to have associated skull fractures than adults
- Extradural haemorrhage in the spinal column can occur as a result of epidural anaesthesia or lumbar puncture

Pathophysiology

Definition

Extradural haematoma (epidural haemorrhage)

Complications

- Neurological deficits (temporary or permanent)
- Death
- Post-traumatic seizures
- Post-concussion syndrome
- Spasticity, neuropathic pain and urinary complications (spinal extradural haematoma)

Management

- ABC approach of resuscitation
- Control of airway in unconscious patient; oxygen may be given
- IV fluids may be required to maintain the circulation and preserve cerebral perfusion
- Stabilise and transfer urgently (with skilled medical and nursing escorts) to a neurosurgical unit
- Measures to decrease raised ICP with IV mannitol or hypertonic saline
- Conservative management for small haematomas
- Surgical intervention with burr holes may be required to evacuate a large haematoma

Prognosis

- Overall mortality rate is approx. 30%
- Those alert on admission rarely die but a low Glasgow Coma Scale (GCS) score worsens the prognosis
- The earlier the intervention, the more likelihood of survival
- Risk factors for poor prognosis include: older age, intradural lesions, increasing volume of haematoma, temporal location, rapid clinical progression, pupillary abnormalities, raised ICP

- **History of trauma** Typically a head strike from sports injury or motor vehicle accident; classically, this is followed by a lucid interval after which the patient deteriorates
- **Loss of consciousness**
- **Severe headache**
- **Nausea/vomiting**
- **Confusion**
- **Evidence of skull fractures, haematomas** or **lacerations**
- **Otorrhoea or rhinorrhoea** Resulting from skull fracture
- **Unequal pupils**
- **Hemiparesis** With brisk reflexes and up-going plantar reflex
- **Other focal neurological deficits** e.g. Aphasia, visual field defects, numbness, ataxia
- **Bradycardia** and **hypertension** Late signs (Cushing reflex)
- **Death** Follows a period of coma and is due to respiratory arrest
- **Spinal cord compression** Produced by a haematoma in the spinal column; features may include: weakness, numbness, alteration in reflexes, urinary incontinence and faecal incontinence

Clinical features

Investigations

- **CT head** Shows haematoma (often biconvex /lens-shaped, see *Fig. 3*); if there is deterioration, CT must be repeated
- **Bloods** FBC, U&Es, coagulation screen (if any suspicion of abnormality of coagulation), group and save
- **Plain skull X-ray head** May be normal or show fracture line crossing the course of the middle meningeal vessels
- **Cervical spine X-ray** Spinal injury must be excluded
- **MRI head** Gives detailed images but may not be suitable for a patient in an unstable condition

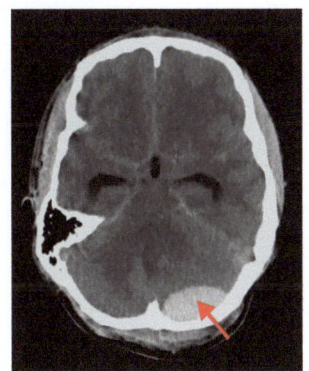

Fig. 3 Extradural haematoma on CT scan

Extradural haematoma (epidural haemorrhage)

Guillain–Barré syndrome (GBS) describes an immune-mediated demyelination of the peripheral nervous system often triggered by an infection. It can lead to life-threatening respiratory failure.

Definition

- History of gastrointestinal or respiratory infection from 1 to 3 weeks prior to the onset of weakness
- Zika virus
- Vaccinations: live and dead vaccines have been implicated
- Malignancy: e.g. lymphomas, especially Hodgkin's disease
- Pregnancy: incidence decreases during pregnancy but increases in the months after delivery

Risk factors

- GBS is usually triggered by an infection: *Campylobacter jejuni*, Epstein–Barr virus (EBV) and cytomegalovirus have all been linked
- It is thought that the infectious organism shares epitopes with an antigen in the peripheral nervous system leading to autoantibody-mediated cell damage
- The suppressor T-cell response is reduced, suggesting a cell-mediated immunological reaction directed at the peripheral nerves; occasionally, serum antibodies to myelin components are detected; nerve damage occurs segmentally; lymphocytes infiltrate the nerve roots and release cytotoxic substances that damage the Schwann cells and myelin
- Correlation between anti-ganglioside antibody (e.g. anti-GM1) and clinical features has been demonstrated; anti-GM1 antibodies are present in approx. 25% of patients

Pathophysiology

Guillain-Barré syndrome

Complications

- Persistent paralysis
- Respiratory failure requiring mechanical ventilation
- Aspiration pneumonia
- Hypotension or hypertension
- Thromboembolism, pneumonia, skin breakdown
- Cardiac arrhythmia
- Urinary retention
- Ileus
- Psychiatric problems e.g. depression, anxiety

Management

- **Plasma exchange** Leads to shorter periods of ventilation and a shorter period until patients are able to walk unaided
- **IV immunoglobulin** If started within 2 weeks from the onset of illness it accelerates recovery as much as plasma exchange
- **DVT prophylaxis** DVT due to immobility; prevent with gradient compression stockings and subcutaneous low molecular weight heparin
- **Admission to ICU** Intubation and assisted ventilation may be required
- **Pain relief** May be required for neuropathic pain

Investigations

- **Lumbar puncture** Most patients have an elevated level of CSF protein, with no elevation in CSF cell counts (the gamma-globulin fraction is usually raised); note: the rise in the CSF protein may not be seen until 1–2 weeks after the onset of weakness
- **Antibody screen** In Miller Fisher syndrome there are often antibodies against GQ1b
- **Spirometry** Forced vital capacity is a major determinant of the need for admission to ICU and then the need for intubation
- **Nerve conduction studies** Abnormal in 85% of patients, even early on in the disease; they show prolonged conduction velocities; repeat after 2 weeks if initially normal
- **ECG** Many different abnormalities may be seen: 2nd-degree and 3rd-degree AV block, T-wave abnormalities, ST depression, QRS widening and a variety of rhythm disturbances
- **Campylobacter serology** Should be performed; positive titres identify a group with a poorer prognosis

- **Weakness**:
  - In 60% of cases, onset occurs approximately 3 weeks after an infection
  - Usually presents with an ascending pattern of progressive symmetrical weakness, starting in the lower extremities
  - This reaches a level of maximum severity 2 weeks after initial onset of symptoms and usually stops progressing after 5 weeks
  - Facial weakness, dysphasia, diplopia or dysarthria may develop
  - In severe cases, muscle weakness may lead to respiratory failure
- **Pain** Neuropathic pain may develop, particularly in the legs; back pain may also occur

- **Reflexes** May be reduced or absent
- **Sensory symptoms** These can include paraesthesia and sensory loss, starting in the lower extremities
- **Autonomic symptoms** Involvement of the autonomic system may present, with reduced sweating, reduced heat tolerance, paralytic ileus and urinary hesitancy; severe autonomic dysfunction may occur
- **Miller Fisher syndrome** (variant of GBS):
  - Associated with ophthalmoplegia, areflexia and ataxia
  - Usually presents as a descending paralysis rather than ascending as seen in other forms of GBS
  - Anti-GQ1b antibodies are present in 90% of cases

Clinical features

Notes

Guillain-Barré syndrome

Migraine is a primary headache disorder which is characterised by episodic severe headaches (often but not always unilateral), with commonly associated symptoms such as photophobia, phonophobia and nausea/vomiting.

- Tiredness, stress
- Alcohol
- Combined oral contraceptive pill
- Lack of food or dehydration
- Cheese, chocolate, red wines, citrus fruits
- Menstruation
- Bright lights

- Severe, often unilateral, throbbing headache
- Aura: 'classic' migraine attacks are precipitated by an aura; these occur in around one-third of migraine patients; typical aura are visual, progressive, last 5–60min and are characterised by transient hemianopic disturbance or a spreading scintillating scotoma
- Nausea/vomiting
- Photophobia
- Phonophobia
- Attacks may last up to 72h

Definition

Common triggers

Clinical features

Migraine

Management

Diagnostic criteria

Acute

- **Paracetamol** e.g. 1g oral QDS; 1st-line treatment for pregnant women as considered safe
- **NSAIDs** e.g. Soluble aspirin 600–900mg (not in children) or ibuprofen 400–600mg
- **Triptans** e.g. Sumatriptan; should be taken as soon as possible after the onset of headache; oral, orodispersible, nasal spray and SC injections are available
- **Anti-emetics** For nausea/vomiting e.g. buccal prochlorperazine or metoclopramide
- Opiate-containing medication, e.g. codeine, should be avoided

Prevention

- Avoid triggers (if possible)
- Prophylaxis should be given if patients are experiencing 2 or more attacks per month
- **Topiramate** or **propranolol** 1st-line for prophylaxis according to the person's preference, comorbidities and risk of adverse events; propranolol should be used in preference to topiramate in women of childbearing age as topiramate may be teratogenic and can reduce the effectiveness of hormonal contraceptives
- **Acupuncture** If above measures fail, NICE recommend a course of up to 10 sessions of acupuncture over 5–8 weeks or gabapentin
- **Riboflavin** May be effective in reducing migraine frequency and intensity for some people
- **Triptans** Frovatriptan or zolmitriptan can be used as a type of 'mini-prophylaxis' for women with predictable menstrual migraine

International Headache Society

The diagnosis of migraine is a clinical diagnosis.

Table 1 International Headache Society diagnostic criteria

Point	Criteria
A	At least 5 attacks fulfilling criteria B–D
B	Headache attacks lasting 4–72h (untreated or unsuccessfully treated)
C	Headache has at least 2 of the following characteristics: • Unilateral location • Pulsating quality (i.e. varying with the heartbeat) • Moderate or severe pain intensity • Aggravation by or causing avoidance of routine physical activity (e.g. walking or climbing stairs)
D	During headache at least one of the following: • Nausea and/or vomiting • Photophobia and phonophobia
E	Not attributed to another disorder (history and examination do not suggest a secondary headache disorder or, if they do, it is ruled out by appropriate investigations or headache attacks do not occur for the first time in close temporal relation to the other disorder)

Table 2 Causes of headaches

	Condition	Notes
Chronic headache	**Tension headache**	• Recurrent, non-disabling, bilateral headache, often described as a 'tight band' • Not aggravated by routine activities of daily living • Not associated with aura, nausea/vomiting or aggravated by routine physical activity • May be associated with stress • Acute treatment: aspirin, paracetamol or an NSAID is 1st-line • Prophylaxis: NICE recommend up to 10 sessions of acupuncture over 5–8 weeks; low-dose amitriptyline is widely used in the UK for prophylaxis against tension-type headache
	Medication overuse headache	• Present for ≥15 days per month • Developed or worsened while taking regular symptomatic medication specifically for headaches • Most common offending drugs are opioids and triptans • There may be a psychiatric comorbidity • Simple analgesics and triptans should be withdrawn abruptly (may initially worsen headaches) • Opioid analgesics should be gradually withdrawn
	Raised intracranial pressure	• e.g. Tumour, idiopathic intracranial hypertension • Typically worse on waking, lying down or bending forward, or with coughing • Associated with vomiting, papilloedema, fits and neurological signs • CT or MRI scan is investigation of choice • Lumbar puncture contraindicated until after imaging
Recurrent acute attacks of headache	**Migraine**	See Mind Map
	Cluster headache	• Intense pain around one eye; recurrent attacks 'always' affect same side • Patient is often restless during an attack due to severity of pain • Pain typically occurs once or twice a day, each episode lasting 15 min to 2 hours with clusters typically lasting 4–12 weeks • Associated eye symptoms include redness, lacrimation, lid swelling • More common in men and smokers • Acute: 100% oxygen, subcutaneous triptan • Prophylaxis: verapamil is 1st-line; a tapering dose of prednisolone can also be considered
	Trigeminal neuralgia	• A unilateral disorder characterised by transient electric shock-like pains, abrupt in onset and termination, limited to one or more divisions of the trigeminal nerve • The pain is commonly triggered by light touch e.g. washing, shaving, talking and brushing the teeth, and frequently occurs spontaneously • Carbamazepine is 1st-line treatment
Subacute onset	**Giant cell arteritis (GCA)**	• Typically patient >60 years old • Usually rapid onset (e.g. <1 month) of unilateral headache • Often associated jaw or tongue claudication • Tender, palpable temporal artery • Raised ESR • See *Ch7: Giant cell arteritis* for further information

Table 2 *(continued)*

	Condition	Notes
Acute single episode	**Subarachnoid haemorrhage**	<ul><li>Sudden onset severe 'thunderclap' headache</li><li>Nausea and vomiting</li><li>Meningism (photophobia, neck stiffness)</li><li>See *Ch6: Subarachnoid haemorrhage* for further information</li></ul>
	Head injury	<ul><li>Headache is common at the site of head injury but it may also be more generalised</li><li>Serious head injury can lead to intracranial bleeds; a CT scan should be done if subdural or extradural haematoma is suspected</li><li>See *Ch6: Subdural haematoma* and *Extradural haematoma* for further information</li></ul>
	Sinusitis	<ul><li>Facial pain: typically frontal pressure pain which is worse on bending forward</li><li>Associated symptoms include nasal discharge and nasal obstruction</li><li>Postnasal drip may produce chronic cough</li><li>Acute sinusitis can be treated with analgesia, intranasal decongestants and antibiotics for severe presentations; intranasal corticosteroids are often useful for recurrent or chronic sinusitis</li></ul>
	Acute glaucoma	<ul><li>Severe pain which may be ocular or headache</li><li>Decreased visual acuity, red eye, haloes, semi-dilated non-reacting pupil, hazy cornea</li><li>Symptoms worse with mydriasis e.g. watching TV in a dark room</li><li>Systemic upset may be seen, such as nausea and vomiting and even abdominal pain</li><li>Requires urgent ophthalmology assessment</li></ul>
	Meningitis/encephalitis	<ul><li>Meningitis: classically presents with fever, photophobia, neck stiffness, headache, purpuric rash</li><li>Encephalitis: classically presents with headache, fever, confusion/odd behaviour, seizures, reduced consciousness</li><li>Requires CT scan followed by lumbar puncture for diagnosis (in absence of raised intracranial pressure)</li></ul>
	Central venous sinus thrombosis	<ul><li>Headache which may be sudden onset</li><li>There may be associated nausea and vomiting, cranial nerve palsies, vision disturbance, seizures</li><li>The diagnosis is usually made with the aid of CT or MRI scan</li><li>Specific treatment involves anticoagulation or thrombolytic treatments</li></ul>

Red flags for headaches

- Immunocompromised e.g. HIV or on immunosuppressive drugs
- Age <20 years and a history of malignancy
- History of malignancy known to metastasise to the brain
- Sudden-onset headache reaching maximum intensity within 5min
- Vomiting without other obvious cause
- Recent (typically within the past 3 months) head trauma
- Worsening headache with fever
- New-onset neurological deficit
- New-onset cognitive dysfunction
- Change in personality
- Impaired level of consciousness
- Headache exacerbated by cough, Valsalva (trying to breathe out with nose and mouth blocked), sneeze or exercise
- Orthostatic headache (headache that changes with posture)
- Symptoms suggestive of GCA (see *Table 2*)
- Symptoms suggestive of acute narrow-angle glaucoma (see *Table 2*)
- A substantial change in the characteristics of patient's headache

Motor neurone disease (MND) is a rare but devastating neurological condition of unknown cause which can present with both upper and lower motor neurone signs. It leads to progressive paralysis and eventual death from respiratory failure.

Definition

Pathophysiology

- MND is a degenerative condition that affects motor neurones, specifically the anterior horn cells of the spinal cord and the motor cranial nuclei
- The cause of the disease is unknown, although 5% of those affected have a familial form of the disease due to a mutation in the superoxide dismutase-1 gene
- It may be caused by abnormality of mitochondrial function causing oxidative stress in motor neurones for which there may be several causes
- It results in lower motor neurone (LMN) and upper motor neurone (UMN) dysfunction, leading to a mixed picture of muscular paralysis, typically with LMN signs predominating

Epidemiology

- MND is relatively uncommon with annual incidence of around 2 cases per 100 000 population
- It can occur at any age but is more common in people aged >50 years
- The male to female ratio is 2:1
- Approximately 5–10% of cases are inherited

Prognosis

- Prognosis is poor with 50% of patients dying within 3 years
- Most patients die of respiratory failure

Motor neurone disease

Management

Riluzole

- A neuroprotective glutamate-release inhibitor; the only drug of proven disease-modifying efficacy
- It is used mainly in ALS
- Prolongs life by approximately 3 months

Other symptomatic treatment

- **Dysarthria** Speech assessment and communication aids
- **Dysphagia** Feeding gastrostomy; cricopharyngeal myotomy
- **Dysphonia** Speech therapists can give expert advice on speech and swallowing difficulties
- **Saliva problems** Consider a trial of antimuscarinic medicine as the 1st-line treatment for sialorrhoea in people with MND
- **Muscle weakness** Physiotherapy, walking aids, splints
- **Muscle cramps** Consider quinine as 1st-line and baclofen as 2nd-line treatment
- **Muscle stiffness, spasticity or increased tone** Consider baclofen, tizanidine, dantrolene or gabapentin
- **Non-invasive ventilation (usually BIPAP)** Used at night; studies have shown a survival benefit of around 7 months

Investigations

There are no specific investigations that will confirm a diagnosis of MND; a range of investigations are carried out to confirm consistent features and exclude other possible pathologies:

- **Nerve conduction studies** Show normal motor conduction and can help exclude a neuropathy
- **EMG** Shows a reduced number of action potentials with an increased amplitude
- **MRI** Usually performed to exclude the differential diagnosis of cervical cord compression and myelopathy

Clinical features/types

- **Amyotrophic lateral sclerosis (ALS)** The most common form of MND; it is a combination of disease of the lateral corticospinal tracts and anterior horn cells producing a progressive spastic tetraparesis and paraparesis with added lower motor neurone signs (muscle wasting and fasciculation)
- **Progressive bulbar palsy and pseudobulbar palsy** Approximately 20% of people with MND have this type; it results from the destruction of the upper (pseudobulbar) and lower (bulbar palsy) motor neurones in the lower cranial nerves; this results in dysarthria, dysphagia with wasting, and fasciculation of the tongue
- **Progressive muscular atrophy** An uncommon form of MND; predominantly lower motor neurone lesion of the spinal cord; the small muscles of the hands and feet are usually first affected, but muscle spasticity is absent
- **Primary lateral sclerosis** Another rare type of MND; it mainly causes weakness in the leg muscles and there is progressive tetraparesis

Multiple sclerosis (MS) is an acquired, chronic, cell-mediated **autoimmune condition** characterised by multiple plaques of **demyelination** in the **central nervous system** that can affect the brain, brainstem and spinal cord.

Definition

- The cause of MS is not completely understood but it is thought to be caused by both genetic and environmental factors
- It is thought to be an autoimmune disease in which exposure of a specific infectious agent e.g. EBV in early life may predispose to the later development of MS in a genetically susceptible host
- The non-self antigen mimics proteins in myelin; this antigen is presented on the surface of macrophages in combination with class 2 MHC causing antibodies produced by B cells and T cells to attack CNS myelin because of molecular mimicry
- This results in inflammation, demyelination and axonal loss leading to plaque formation; this slows or blocks the transmission of signals to and from the brain and spinal cord (see *Fig. 1*); in this way movement and sensation may be impaired
- The lesions are disseminated in both 'space and time' i.e. episodes occur months or years apart and affect different anatomic locations

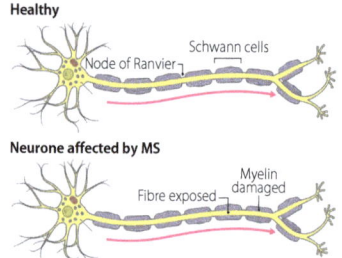

Fig. 1 Healthy neurone vs neurone in MS

Pathophysiology

Good prognosis features:
- Female sex
- Young age of onset (i.e. 20s or 30s)
- Relapsing-remitting disease
- Sensory symptoms only
- Long interval between first two relapses
- Complete recovery between relapses

Prognosis

Multiple sclerosis

Management

Pharmacological

Managing acute relapse:

High-dose steroids (e.g. oral or IV methylprednisolone) may be given for 5 days to shorten the length of an acute relapse

Note: steroids shorten the duration of a relapse and do not alter the degree of recovery i.e. whether a patient returns to baseline function

Disease-modifying drugs:

- **Beta interferon:** shown to reduce the relapse rate of MS; it is given by SC or IM injection; the most common side effect is flu-like symptoms
- **Glatiramer acetate:** licensed for reducing the frequency of relapses in ambulatory patients with relapsing-remitting MS who have had at least 2 clinical relapses in the previous 2 years;

it is an immunomodulating drug designed to mimic the effects of the main proteins in myelin; it is given daily by SC injection
- **Dimethyl fumarate:** an option for treating adults with active relapsing-remitting MS (2 clinically significant relapses in the previous 2 years) but only if they do not have highly active or rapidly evolving severe relapsing-remitting MS
- **Alemtuzumab:** an option for treating adults with active relapsing-remitting MS; it is a monoclonal antibody that binds to CD52, a protein present on the surface of mature lymphocytes
- **Natalizumab:** 2nd-line treatment for MS; it is a recombinant monoclonal antibody that antagonises alpha-4 beta-1-integrin found on the surface of leucocytes, thus inhibiting their migration across the endothelium across the blood–brain barrier; it is given monthly by IV infusion
- **Fingolimod:** 2nd-line treatment for MS; it is a sphingosine 1-phosphate receptor modulator, and prevents lymphocytes from leaving lymph nodes; an oral formulation is available

Tackling other specific problems

- **Fatigue:** trial of amantadine once other causes have been excluded
- **Spasticity:** baclofen and gabapentin are 1st line; other options include diazepam, dantrolene and tizanidine; botulinum toxin and cannabis (Sativex spray) can be considered if not responding to other treatments
- **Neuropathic pain:** can be treated with carbamazepine, gabapentin, or using antidepressants such as amitriptyline
- **Bladder dysfunction:** anticholinergics may improve urinary frequency if there is no residual volume on US scan; intermittent self-catheterisation can be used for urine retention

Non-pharmacological

- Access to multidisciplinary team including physiotherapy and occupational therapy
- Referral to speech and language therapist for dysarthria
- Mindfulness training and CBT for fatigue; aerobic exercise or yoga may also be beneficial
- Inform patients of their legal obligation to notify the DVLA of their condition

Epidemiology

- 3 times more common in women
- Most commonly diagnosed in people aged 20–40 years
- It is the most common cause of neurological disability in young adults

Types

Relapsing-remitting disease

- Most common form (in around 85% of patients)
- Acute attacks (e.g. last 1–2 months) followed by periods of remission and periods of stability

Secondary progressive disease

- Describes relapsing-remitting patients who have deteriorated and have developed neurological signs and symptoms between relapses
- Approximately 65% of patients with relapsing-remitting disease go on to develop secondary progressive disease within 15 years of diagnosis
- Gait and bladder disorders are typically seen

Primary progressive disease

- Accounts for 10% of patients
- Progressive deterioration from onset
- More common in older individuals

Clinical features

Visual

- Optic neuritis: common presenting feature; usually unilateral
- Optic atrophy
- Internuclear ophthalmoplegia
- Uhthoff's phenomenon: worsening of vision following rise in body temperature

Sensory

- Pins/needles
- Numbness
- Trigeminal neuralgia
- Lhermitte's sign: paraesthesia in limbs on neck flexion

Motor

- Spastic weakness: most commonly seen in the legs

Cerebellar

- Ataxia
- Tremor
- Dysarthria
- Vertigo

ENT

- Deafness
- Taste and smell disturbance

Urogenital

- Urinary incontinence
- Sexual dysfunction

Complications

- Urinary incontinence
- Bowel incontinence
- Depression
- Epilepsy
- Paralysis

Investigations

Bloods

FBC, CRP/ESR, U&Es, LFT, TFT, glucose, HIV serology, calcium and B_{12} levels to exclude other causes

Electrophysiology

Visual, auditory and somatosensory evoked potentials may be prolonged

MRI brain and spinal cord

The investigation of choice for diagnosis and shows plaques particularly in the periventricular area and brainstem (see *Fig. 2*)

Lumbar puncture

Shows rise in total protein with increase in immunoglobulin concentration with presence of oligoclonal bands

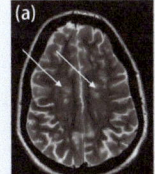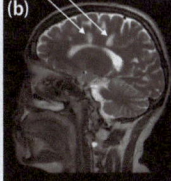

Fig. 2 Radiological appearance of MS plaques in **(a)** T2W axial and **(b)** sagittal MRI images

Definition

Myasthenia gravis (MG) is an acquired autoimmune disorder resulting in insufficient functioning acetylcholine receptors. It is characterised by weakness, typically of the periocular, facial, bulbar and girdle muscles.

Pathophysiology

- MG is an **autoimmune disease** in which antibodies result in a loss of muscle **acetylcholine receptors (AChRs)**
- In 85% of cases the antibodies bind to the AChRs themselves and in the remaining cases the antibodies bind to a different muscle membrane target
- There are associations between MG and **thymic hyperplasia** (75% of cases) and **thymoma** (15%)

Epidemiology

- MG is more common in women (2:1)
- It can occur in any age but peaks occur in the 20–30s and 60–80s

Myasthenia gravis

Complications

- Aspiration pneumonia due to throat muscle weakness
- Acute respiratory failure during an exacerbation

Management

- **Long-acting anticholinesterase inhibitors** Pyridostigmine is the preferred symptomatic treatment
- **Immunosuppression** Prednisolone initially
- **Plasmapheresis and IV immunoglobulin** Used for myasthenic crisis
- **Thymectomy** Important if a thymoma is present but may be beneficial even without one

Triggers

- Emotional stress
- Pregnancy
- Menses
- Secondary illness
- Thyroid dysfunction
- Trauma
- Temperature extremes
- Hypokalaemia
- Drugs: aminoglycosides, beta blockers, calcium channel blockers, quinidine, procainamide, chloroquine, lithium, macrolides, tetracycline, penicillamine, succinylcholine, magnesium, ACE inhibitor
- Surgery

Associations

- Thymomas in 15%
- Autoimmune disorders: pernicious anaemia, autoimmune thyroid disorders, rheumatoid, SLE
- Thymic hyperplasia in 50–70%

The key feature is **muscle fatigability** – muscles become progressively weaker during periods of activity and slowly improve after periods of rest:
- Extraocular muscle weakness: diplopia
- Proximal muscle weakness: face, neck, limb girdle
- Ptosis (see *Fig. 1*)
- Bulbar involvement: dysphagia, dysphonia, dysarthria

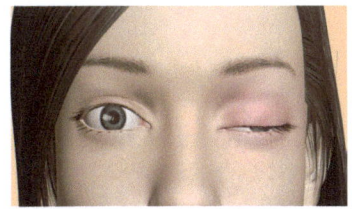

Fig. 1 Myasthenia gravis illustration showing left-sided ptosis

Clinical features

- **Autoantibodies** Around 85–90% of patients have antibodies to acetylcholine receptors; in the remaining patients, about 40% are positive for anti-muscle-specific tyrosine kinase antibodies
- **CK** Normal
- **EMG (single fibre)** High sensitivity (92–100%)
- **CT or MRI thorax** To exclude thymoma
- **Tensilon test** IV edrophonium reduces muscle weakness temporarily (rarely used any more due to the risk of cardiac arrhythmia)

Investigations

Notes

Myasthenia gravis

Myasthenic crisis

- A reversible life-threatening neurological emergency that affects 20–30% of myasthenic patients, usually within the first year of illness; it may be the first indication of the disease
- Results in weakness of respiratory muscles; facial muscles may be slack, and face may be expressionless; patient may be unable to support the head, which will fall onto the chest while the patient is seated; jaw is slack; voice has a nasal quality; body is limp
- Often triggered by medications e.g. aminoglycosides, beta blockers
- Gag reflex is often absent, and such patients are at risk for aspiration of oral secretions
- Management: monitor forced vital capacity, ventilatory support, plasmapheresis or IV immunoglobulins

Neurofibromatosis (NF) refers to a group of genetic disorders that primarily affect the cell growth of neural tissues. There are two types:
- **Neurofibromatosis type 1 (NF1)**, also known as von Recklinghausen's disease
- **Neurofibromatosis type 2 (NF2)**

Definition

Pathophysiology

NF1
- NF1 is a **dominantly inherited** genetic disorder that results from a germline mutation in the *NF1* tumour-suppressor gene, **neurofibromin**, which is located on chromosome 17q11.2
- About 50% of individuals with NF1 have no family history of the disease and the disease is due to *de novo* mutations

NF2
- NF2 is caused by a mutation in the gene encoding for the **protein merlin** or **schwannomin** on chromosome 22
- It is also **autosomal dominant** although around 50% are *de novo* with mosaicism in some

Neurofibromatosis

Management

NF1
- Multidisciplinary team involvement including geneticist, neurologist, surgeon and physiotherapist, coordinated by a GP
- Comprehensive examination each year in children e.g. detailed skin examination, eye tests, and assessment of bone, behaviour, blood pressure, physical ability and progress at school
- Neurofibromas should not be excised unless they show evidence of malignancy or are causing symptoms
- Other options include chemotherapy or radiation if a tumour has turned malignant or cancerous
- Plexiform neurofibromas may be treated with plastic surgery but there is risk of paralysis especially if the cranial nerves are involved superficially
- Cranial and spinal neurofibromas are amenable to corrective surgery
- Any gliomas or meningiomas should usually be extirpated, partially or completely, once intracranial pressure is raised
- Genetic counselling

NF2
- Annual monitoring usually involving hearing tests, an MRI brain scan and eye testing
- Hearing aids and management of tinnitus may be required
- Surgery and radiotherapy (less common) are options for brain tumours depending on size
- Genetic counselling

Complications

NF1
- Mild learning disability
- Nerve root compressions caused by neurofibromas
- GI bleeds/obstruction
- MSK complications: bone-cystic lesions, scoliosis, pseudarthrosis
- Hypertension (from renal artery stenosis)
- Phaeochromocytoma
- Malignancy
- Optic glioma
- Increased risk of epilepsy
- Carcinoid syndrome (rare)

NF2
- Partial/total deafness and tinnitus
- Facial nerve damage
- Visual disturbance
- Schwannomas
- Weakness or numbness in the extremities
- Multiple benign brain tumours

Diagnosis is made if at least 2 of the following are found (in the absence of alternative diagnoses):

1. **≥6 Café-au-lait spots** or **hyperpigmented macules** >5mm in diameter in prepubertal children and >15mm postpubertal (see *Fig. 1*)
2. **Axillary or inguinal freckles**
3. ≥2 Typical neurofibromas (see *Fig. 2*) or 1 plexiform neurofibroma
4. **Optic nerve glioma**
5. **≥2 Iris hamartomas (Lisch nodules)**: often only through slit-lamp examination by an ophthalmologist (see *Fig. 3*)
6. **Sphenoid dysplasia** or **typical long-bone abnormalities** such as pseudarthrosis
7. **1st-degree relative** (e.g. mother, father, sister, brother) with NF1

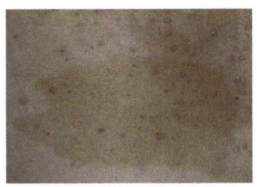

Fig. 1 Café-au-lait macules

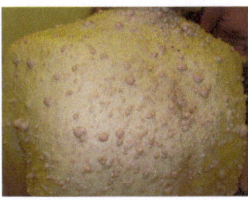

Fig. 2 Neurofibromas

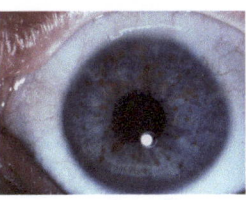

Fig. 3 Lisch nodules

Diagnosis requires at least 1 of the following clinical scenarios:
1. Bilateral vestibular schwannomas
2. A 1st-degree relative with NF2 *and*
   - Unilateral vestibular schwannoma *or*
   - Any 2 of: meningioma, schwannoma, glioma, neurofibroma, posterior subcapsular lenticular opacities
3. Unilateral vestibular schwannoma *and*
   - Any 2 of: meningioma, schwannoma, glioma, neurofibroma, posterior subcapsular lenticular opacities
4. Multiple meningiomas *and*
   - Unilateral vestibular schwannoma *or*
   - Any 2 of: schwannoma, glioma, neurofibroma, cataract

Clinical features/diagnostic criteria

Notes

Neurofibromatosis

Definition

Parkinsonism is an umbrella term for the clinical syndrome involving bradykinesia plus at least one of tremor, rigidity and/or postural instability. **Parkinson's disease (PD)** is an idiopathic progressive neurodegenerative condition caused by degeneration of dopaminergic neurones in the substantia nigra of the basal ganglia.

Causes

- PD (most common cause)
- Drug induced: antipsychotics, metoclopramide, phenothiazines e.g. chlorpromazine
- Progressive supranuclear palsy or Steele–Richardson–Olszewski syndrome
- Multiple system atrophy (previously Shy–Drager syndrome)
- Wilson's disease
- Post encephalitis
- Dementia pugilistica or chronic traumatic encephalopathy (secondary to chronic head trauma e.g. boxing)
- Toxins: carbon monoxide, MPTP, copper

Pathophysiology

- The 2 major neuropathological findings in PD:
  - Loss of pigmented dopaminergic neurones in the pars compacta of the substantia nigra
  - The presence of Lewy bodies and Lewy neurites
- Approximately 60–80% of dopaminergic neurones are lost before the motor signs of PD emerge

Parkinsonism

Complications

- Infections, most commonly aspiration pneumonia
- Bed sores
- Poor nutrition
- Falls
- Contractures
- Bowel and bladder disorders
- Acute akinesia

Management

Conservative

- Education and support, notifying DVLA, carer support, access to a multidisciplinary team

Pharmacological (see *Notes*)

- **Dopamine receptor agonists**
- **Levodopa**
- **MAO-B (monoamine oxidase B) inhibitors**
- **COMT (catechol-*O*-methyltransferase) inhibitors**
- **Amantadine**
- **Antimuscarinics**

Deep brain stimulation/surgery

- Considered for people with advanced PD who fail to be controlled by medical therapy, are biologically fit, are levodopa responsive and have no mental health problems

Motor (see *Fig. 1*)

- **Tremor** Worse at rest and usually improves with movement; asymmetrical onset; often 'pill rolling' of thumb over fingers (4–6 cycles/sec)
- **Rigidity/↑tone** Lead-pipe and cog-wheel rigidity
- **Bradykinesia/hypokinesia** Slow to initiate movements, expressionless face
- **Postural instability** May cause falls
- **Gait disorder** ↓Arm swing, festinating (shuffling steps difficult to stop with flexed trunk), freezing

Non-motor

- Sense of smell reduced
- Constipation
- Psychosis: complex visual hallucinations and paranoid ideation
- Frequency/urgency
- Dribbling of saliva
- Sweating
- Sleep disorders
- Swallowing difficulties
- Depression
- Dementia

Clinical features

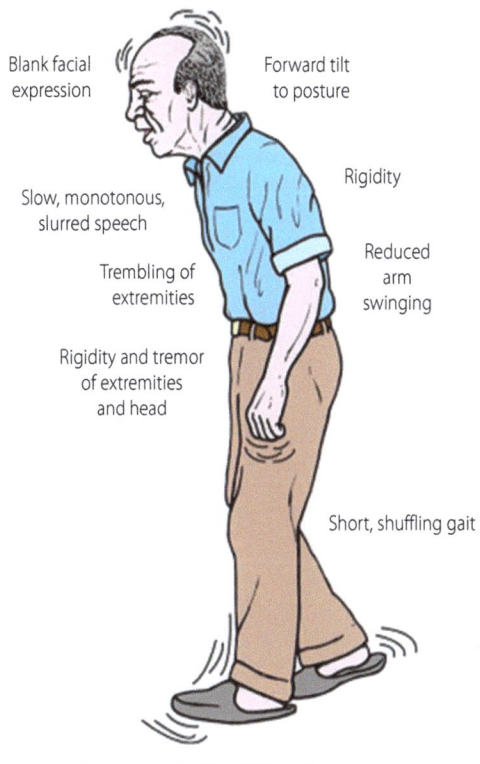

Blank facial expression

Forward tilt to posture

Slow, monotonous, slurred speech

Rigidity

Trembling of extremities

Reduced arm swinging

Rigidity and tremor of extremities and head

Short, shuffling gait

Fig. 1 Typical appearance of parkinsonism

Parkinson-plus syndromes

A group of neurodegenerative diseases featuring the classical features of PD with additional features that distinguish them from simple idiopathic PD:

- **Progressive supranuclear palsy** Impairment of vertical gaze (patients may complain of difficulty reading or descending stairs), early postural instability, symmetrical onset, speech and swallowing problems, little tremor
- **Multiple system atrophy** Early autonomic disturbance (postural hypotension, impotence/incontinence) and cerebellar signs
- **Lewy body dementia** Fluctuating cognition with visual hallucinations and early dementia
- **Corticobasal degeneration** Akinetic rigidity affecting one limb, cortical sensory loss, apraxia
- **Vascular parkinsonism** Pyramidal signs (legs), e.g. in diabetic/hypertensive patients who fall or have gait problems

Investigations

Note: diagnosis is clinical, and investigations mainly focus on excluding other causes of the presentation:

- **CT** or **MRI brain** For patients who do not respond to levodopa; MRI can be used to exclude secondary causes of parkinsonism e.g. tumours
- **PET, SPECT, DaT scan** Used to measure basal ganglia dopaminergic function where diagnosis is unclear
- **Genetic testing** e.g. Huntington's gene; <5% of all PD cases are caused by known single-gene mutations
- **Olfactory testing**
- **Caeruloplasmin levels** (rule out Wilson's disease) and **syphilis serology** (rule out syphilis) For young-onset or atypical disease

Parkinsonism notes

Pharmacological management

Levodopa
- Levodopa (L-dopa) should be offered to people in the early stages of PD whose motor symptoms impact on their quality of life
- It crosses the blood–brain barrier where it is converted to dopamine
- Usually combined with a decarboxylase inhibitor (e.g. carbidopa or benserazide) to prevent peripheral metabolism of L-dopa to dopamine
- Effectiveness reduces with time (usually by 2 years)
- Side effects include: dyskinesia, dry mouth, 'on-off' effect, drowsiness, anorexia, palpitations, postural hypotension, psychosis

Dopamine receptor agonists
- Dopamine agonists may be used 1st line as a symptomatic treatment for people with early PD
- Can also be used in advanced disease in conjunction with L-dopa to control fluctuations in response
- May be ergot derived or non-ergot derived
- Non-ergot-derived dopamine agonists are preferred (pramipexole and ropinirole) due to fewer adverse effects
- Ergot-derived drugs (e.g. bromocriptine, cabergoline, lisuride) should not be offered as 1st-line treatment for PD because of the risk of pulmonary, retroperitoneal and cardiac fibrosis; echocardiogram, ESR, creatinine and CXR should be obtained prior to treatment and patients should be closely monitored
- Side effects include: impulse control disorders, excessive daytime somnolence, hallucinations, postural hypotension, nasal congestion

MAO-B (monoamine oxidase B) inhibitors
- e.g. Selegiline, rasagiline
- Inhibit the breakdown of dopamine secreted by the dopaminergic neurones
- May be used as a symptomatic treatment for people with early PD or in advanced Parkinson's to reduce motor fluctuations

COMT (catechol-O-methyltransferase) inhibitors
- e.g. Entacapone, tolcapone
- Used as a 2nd-line treatment for PD
- Used as an adjunct to L-dopa as increases half-life of the drug

Amantadine
- May be used as a treatment for people with early PD but should not be used 1st line as response rate is low and tolerance occurs
- Mechanism of action is not entirely understood; it probably increases dopamine release and inhibits its uptake at dopaminergic synapses
- Side effects include: ataxia, slurred speech, confusion, dizziness and livedo reticularis

Antimuscarinics
- e.g. Procyclidine, benzatropine, trihexyphenidyl
- Block cholinergic receptors
- Used more to treat drug-induced parkinsonism rather than idiopathic PD; help with tremor and rigidity
- Side effects include: dry mouth, constipation, urinary retention, blurred vision

Apomorphine
- A potent dopamine agonist
- Useful in patients with severe motor complications to decrease 'off' periods and dyskinesia
- Two main treatment options: intermittent subcutaneous rescue injections or via a continuous infusion

Beta blockers
- Propranolol may be used as an adjunct for the symptomatic treatment of postural tremor in PD

- The pathophysiology of polyneuropathy depends on the underlying cause
- It is usually symmetrical and widespread with distal weakness and sensory loss: 'glove and stocking' (see *Fig. 1*)
- Two pathological processes predominate in diseases of peripheral nerves:
  - **Axonal degeneration** The most common pathology seen in systemic, metabolic, toxic and nutritional causes
  - **Segmental demyelination** Primary destruction of the myelin sheath leaving the axon intact (note: axonal degeneration may also be present in demyelinating neuropathies and vice versa); an example is GBS

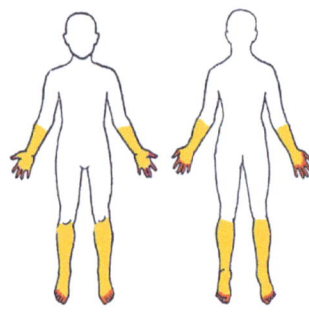

Fig. 1 Typical 'glove and stocking' pattern of peripheral neuropathy

Peripheral polyneuropathy is an acute or chronic, diffuse, often symmetrical, disease and may involve motor, sensory, or autonomic nerves, either alone or in combination.

Definition

Pathophysiology

Polyneuropathies

Management

Treat underlying cause

For example, good diabetes control, treat nutritional deficiencies e.g. vitamin B$_{12}$/folate, treat underlying malignancy, alcohol cessation, IV immunoglobulins in GBS (see *Ch6: Guillain–Barré syndrome*)

Supportive management

- Physio/occupational therapy involvement for mobility, muscle strengthening and home adaptation
- Walking aids, e.g. a stick or Zimmer frame, for support
- Foot care and shoe choice are very important in sensory neuropathies to minimise trauma

Management of neuropathic pain

► **Non-pharmacological**

- **Acupuncture**
- **Transcutaneous electrical nerve stimulation (TENS)** Non-invasive therapeutic option which uses peripheral nerve electrical stimulation by means of electrodes placed on the skin surface at known well-tolerated intensities
- **Percutaneous electrical nerve stimulation (PENS)** Uses needle-like electrodes (similar to those used in acupuncture) located in soft tissues or muscles at the corresponding dermatomes for that local pathology

► **Pharmacological**

- Neuropathic-specific analgesics such as duloxetine, amitriptyline, gabapentin, or pregabalin
- Other options include tramadol (short term) and capsaicin cream (for people with localised neuropathic pain who wish to avoid or cannot tolerate oral treatments)

- **Metabolic** Diabetes mellitus, renal failure, hypothyroidism, hypoglycaemia
- **Vasculitides** Polyarteritis nodosa, rheumatoid arthritis, Wegener's granulomatosis
- **Malignancy** Paraneoplastic syndrome, polycythaemia rubra vera
- **Inflammatory** Guillain–Barré syndrome (GBS), sarcoidosis, chronic inflammatory demyelinating polyneuropathy (CIDP)
- **Nutritional** ↓Vitamin B_1, B_{12}, vitamin E, folate
- **Inherited** Charcot–Marie–Tooth (CMT), porphyria, Refsum syndrome, leucodystrophy
- **Toxins/drugs** Alcohol, vincristine, nitrofurantoin, phenytoin, metronidazole, lead, arsenic
- **Others** Amyloidosis, paraproteinaemias

Causes

Polyneuropathies can be classified by time course (**acute** vs **chronic**), underlying pathology (**demyelination** vs **axonal degeneration**) or by affected function (**motor** vs **sensory**)

Predominantly motor

- GBS
- Porphyria
- Lead poisoning
- Hereditary sensorimotor neuropathy (HSMN): CMT
- CIDP
- Diphtheria

Predominantly sensory

- Diabetes
- Alcoholism
- Vitamin B_{12} deficiency
- Uraemia
- Leprosy
- Amyloidosis

Classification

Clinical features

Investigations

- **Urine** Dipstick (for glucose, protein), urine ACR and Bence Jones proteins
- **Bloods** FBC, ESR, vitamin B_{12}, folate, fasting glucose/HbA1c, U&Es, LFTs, TFTs, serum electrophoresis, RF, ANA, anti-ganglioside antibodies, anti-Ro and anti-La antibodies, anti-neuronal antibodies (Hu, Yo)
- **Nerve conduction studies** Helpful in differentiating primary demyelination from axonal degeneration
- **Lumbar puncture** Helps to diagnose GBS and CIDP
- **Genetic testing** e.g. For CMT
- **Nerve biopsy** May be required

Sensory symptoms

- Numbness, tingling, pins and needles in the hands and feet
- Burning sensations
- Pain in the extremities
- Sensations of 'walking on cotton wool'
- Band-like sensations around the wrists or ankles
- Unsteadiness on the feet, or stumbling

Motor symptoms

- Weakness or clumsiness of the limbs
- Difficulty walking (including falls and stumbling)
- Wasting of affected muscles
- Reduced/absent reflexes
- Respiratory difficulty

Autonomic neuropathy

- Postural hypotension
- Erectile dysfunction
- Anhidrosis
- Constipation or diarrhoea
- Urinary retention
- Horner syndrome
- Cardiac arrhythmias
- Holmes–Adie pupil

Transient ischaemic attack, sometimes referred to as 'mini stroke', refers to transient (**<24h**) neurological dysfunction caused by focal brain, spinal cord or retinal ischaemia, without evidence of acute infarction.

- The cause is usually **embolic**; it may be **thrombotic**, and occasionally **haemorrhagic**
- The most common source of emboli is the carotids, usually at the bifurcation; they may originate in the heart (particularly in AF); the vertebrobasilar arteries may also be a source

Definition

Causes

Transient ischaemic attack

Management

Investigations

Initial

- **Aspirin 300mg** Unless contraindicated should be given immediately; if the patient is already taking low-dose aspirin regularly it should be continued on the current dose until reviewed by a specialist
- **Specialist assessment by stroke physician** Within 24h if the patient has had a suspected TIA <7 days ago and within 7 days if they have had suspected TIA >7 days ago

Long-term

- **Control risk factors** e.g. HTN and diabetes, obesity, smoking cessation
- **Antiplatelet long term** Clopidogrel is recommended 1st line 75mg OD; aspirin + dipyridamole should be given to patients who cannot tolerate clopidogrel
- **Anticoagulate** In AF (see *Ch1: Atrial fibrillation*)
- **Long-term statin** e.g. Atorvastatin 20–80mg daily
- **Carotid endarterectomy** Consider if carotid stenosis >70% according to ECST criteria or > 50% according to NASCET criteria
- **Driving** Must not drive for 1 month following a TIA; if multiple TIAs over a short period, require 3 months free from further attacks before resuming driving, and DVLA should be notified

- **Bloods** FBC, ESR/CRP, U&Es, glucose, LFTs, TFTs, cholesterol, clotting and antiphospholipid antibodies
- **ECG/24-h ECG** Look for arrhythmias e.g. AF/paroxysmal AF
- **CT brain** To primarily rule out haemorrhage
- **MRI brain** To determine the region of ischaemia, rule out haemorrhage or other pathologies
- **Carotid imaging** Carotid Doppler and duplex US to look for atheroma and stenosis; MRI or CT angiography may be required
- **Transoesophageal/transthoracic ECHO** To rule out transmural thrombus or valvular heart disease

Risk factors

Lifestyle factors

- Smoking
- Alcohol misuse and drug abuse e.g. cocaine, methamphetamine
- Physical inactivity
- Poor diet

Established cardiovascular disease

- Hypertension
- AF (causes more than 20% of ischaemic strokes)
- Ischaemic heart disease
- Infective endocarditis
- Valvular heart disease
- Congestive heart failure
- Congenital or structural heart disease

Other factors

- Increasing age
- Gender: men, ↑risk at younger age; women, ↑stroke risk linked to oral contraceptives, migraine with aura, the immediate postpartum period and pre-eclampsia
- Peripheral vascular disease
- Hyperlipidaemia
- Diabetes mellitus
- Sickle cell disease
- Antiphospholipid syndrome and other hypercoagulable disorders
- Chronic kidney disease
- Obstructive sleep apnoea

Clinical features

Carotid territory symptoms

- Amaurosis fugax
- Aphasia
- Hemiparesis
- Hemisensory loss
- Hemianopic visual loss

Vertebrobasilar territory symptoms

- Diplopia
- Vertigo
- Vomiting
- Choking and dysarthria
- Ataxia
- Hemisensory loss
- Hemianopic or bilateral visual loss
- Tetraparesis
- Loss of consciousness

Differential diagnosis

- Stroke
- Hypoglycaemia
- Migraine with aura
- Focal epilepsy
- Intracranial lesion e.g. tumour or haemorrhage
- Hyperventilation
- Retinal or vitreous haemorrhage
- Labyrinth disorder
- Malignant hypertension

ABCD$_2$ score

Estimates stroke risk after suspected TIA but should not be used any more for deciding management:

- **Age** ≥60 years (1 point)
- **Blood pressure** ≥140/90mmHg (1 point)
- **Clinical features** Unilateral weakness (2 points), speech disturbance without weakness (1 point)
- **Duration of symptoms** ≥60 min (2 points), 10–59 min (1 point)
- **Diabetes** Presence of diabetes (1 point)
(**low risk:** 1–3, **moderate risk:** 4–5, **high risk:** 6–7)

Causes

Ischaemic stroke (85%)

Occurs when large arteries (such as the extracranial carotid or vertebral arteries), intracranial arteries or small penetrating arteries (lacunar) are occluded by:

- **Thrombus** due to atherosclerosis *or*
- **Embolus** of fatty material from an atherosclerotic plaque or a clot in a larger artery or the heart (often due to AF or atherosclerosis of the carotid arteries)

Haemorrhagic stroke (15%)

- **Intracerebral haemorrhage** (main cause is hypertension)
- **Subarachnoid haemorrhage**

Rarer causes

- **Cerebral venous thrombosis:** more common in patients in pro-thrombotic state e.g. related to pregnancy, infection, dehydration or malignancy
- **Carotid artery dissection:** more common in younger people and may be preceded by neck trauma
- **Genetic conditions** such as Fabry's disease and CADASIL (cerebral autosomal dominant arteriopathy with subcortical infarcts and leucoencephalopathy)

Definition

A clinical syndrome characterised by sudden onset of rapidly developing focal or global neurological disturbance which lasts more than 24h or leads to death.

Risk factors

Same as TIA (see *Ch6: Transient ischaemic attack*)

Stroke

Management

Acute stroke management

- Arrange **urgent CT head** (see *Fig. 1*) or **MRI scan**
- Blood glucose, hydration, oxygen saturations and temperature should be maintained within normal limits; (hypertension and labile BP are common on presentation and should not be acutely corrected)
- Give **aspirin 300mg** orally or rectally (if unable to swallow) ASAP if a haemorrhagic stroke has been excluded
- Admit to stroke unit
- NBM if swallowing deemed unsafe with SALT assessment and support with feeding
- Prevention of DVT with early mobilisation and TED stockings

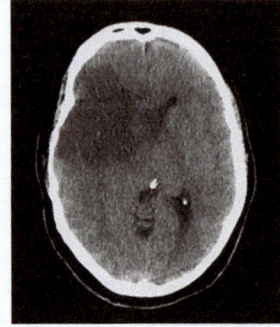

Fig. 1 Axial non-contrast CT head showing right middle cerebral artery infarct (darker area)

Thrombolysis

Alteplase should only be given if administered <4.5h from onset of stroke symptoms and haemorrhage has been definitively excluded (see *Notes: Thrombolysis contraindications*).

Thrombectomy

Mechanical thrombectomy is a relatively new treatment option for patients with an acute ischaemic stroke. All decisions about thrombectomy should take into account a patient's overall clinical status.

Neurosurgery

This is for patients with haemorrhagic stroke.

Long-term stroke management (see *Notes*)

Cerebral hemisphere infarcts (approx. 50%)

Most commonly due to infarction of the internal capsule due to occlusion of a branch of the middle cerebral artery:
- Contralateral hemiplegia
- Contralateral hemisensory loss
- Homonymous hemianopia
- Dysphasia: if the site of the lesion is in the left (usually the dominant cerebral hemisphere) then language functions will be affected
- Upper motor neurone signs, including facial weakness
- In right-sided cerebral infarcts there is likely to be neglect of the contralateral limbs, constructional or dressing apraxia, and topographical agnosia

Lacunar infarcts (approx. 25%)

Caused by small infarcts that produce localised deficits:
- Pure sensory, pure motor or mixed motor and sensory deficit
- Sudden-onset unilateral cerebellar ataxia and sudden dysarthria with a clumsy hand are typically caused by single lacunar infarct

Brainstem infarcts (approx. 25%)

Cause complex patterns of dysfunction and depend on the site involved:
- **Lateral medullary syndrome** (most common form) Caused by posterior cerebellar artery occlusion; presents with sudden vomiting and vertigo, ipsilateral Horner syndrome, facial numbness, cerebellar signs and palatal paralysis with diminished gag reflex; there may be pain and loss of temperature sensation on the contralateral side
- **Coma** Due to involvement of reticular activating system
- **The locked-in syndrome** Caused by upper brainstem infarction; all voluntary muscles are paralysed except those that control eye movement
- **Pseudobulbar palsy** Caused by lower brainstem infarction

Clinical features

Investigations

Same as TIA (see *Ch6: Transient ischaemic attack*)

Complications

Acute

- Haemorrhagic transformation of ischaemic stroke
- Cerebral oedema
- Seizures
- Venous thromboembolism: pulmonary embolism
- Cardiac complications: MI, heart failure, AF and arrhythmias are common
- Infection: including aspiration pneumonia, UTI and cellulitis from infected pressure sores

Long-term

- Mobility problems: hemiparesis or hemiplegia, ataxia, falls, spasticity and contractures
- Sensory deficits
- Urinary and faecal incontinence
- Long-term pain (neuropathic or musculoskeletal)
- Fatigue
- Dysphagia, poor oral hygiene, dehydration and malnutrition
- Sexual dysfunction
- Pressure sores
- Visual problems: altered acuity, hemianopia, diplopia, nystagmus and blurred vision
- Cognitive problems
- Difficulties with activities of daily living (ADL)
- Anxiety and depression
- Communication problems: dysphasia and dysarthria

Assessment tools

FAST (for general public use)

- **F**acial weakness Can they smile? Has their mouth or eye drooped?
- **A**rm weakness Can they raise both arms?
- **S**peech problems Can they speak clearly and can they understand what you're saying?
- **Time** It is time to call 999 immediately if you see any of these symptoms

Rosier score (for medical professionals)

Exclude hypoglycaemia first, then assess the following (a stroke is likely if >0):
- **Loss of consciousness** or **syncope** (−1 point)
- **Seizure activity** (−1 point)
- New, acute onset of:
  - **Weakness** Asymmetric facial weakness (+1 point), asymmetric arm weakness (+1 point), asymmetric leg weakness (+1 point)
  - **Speech disturbance** (+1 point)
  - **Visual field defect** (+1 point)

Thrombolysis contraindications

Absolute	Relative
• Previous intracranial haemorrhage • Seizure at onset of stroke • Intracranial neoplasm • Suspected subarachnoid haemorrhage • Stroke or traumatic brain injury in preceding 3 months • Lumbar puncture in preceding 7 days • GI haemorrhage in preceding 3 weeks • Active bleeding • Pregnancy • Oesophageal varices • Uncontrolled hypertension >200/120mmHg	• Concurrent anticoagulation (INR >1.7) • Haemorrhagic diathesis • Active diabetic haemorrhagic retinopathy • Suspected intracardiac thrombus • Major surgery/trauma in the preceding 2 weeks

Long-term management of stroke

Secondary prevention

- **Control risk factors** e.g. HTN and diabetes, obesity, smoking cessation
- **Antiplatelet long term** Clopidogrel is recommended 1st line 75mg OD long term; aspirin + dipyridamole should be given to patients who cannot tolerate clopidogrel
- **Anticoagulate** in AF (see *Ch1: Atrial fibrillation*)
- **Long-term statin** e.g. Atorvastatin 20–80mg daily
- **Carotid endarterectomy** Should be considered if carotid stenosis >70% according to ECST criteria or >50% according to NASCET criteria

Stroke neurorehabilitation

- Optimal treatment is on a stroke rehabilitation unit that provides multidisciplinary service
- Early **physiotherapy** is particularly useful in the first few months in reducing spasticity, relieving contractures and helping with walking aids
- **Occupational therapists** play a vital role in assessing the requirement for and arranging various aids and home modification

Management of long-term complications

- **Swallowing or speech difficulty** Assessment and ongoing management by speech and language therapist
- **Nutrition and hydration** Refer to a dietitian if oral intake of nutrition and fluids is inadequate, or if food or fluid consistency needs to be modified
- **Incontinence** Ongoing incontinence should be followed up by community continence services
- **Cognitive dysfunction** Consider screening for cognitive impairment and referring for a neuropsychological assessment if this is suspected
- **Depression and anxiety** Screen all patients for this and treat appropriately
- **Mouth care** Advise people with stroke (particularly those who are tube fed or have swallowing problems) and their carers to carry out mouth care at least 3 times a day
- **Visual problems** Patients should be referred to an orthoptist or ophthalmologist specialising in stroke if there are any visual complications
- **Long-term pain** Treat people with central post-stroke pain with amitriptyline, gabapentin or pregabalin; people with ongoing musculoskeletal pain should initially be treated with simple analgesic drugs such as paracetamol and NSAIDs
- **Sexual dysfunction** Patients should be screened for sexual dysfunction
- **Spasticity and contractures** Spasticity and development of contractures are common following stroke and can lead to discomfort and pain; splinting and physiotherapy may be useful
- **End of life** Those with stroke who are nearing the end of life should have access to the specialist palliative care team when needed

Driving

- Patients who are group 1 vehicle drivers cannot drive for 1 month after a stroke provided there are no residual deficits; they do not need to inform the DVLA
- Patients who drive large goods vehicles or passenger-carrying vehicles must inform the DVLA

Barthel index for ADL

Assesses functional independence in stroke patients:

Bowels	0	Incontinent
	5	Occasional accident
	10	Continent
Bladder	0	Incontinent
	5	Occasional accident
	10	Continent
Grooming	0	Needs help with personal care
	5	Independent (face, hair, teeth, shaving)
Toilet use	0	Dependent
	5	Needs some help (can do some things alone)
	10	Independent (on and off dressing and wiping)
Feeding	0	Unable
	5	Needs help with cutting, spreading butter etc.
	10	Independent
Transfer (bed to chair and back)	0	Unable, no sitting balance
	5	Major help needed (physical, 1–2 people), can sit
	10	Minor help needed (verbal or physical)
	15	Independent
Mobility (on level surfaces)	0	Immobile
	5	Wheelchair independent, including corners
	10	Walks with help of 1 person
	15	Independent
Dressing	0	Dependent
	5	Needs some help but can do some things alone
	10	Independent (including buttons, zips, laces)
Stairs	0	Unable
	5	Needs help (verbal, physical, carrying aid)
	10	Independent
Bathing/ showering	0	Dependent
	5	Independent

Interpretation:

80–100 Independent
60–79 Minimally dependent
40–59 Partially dependent
20–39 Very dependent
<20 Totally dependent

Definition

Subarachnoid haemorrhage (SAH) is bleeding into the subarachnoid space and is a medical emergency. It is usually as a result of bleeding from an aneurysm in the circle of Willis (see *Fig. 1*).

Causes

- Spontaneous rupture of **berry aneurysms** (85%): conditions associated with berry aneurysms include adult polycystic kidney disease, Ehlers–Danlos syndrome and coarctation of the aorta
- AV malformations
- Trauma
- Tumours

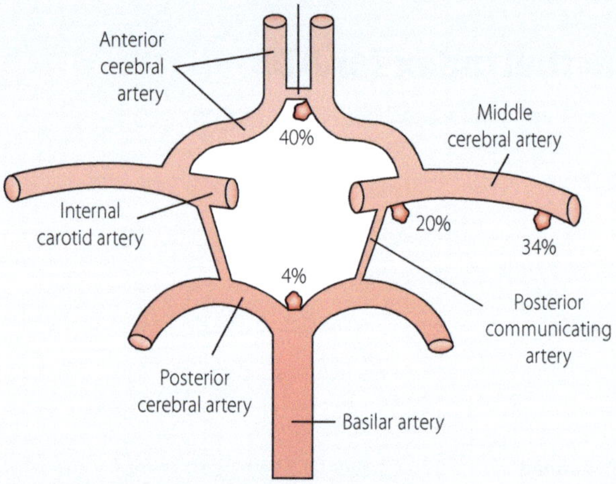

Fig. 1 The main cerebral arteries showing the circle of Willis and the most common sites for berry aneurysms

Subarachnoid haemorrhage

Complications

- Re-bleeding (in 30%)
- Obstructive hydrocephalus (due to blood in ventricles)
- Cerebral ischaemia
- Death

Management

- Bed rest and supportive measures with cautious control of hypertension
- Nimodipine, e.g. 60mg 4-hourly orally or by IV infusion, has been shown to reduce the severity of neurological deficits but does not reduce re-bleeding
- Neurosurgical opinion: no clear evidence over early surgical intervention against delayed intervention

Investigations

- **CT head scan** The investigation of choice and should be done as soon as possible; detects SAH in 95% of cases with scanning within 24h of haemorrhage; the sensitivity decreases with time (see *Fig. 2*)
- **Bloods** FBC (check platelet count prior to lumbar puncture), U&Es, clotting screen
- **ECG** Peaked P and T waves, short PR interval, prolonged QT interval, tall U waves
- **Lumbar puncture** If the CT head is normal. A lumbar puncture must not be performed if there are features of raised intracranial pressure; if performed within 6–12h then CSF is uniformly bloodstained; if performed between 12h and 2 weeks after initial headache then the CSF is xanthochromic
- **CT/MR angiography** Usually performed to establish the source of bleeding in all patients potentially fit for surgery

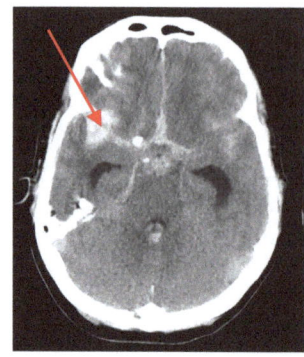

Fig. 2 Left temporal lobe subarachnoid haemorrhage on CT scan

- Hypertension
- Smoking
- Cocaine use
- Excessive alcohol
- Linked genetic disorders include autosomal dominant adult polycystic disease, Ehlers–Danlos syndrome type IV and neurofibromatosis type 1, Marfan syndrome
- 1st-degree relatives have a 3–7× relative risk compared with the general population

The Hunt and Hess Classification of Subarachnoid Haemorrhage
Classifies severity of subarachnoid haemorrhage to predict mortality:
- **Grade 1** Asymptomatic, mild headache, slight nuchal rigidity
- **Grade 2** Moderate–severe headache, nuchal rigidity, no neurological deficit other than cranial nerve palsy
- **Grade 3** Drowsiness/confusion, mild neurological deficit
- **Grade 4** Stupor, moderate–severe hemiparesis
- **Grade 5** Coma, decerebrate posturing

Risk factors

Classification

Clinical features

- Headache: 'sudden onset', 'worst ever', 'thunderclap'
- Vomiting
- Neck stiffness and positive Kernig's sign
- Photophobia
- Drowsiness
- Confusion
- Unilateral eye pain
- Loss of consciousness
- Seizure
- Coma
- Reactive hypertension
- Focal neurological signs
- Fundoscopy: subhyaloid haemorrhages, with or without papilloedema

Notes

Subarachnoid haemorrhage

An acute SDH is usually caused by:

- Tearing of bridging veins from the cortex to one of the draining venous sinuses – typically occurring when bridging veins are sheared during rapid acceleration–deceleration of the head
- Bleeding from a damaged cortical artery
- Blunt head trauma is the usual mechanism of injury but spontaneous SDH can arise as a consequence of clotting disorder, arteriovenous malformations/aneurysms or other conditions
- In the subacute phase, the collection of clotted blood liquefies; in the chronic phase it becomes a collection of serous fluid in the subdural space

- **Acute** This phase begins less than 3 days after initial injury
- **Subacute** This phase begins 3–7 days after the initial injury
- **Chronic** This phase begins 2–3 weeks after the initial injury
- **Simple SDH** There is no associated parenchymal injury
- **Complicated SDH** There is associated underlying parenchymal injury, such as contusion

A subdural haematoma (SDH) is a collection of blood deep in the dural layer of the meninges.

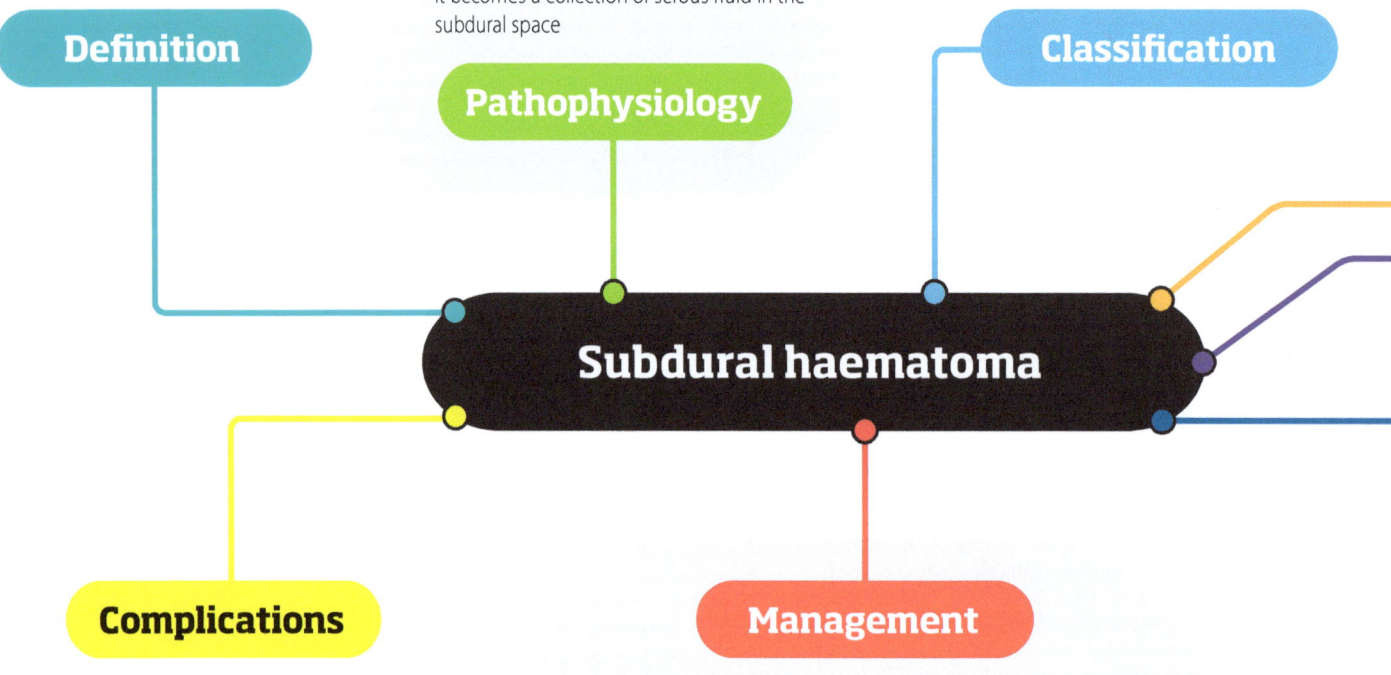

Definition

Pathophysiology

Classification

Subdural haematoma

Complications

Management

- Death due to cerebellar herniation
- Raised intracranial pressure
- Cerebral oedema
- Recurrent haematoma formation during recovery
- Seizures
- Wound infection, subdural empyema, meningitis
- Permanent neurological or cognitive deficit due to pressure effects on the brain
- Coma/persistent vegetative state

- ABC approach of resuscitation
- Intubation and assisted ventilation may be needed depending on level of consciousness
- In cases of severe trauma, the cervical spine should be immobilised and the trauma team should be alerted
- If suspected or confirmed by investigation, refer urgently to the neurosurgical team
- Treat any coagulopathy, e.g. vitamin K, fresh frozen plasma, for reversing the effects of warfarin
- Measures to decrease raised intracranial pressure include IV mannitol or hypertonic saline
- Burr holes may be considered if there is rapid deterioration
- For a small asymptomatic acute SDH, this can be managed by observation, serial examinations and serial CT scanning
- Surgery is needed if there are focal signs, deterioration, a large haematoma, raised intracranial pressure or midline shift
- SDH is treated by emergency craniotomy and clot evacuation
- The use of a drain can reduce the risk of recurrence

- Any factor that stretches the bridging veins:
  - Cerebral atrophy, e.g. elderly
  - Low CSF pressure after shunting, e.g. for long-standing hydrocephalus or a fistula
- Alcoholism
- Coagulation disorder or anticoagulation therapy e.g. warfarin

- **History of trauma:** often minor and the latent interval between injury and symptoms may be weeks or months
- **Fluctuating conscious level:**
  - There may be a history of gradual-onset of headaches, memory loss, personality change, confusion and drowsiness
  - Symptoms vary from day to day with intervening lucid periods
- **Focal neurological signs:** often, hemiparesis
- **Aphasia:** if the lesion is on the left side

Risk factors

Clinical features

Investigations

Bloods

- FBC, U&Es and LFTs may reveal alternative causes of impaired consciousness; thrombocytopenia may indicate a bleeding diathesis
- Coagulation screen: to screen for coagulopathy
- Group and save/cross-match if SDH seems likely, in anticipation of operative intervention

Imaging

- **CT head** 1st-line investigation; shows a crescentic collection, not limited by suture lines; acute subdural haematomas will appear hyperdense (bright) in comparison with the brain (see *Fig. 1*); chronic SDHs are hypodense (dark) compared with the substance of the brain (see *Fig. 2*)
- **Skull X-ray** May reveal skull fracture
- **MRI head** Can be used to detect SDH

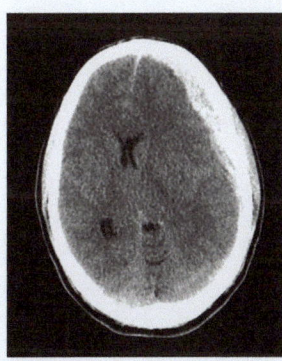

Fig. 1 Left acute subdural haematoma on CT scan

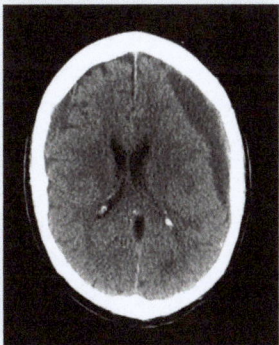

Fig. 2 Left chronic subdural haematoma on CT scan

Chapter 7

Rheumatology

Definition

Ankylosing spondylitis (AS) is a chronic **seronegative spondyloarthropathy** which primarily involves the sacroiliac (SI) joints and the spine. Other clinical features include peripheral arthritis, enthesitis and extra-articular organ involvement.

Pathophysiology

- Both genetic and environmental factors contribute to AS
- **HLA-B27** is the most common predisposing gene in AS
- The disease is first characterised by inflammation of the SI joints; in the later stages the annulus fibrosus starts to calcify, creating a bony bridge between the vertebral bodies (syndesmophytes)
- These may then fuse with the vertebral body above causing ankyloses (see *Fig. 1*).

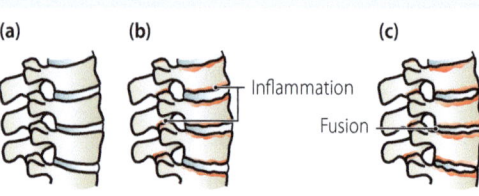

Fig. 1 (a) Normal spine, **(b)** early AS, **(c)** advanced AS

Ankylosing spondylitis

Management

Conservative

- Patient education
- Exercise
- Physiotherapy
- Hydrotherapy and swimming are excellent activities to maintain mobility and fitness

Pharmacological

- **NSAIDs** 1st line for pain and stiffness
- **Other analgesics** When NSAIDs are insufficient e.g. paracetamol and codeine
- **Steroids** Local corticosteroid injections are useful for symptomatic sacroiliitis, peripheral enthesitis and arthritis; oral corticosteroids can be used for short-term relief of symptoms
- **Anti-TNF-alpha therapy** e.g. Etanercept and adalimumab are effective in AS that is poorly controlled with NSAIDs
- **Bisphosphonates** Often used to treat osteoporosis and reduce the risk of fractures in AS

Surgical

- **Vertebral osteotomy** May be performed to correct spinal deformities, but may cause significant neurological complications.
- **Joint replacement** Patients may need total hip replacement and, occasionally, total shoulder replacement.

Risk factors

- HLA-B27 gene: 90% of AS patients are carriers
- Men (3:1)
- Age 17–35 years
- Northern European

Clinical features

Articular

- **Back pain and stiffness** Typically radiating from the SI joints to the hips/buttocks
- **Reduced motion** In the lumbar and cervical spine
- **Loss of lumbar lordosis**
- **Reduced chest expansion**
- **Thoracic kyphosis** and **neck hyperextension** 'Question mark posture'
- **Peripheral synovitis** Typically asymmetrical oligoarthritis (most commonly affects the hip and knee)

Extra-articular (The 'A' factors)

- **A**tlanto-axial subluxation
- **A**nterior uveitis
- **A**pical lung fibrosis
- **A**ortic valve incompetence
- **A**trioventricular node block
- **A**chilles tendonitis
- **A**myloidosis (rare and late complication)

The modified Schober's test examines the degree of flexion of the spine (see *Fig. 2*):

1. An inferior mark at the level of the posterior superior iliac spine is drawn and a 10-cm segment above this is marked
2. The increase in distance on maximum forward flexion with locked knees is measured
3. The measured distance should increase from 10cm to at least 13.5–15cm in a healthy adult

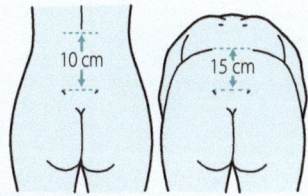

Fig. 2 Modified Schober's test

Investigations

Imaging

- **X-rays:**
  - *Early stages*: may be normal or there may be bony erosions, widening of SI joints and squaring of vertebral bodies with shiny corners (Romanus lesions)
  - *Later stages*: ossification of the longitudinal ligaments of the spine (syndesmophytes) giving the spine a bamboo appearance (see *Fig. 3*)
- **MRI**: of the sacroiliac joints is more sensitive than either plain X-ray or CT scan in demonstrating sacroiliitis
- **Ultrasound**: Can help in diagnosing enthesitis

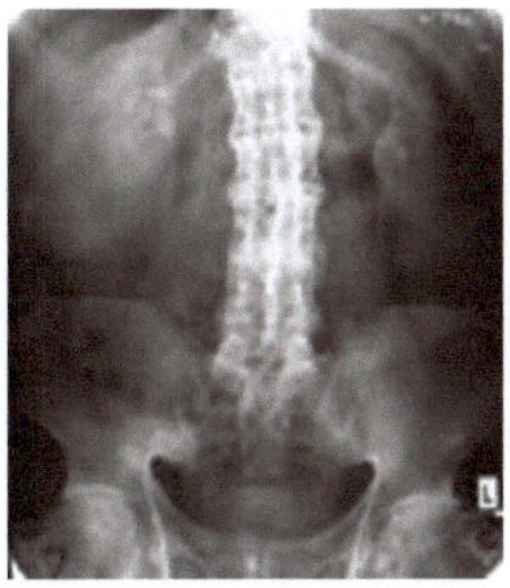

Fig. 3 X-ray of a 'bamboo spine' in AS

Bloods

- **FBC** Usually normal
- **ESR/CRP** ↑ In active disease
- **ANA/RF** Negative
- **ALP** Often elevated
- **HLA-B27** +ve in 90% of patients but has little role in diagnosis. It may indicate AS predisposition in appropriate clinical context

Notes

Ankylosing spondylitis

Fibromyalgia is a syndrome of chronic pain and the presence of **hyperalgesic points** at specific anatomical sites, as well as a range of other physical and psychological symptoms with no identifiable organic cause. It is not a diagnosis of exclusion and can occur in patients with other conditions such as inflammatory arthritis and osteoarthritis.

- The cause of fibromyalgia is poorly understood but abnormal central and peripheral pain processing is thought to be responsible for reduced pain threshold, **hyperalgesia** (amplification of pain) and **allodynia** (pain produced by non-noxious stimuli)

- The nociceptive system has links with the stress-regulating, immune and sleep systems which may explain some of the clinical features
- Genetic and environmental factors may play a role in fibromyalgia as it is more common in the relatives of affected patients

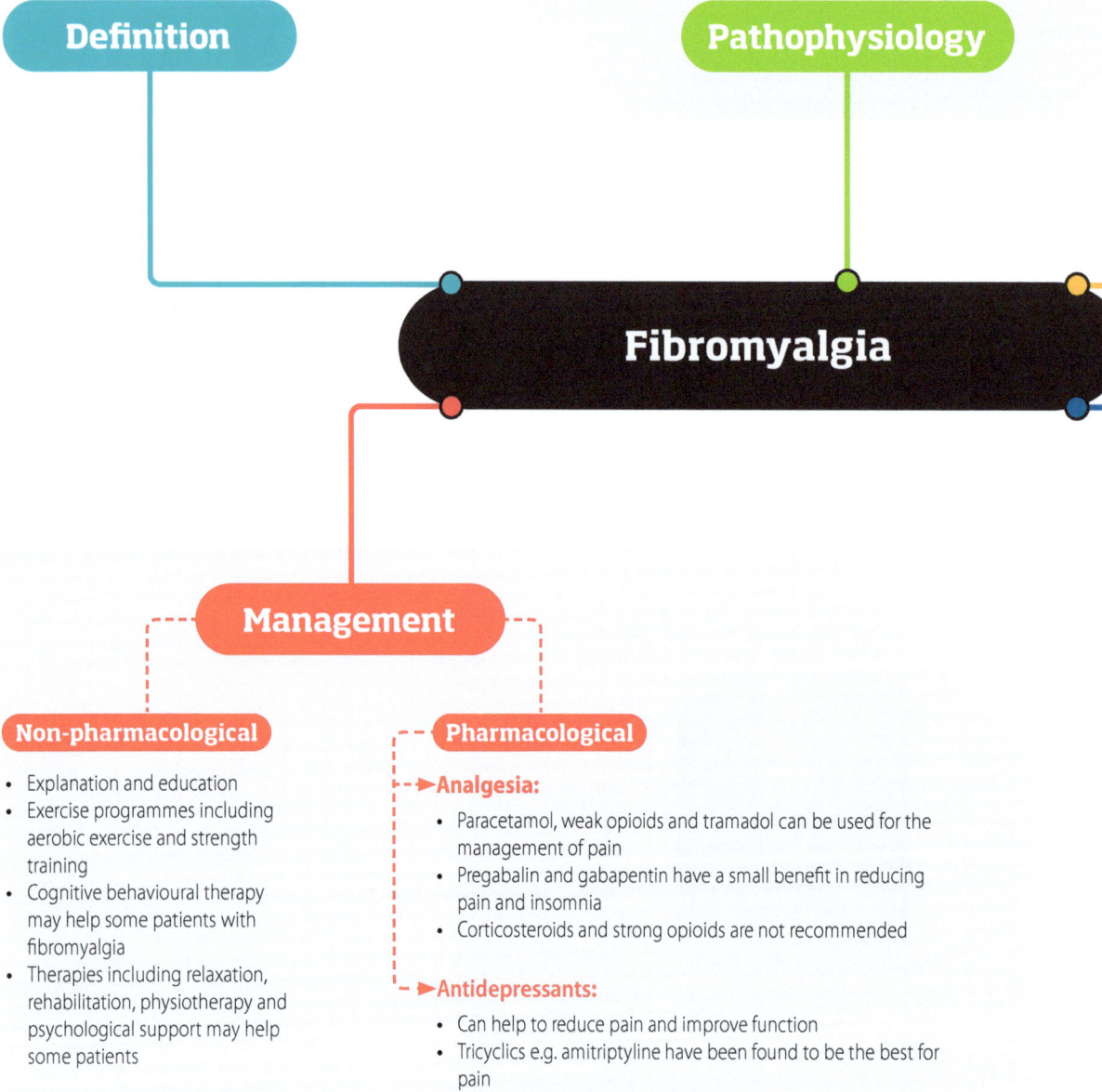

Definition

Pathophysiology

Fibromyalgia

Management

Non-pharmacological

- Explanation and education
- Exercise programmes including aerobic exercise and strength training
- Cognitive behavioural therapy may help some patients with fibromyalgia
- Therapies including relaxation, rehabilitation, physiotherapy and psychological support may help some patients

Pharmacological

Analgesia:

- Paracetamol, weak opioids and tramadol can be used for the management of pain
- Pregabalin and gabapentin have a small benefit in reducing pain and insomnia
- Corticosteroids and strong opioids are not recommended

Antidepressants:

- Can help to reduce pain and improve function
- Tricyclics e.g. amitriptyline have been found to be the best for pain
- SNRIs, e.g. venlafaxine and duloxetine, may be useful in treating pain and low mood
- SSRIs, e.g. fluoxetine, for low mood

- Female: 10× more likely to be affected
- Age: common in individuals aged 20–50 years but it can occur in any age
- Physical trauma: e.g. whiplash-type injuries to the neck and trunk
- Stress, anxiety and depression
- Life events: failing to complete education, low income, divorce
- Viral infections: may occur as a post-viral syndrome

Risk factors

- Pain at multiple sites
- Fatigue
- Insomnia
- Morning stiffness
- Paraesthesia
- Feeling of swollen joints (with no objective swelling)
- Problems with cognition (e.g. memory disturbance, difficulty with word finding)
- Headaches
- Light-headedness or dizziness
- Fluctuations in weight
- Anxiety and depression

(Symptoms are generally reported as worse in cold, humid weather and under times of stress)

Clinical features

Notes

Fibromyalgia

Investigations

All investigations including blood tests and imaging are normal. The American College of Rheumatology criteria for the classification of fibromyalgia include:
- **Widespread pain:** above and below the waist as well as the axial skeleton for at least 3 months
- Presence of **11/18 tender points** shown in *Fig. 1*

Note: The thumb should be used for digital palpation of tender points; the pressure applied should be just enough to blanch the examiner's thumbnail. In the absence of fibromyalgia, the palpation would not be enough to cause pain.

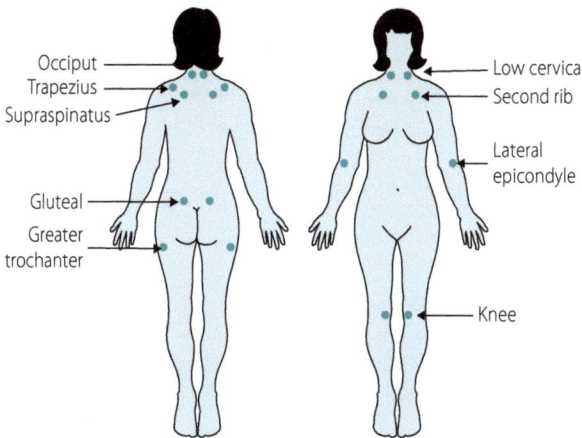

Occiput
Trapezius
Supraspinatus

Low cervical
Second rib

Lateral epicondyle

Gluteal

Greater trochanter

Knee

Fig. 1 Common distribution of hyperalgesic tender points in fibromyalgia

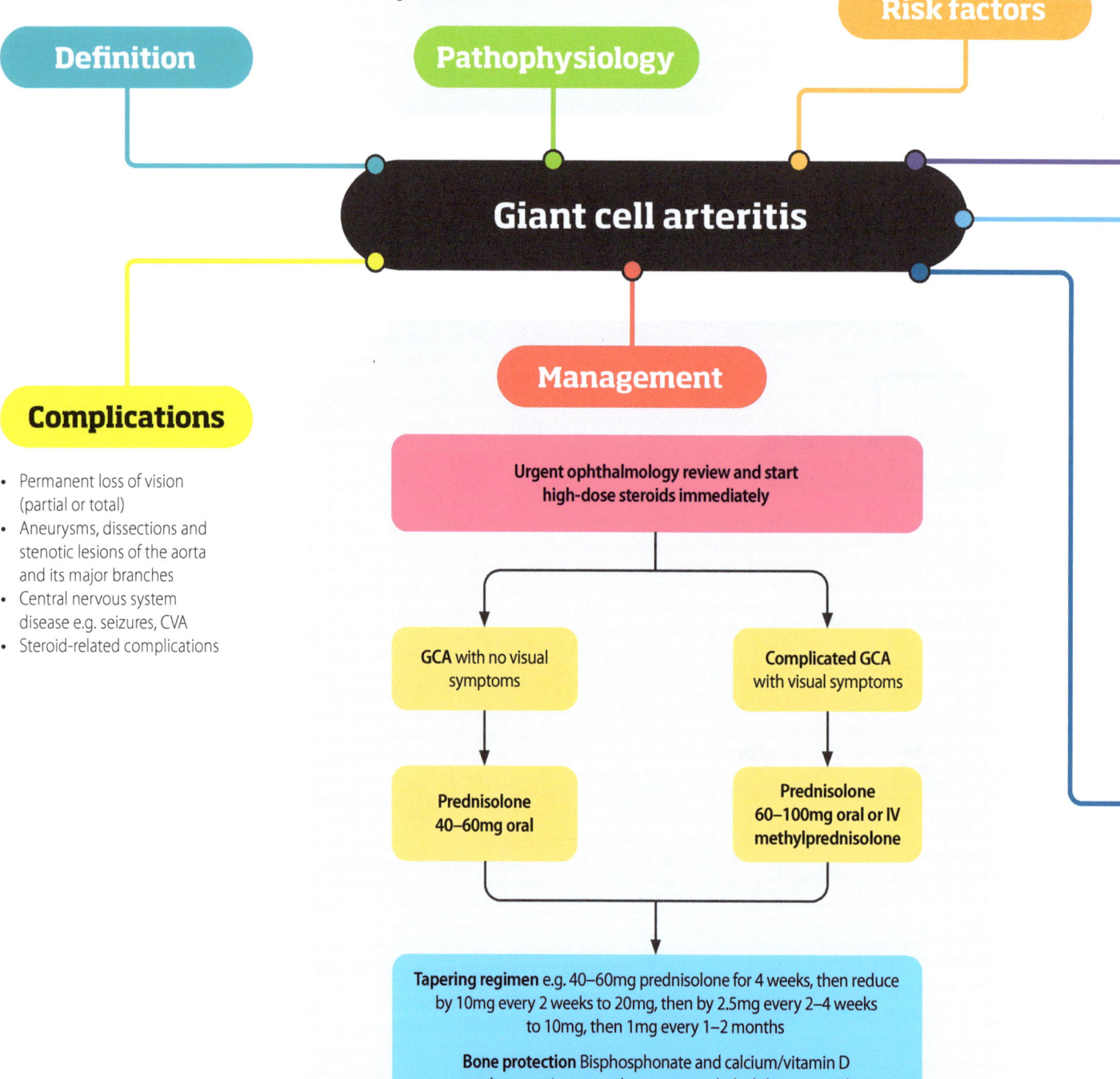

Definition

Giant cell arteritis (GCA) is a **systemic immune-mediated vasculitis** affecting medium- and large-sized arteries, particularly the carotid artery and its extracranial branches. GCA can cause sudden vision loss and is therefore a medical emergency.

Pathophysiology

- GCA is an autoimmune disorder where exposure to an unknown environmental trigger causes breakdown of immune tolerance, resulting in an autoimmune reaction against the arterial wall
- GCA mainly affects the extracranial branches of the carotid artery, specifically the **temporal artery**
- The histopathological hallmark of GCA is the predominance of mononuclear infiltrates of **granulomas** consisting of mainly multinucleated giant cells

Risk factors

- **Polymyalgia rheumatica (PMR):** 50% of patients with GCA have PMR
- Age: almost exclusively in patients **>50 years**
- Females: 3× more common than males
- Caucasians

Complications

- Permanent loss of vision (partial or total)
- Aneurysms, dissections and stenotic lesions of the aorta and its major branches
- Central nervous system disease e.g. seizures, CVA
- Steroid-related complications

Giant cell arteritis

Management

Urgent ophthalmology review and start high-dose steroids immediately

GCA with no visual symptoms

Prednisolone 40–60mg oral

Complicated GCA with visual symptoms

Prednisolone 60–100mg oral or IV methylprednisolone

Tapering regimen e.g. 40–60mg prednisolone for 4 weeks, then reduce by 10mg every 2 weeks to 20mg, then by 2.5mg every 2–4 weeks to 10mg, then 1mg every 1–2 months

Bone protection Bisphosphonate and calcium/vitamin D supplementation strongly recommended while on steroids to prevent osteoporosis

Symptoms

- **Headache** (85%) Usually one-sided (often in the temporal or occipital region), commonly worse at night and tender to touch
- **Visual symptoms** Amaurosis fugax (sudden transient loss of vision in one eye), blurred vision, diplopia, partial or complete loss of vision
- **Jaw and tongue claudication** (65%)
- **Systemic features of PMR** Muscle ache, fever, fatigue, weight loss

Signs

- Scalp tenderness/tenderness over the temporal artery
- Decreased temporal artery pulse
- Swollen temporal artery (see *Fig. 1*).
- Carotid bruits (may be heard on auscultation)
- Muscle/joint tenderness (if PMR also present)
- Abdominal bruits or abnormal pulsatile aneurysm swelling
- Pale optic disc

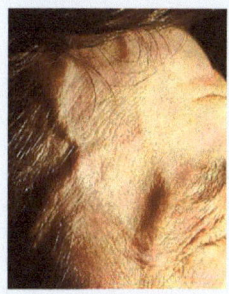

Fig. 1 Swollen temporal artery in a patient with GCA

Clinical features

Notes

Diagnostic ACR criteria (NEAT)

1. **N**ew-onset headache (localised pain in head)
2. **E**levated ESR (≥50mm/h)
3. **A**bnormal artery biopsy: mononuclear cell infiltration or granulomatous lesions (usually with multinucleated giant cells)
4. **A**ge of onset ≥50 years
5. **T**emporal artery abnormality (tenderness on palpation or ↓pulsation)

(3/5 → high risk of GCA)

Investigations

- **Bloods** ESR elevated (typically >50mm/h but <30mm/h in 10% of patients); CRP may be elevated; FBC: may show normocytic normochromic anaemia, thrombocytosis may be present
- **Colour duplex US** Shown to be relatively accurate at diagnosing GCA
- **Temporal artery biopsy** May show a typical appearance of intermittent inflammation ('skip lesions'); may be negative in approximately 20–30% of cases

Gout is a disorder of purine metabolism characterised by a raised uric acid level in the blood (**hyperuricaemia**) and the deposition of urate crystals in joints and other tissues, such as soft connective tissues or the urinary tract. Gouty arthritis is arthritis due to urate crystals in joints.

- There is a strong association between gouty arthropathy and hyperuricaemia which is often asymptomatic for years before the initial attack
- The build-up of urate crystals can be caused by decreased renal excretion e.g. chronic kidney disease, diuretics and overproduction of uric acid e.g. myeloproliferative disorders or overconsumption of purine-rich food that are metabolised to urate
- When these crystals deposit in the synovial fluid of joints they cause gouty arthritis

- Male gender: 4:1
- Diet: meat, seafood, oily fish and yeast products
- Alcohol
- Drugs: e.g. diuretics, chemotherapy
- Obesity
- Hypertension
- Coronary heart disease
- Diabetes mellitus
- Chronic kidney disease
- High triglycerides
- Heart failure
- Psoriasis
- Lesch–Nyhan syndrome

Definition

Pathophysiology

Risk factors

Gout

Complications

- Chronic urate nephropathy
- Severe degenerative arthritis
- Secondary infections
- Recurrent painful episodes
- Carpal tunnel syndrome (rare)
- Nerve or spinal cord impingement

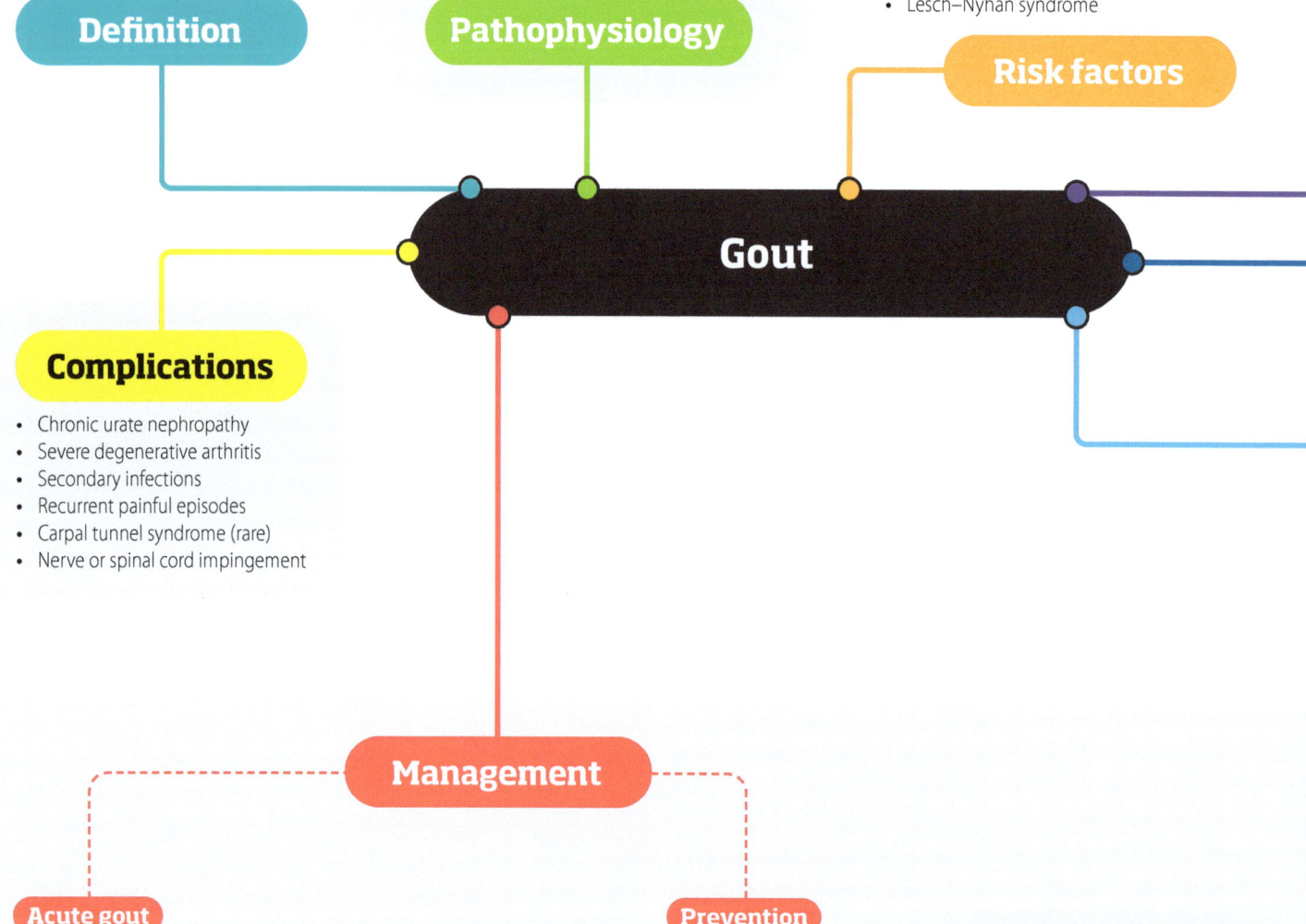

Management

Acute gout

- **NSAIDs** 1st-line treatment for acute gout in the absence of contraindications
- **Colchicine** Used if NSAIDs are contraindicated, not tolerated or have previously been ineffective
- **Corticosteroids** If NSAIDs and colchicine are contraindicated e.g. in renal impairment; a course of oral corticosteroids or intra-articular steroids can be given
- **Canakinumab** A recombinant monoclonal antibody licensed for use in patients whose condition has not responded adequately to treatment with NSAIDs or colchicine, or who are intolerant of them
- **Paracetamol** With/without codeine in addition to drugs above, solely for pain relief

Prevention

- **Lifestyle changes** Lose weight, ↓excessive consumption of food rich in purines e.g. meat and seafood, ↓alcohol consumption, regular exercise, smoking cessation, stop offending drugs if possible
- **Allopurinol** 1st line; recommended for recurrent attacks (≥2 attacks in 12 months), tophi, renal disease, uric acid renal stones and prophylaxis if on cytotoxics or diuretics; start 1–2 weeks after acute gout attack has resolved; co-prescribe NSAID or low-dose colchicine for at least 1 month to prevent gout attack; avoid stopping allopurinol in subsequent gout attacks
- **Febuxostat** 2nd-line therapy if allopurinol is contraindicated/not tolerated
- **Uricosurics** e.g. Sulfinpyrazone, work by increasing renal urate excretion

Acute gout

- Presents as an excruciatingly painful red joint that is tender and warm to touch (see *Fig. 1*)
- Most commonly affects the metatarsophalangeal joint (podagra) in about 70% of cases
- Other common sites include small joints of the foot (mid-tarsal), hands, ankle, knee and elbow

Chronic gout

- Usually affects more than one joint (polyarthritis)
- Tophi (subcutaneous deposition of uric acid crystals) (see *Fig. 2*)
- Fever and malaise may be present (uncommon)
- Uric acid kidney stones may also develop

Clinical features

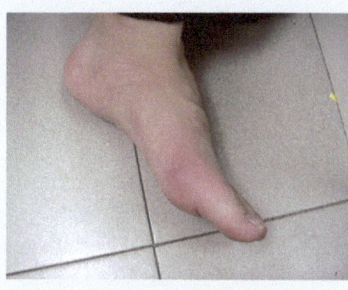

Fig. 1 Gout of the big toe

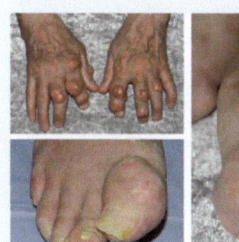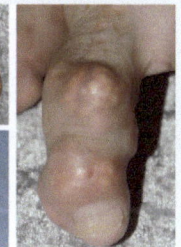

Fig. 2 Chronic tophaceous gout

Pseudogout

- The deposition of **calcium pyrophosphate crystals** in the joint space
- Presents in a similar way to gout but usually affects larger joints e.g. knee, wrist and ankle
- X-ray may show **chondrocalcinosis** (calcification of cartilage) and OA changes
- Aspiration of the joint and synovial fluid analysis → **positively birefringent rhomboid-shaped crystals** under polarised light microscopy
- Acute attacks are as per gout, but allopurinol has no role in prevention of pseudogout

Investigations

Bloods

- Serum urate is often ↑ but may fall during an acute attack; useful for monitoring response to treatment
- Fasting glucose and lipids to rule out hyperglycaemia and hyperlipidaemia, as gout is commonly associated with metabolic syndrome

X-ray

- Early: soft tissue swelling
- Later: punched-out erosions, areas of sclerosis, tophi
- US/CT/MRI: can identify urate deposition, structural joint damage and joint inflammation in gout

Joint aspiration and synovial fluid analysis

- Used to rule out septic arthritis as a differential diagnosis
- Provides definitive diagnosis of gout characterised by presence of **negatively birefringent crystals** under polarised light microscopy

Osteoarthritis (OA) is the most common form of arthritis and is the major cause of impaired mobility. It is a condition characterised by cartilage damage and joint space narrowing resulting in pain, functional limitation and impaired quality of life. It can affect any joint but the hip, knee, lumbar/cervical spine and wrist joints are most commonly affected.

- OA occurs when there is an imbalance between joint breakdown and sufficient repair process
- Normal articulating cartilage (hyaline cartilage) undergoes turnover in which 'worn out' collagen and other matrix components are degraded and replaced by chondrocyte cells
- Both genetic and environmental factors can stimulate apoptosis of chondrocytes therefore disrupting the normal cartilage repair mechanism
- Certain cytokines, e.g. IL-1 and TNF-alpha, as well as protease enzymes, e.g. metalloproteinase, are found to be increased in the cartilage of patients with OA triggering direct cartilage damage
- Eventually cartilage destruction exposes underlying bone

Definition

Pathophysiology

Osteoarthritis

Investigations

Management

Non-pharmacological

- Education and advice
- Exercise
- Weight loss
- Physiotherapy
- TENS
- Aids and devices

Pharmacological

- Paracetamol and/or topical NSAIDs/capsaicin
- Addition of weak opioid e.g. codeine
- Oral NSAID + proton pump inhibitor
- Intra-articular corticosteroid injections

Surgical

- Joint replacement: most commonly hip, knee and base of thumb joints; the ankle joint can be fused or replaced
- Arthroscopy lavage and debridement: should only be referred if they have OA of the knee with a clear history of mechanical locking

- **X-ray** (**LOSS**, see *Fig. 2*):
  - **L**oss of joint space
  - **O**steophytes
  - **S**ubchondral cysts
  - **S**ubchondral sclerosis
- **Bloods** FBC (usually normal), CRP/ESR (usually normal), RF/anti-CCP (negative)
- **MRI** Can demonstrate early thinning of the cartilage
- **Arthroscopy** Cartilage loss and erosion
- **Joint aspiration** May be considered for swollen joints to exclude other causes such as septic arthritis and gout; in OA there is sterile viscous fluid, WCC may slightly elevated

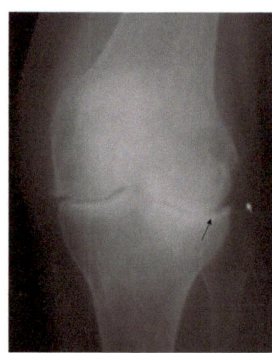

Fig. 2 X-ray changes associated with OA characterised by the loss of joint space (arrow), osteophytes and subchondral sclerosis

Risk factors

Systemic

- **Age** Risk increases with age
- **Gender** Polyarticular OA is more common in women
- **Family history** 40–60% of 'common OA' is thought to have a hereditary component
- **Bone density** Increased bone density, e.g. Paget's disease, increases risk of OA; reduced bone density, e.g. osteoporosis, reduces risk of OA

Mechanical

- **Obesity** Places mechanical stress on joint cartilage
- **Injury** Ligament damage or fractures can lead to abnormal stress on joint cartilage
- **Joint damage** Due to underlying disease, e.g. RA, Paget's disease
- **Joint site** Weight-bearing joints are at increased risk of OA, e.g. hip and knee joint
- **Occupation** Cleaners have increased risk of hip, knee and shoulder OA; hairdressers have increased risk of hand OA; farmers have increased risk of hip OA

Clinical features

Symptoms

- Joint pain: typically worse on movement, load bearing and at the end of the day
- Joint stiffness: typically in the morning or after rest <30 min
- Reduced joint function
- Joint instability

Signs

- Periarticular tenderness
- Crepitus
- ↓Range of movement
- Muscle wasting

- Joint deformity and instability
- Squaring of the thumb
- Swelling of the proximal interphalangeal (PIP; Bouchard's nodes) and distal interphalangeal (DIP; Heberden's nodes) joints (see *Fig. 1*)
- Effusion

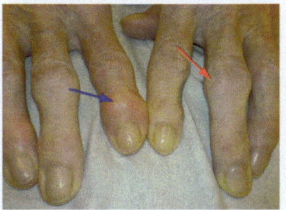

Fig. 1 Heberden's nodes (DIP joints) (blue arrow on left) and Bouchard's nodes (PIP joints) (red arrow on right) due to osteophyte formation

Notes

Osteoarthritis

Definition

Osteoporosis is a progressive **systemic skeletal disorder** characterised by **low bone mass** and micro-architectural deterioration of bone tissue with resultant increase in **bone fragility** and susceptibility to fracture. It exists when bone mineral density (BMD) values are reduced by >2.5 standard deviations below that observed in young healthy adults.

Pathophysiology

- Osteoporosis develops when there is excessive bone resorption by **osteoclast cells** at a rate that exceeds bone formation by **osteoblast cells**
- This results in decreased bone mass and incomplete bone remodelling resulting in increased bone fragility and susceptibility to fracture

Causes

Primary

- **Type 1**: **postmenopausal (most common)** ↑Osteoclast activity; distal radius and vertebral fractures common
- **Type 2**: **age-related 'senile' osteoporosis** ↓Osteoblast activity; neck of femur fractures common

Secondary

Underlying cause present: hormonal, nutritional, drug related or inherited

Osteoporosis

Management

Conservative measures

- Smoking cessation
- Alcohol reduction
- Diet: food rich in vitamin D/calcium
- Weight-bearing exercises
- Physiotherapy
- Reducing fall risk and home assessment
- Hip protectors

Pharmacological

- **Calcium/vitamin D supplements**
- **Bisphosphonates** Usually 1st-line; can be taken once weekly (alendronate), once monthly (risedronate) or yearly IV injections (zoledronate)
- **Denosumab** A monoclonal antibody that reduces osteoclast activity which is given by 6-monthly SC injections; it may be a suitable option in women who are unable to comply with instructions for bisphosphonates
- **Strontium ranelate** Used for the prevention of osteoporotic fractures in postmenopausal women with osteoporosis but where other medications are not tolerated; it is less commonly used as there are increased risks such as venous thromboembolism (VTE), PE and MI
- **Teriparatide** A parathyroid hormone analogue; intermittent exposure activates osteoblasts resulting in new bone formation; it is reserved for severe cases
- Others: raloxifene (selective oestrogen receptor modulator), hormone replacement therapy (HRT) and calcitonin are less commonly used

Note: The FRAX® tool helps to identify people who may be at risk of developing osteoporosis. It uses risk factors with DEXA measurements to estimate 10-year probability of a fracture. It is useful in aiding clinical decision-making about the use of pharmacological therapies in patients with reduced BMD.

Surgical

- Fixation of fractures or hip replacements (for neck of femur fractures)
- Kyphoplasty: balloon or cement for restoration of vertebral height

Female sex, family history and
SHATTERED:
- **S**teroid use, **S**moking
- **H**yperthyroidism
- **A**ge >50, **A**lcohol
- **T**hin (BMI <22)
- **T**estosterone deficiency
- **E**arly menopause
- **R**enal failure and liver failure
- **E**rosive bone disease e.g. RA, myeloma
- **D**eficiency of calcium or vitamin **D**, **D**iabetes

Usually asymptomatic unless a fracture is present:
- **Vertebral fracture** → Back pain, reduced height, kyphosis, respiratory difficulty
- **Hip fracture** → Painful, shortened and externally rotated hip
- **Wrist fracture** → Pain and deformity

Risk factors

Clinical features

Investigations

Bloods

- FBC: ↑WCC in inflammatory disease e.g. RA, myeloma
- CRP/ESR: ↑ in inflammatory disease e.g. RA, myeloma
- U&Es: renal failure is a risk factor for osteoporosis
- LFTs: liver failure is a risk factor for osteoporosis
- TFTs: rule out hypo/hyperthyroidism
- PTH: ↑ in hyperparathyroidism
- Vitamin D: deficiency is a risk factor
- Calcium: normal
- Phosphate: normal
- ALP: normal
- FSH: ↑ in menopause
- Testosterone: to rule out testosterone deficiency in men

X-ray

- To confirm suspected fractures
- Can comment whether bones appear osteopenic but cannot determine osteoporosis from X-rays

DEXA scan

The gold standard for diagnosing osteoporosis; dual-energy X-ray absorptiometry is a means of measuring bone mineral density; two scores are calculated:

1. T-score:
- Diagnostic of osteoporosis
- Gives the number of standard deviations of the BMD below that of a young healthy adult
- Interpretation:
  - **>0** BMD better than reference population
  - **0 to –1** No evidence of osteoporosis
  - **–1 to –2.5** Osteopenia
  - **–2.5 or below** Osteoporosis
  - **–2.5 or below plus fragility fracture** Established osteoporosis

1. Z-score:
- Compares an individual's results to others of the same age and gender; a Z-score of <–1.5 raises concerns of factors other than ageing and gender contributing to osteoporosis

Paget's disease is a common bone disease characterised by focal increases in bone remodelling resulting in the abnormal production of bone which is mechanically weak. The most commonly affected bones include the pelvis, spine, skull, femur and tibia.

- Both genetic and environmental factors are thought to play a role
- Autosomal dominant inheritance has also been described in some families
- Sequestosome1 (*SQSTM1*) is the most important gene mutation involved
- Mechanical stress and infections from viruses, e.g. paramyxoviruses, may play a role
- There are thought to be 3 phases involved in the pathophysiology:
  - **Lytic phase** Transient ↑osteoclast activity causing ↑bone resorption and marked ↑ in ALP
  - **Mixed phase** Both osteoclastic and osteoblastic activity, with ↑ levels of bone turnover leading to deposition of structurally abnormal bone
  - **Sclerotic phase** A chronic sclerotic phase, during which bone formation outstrips bone resorption

- The mean age of onset is approximately 55 years
- The highest prevalence is in England, USA, Australia and New Zealand; it is rare in Asia, Scandinavia and most of Latin America
- The male to female ratio is approx. 3:2

Definition

Pathophysiology

Epidemiology

Paget's disease

Complications

Common

- Bone pain (most common)
- Bone deformity and enlargement: typically the pelvis, lumbar spine, skull, femur and tibia
- ↑Temperature over affected bone due to hypervascularity
- Pathological fractures
- 2° OA due to Paget's disease surrounding the joint
- Hearing loss and tinnitus if Paget's disease affects the skull bones and compresses the vestibulocochlear nerve

Rarer

- Spinal stenosis
- Nerve compression syndromes and cauda equina syndrome
- Hypercalcaemia
- High-output cardiac failure
- Paraplegia
- Osteosarcoma

Management

Conservative

- Orthotic devices, sticks and walkers may be useful for Paget's disease of the legs
- Adequate intake of calcium and vitamin D

Pharmacological

- Bisphosphonates to reduce bone turnover, e.g. oral risedronate or IV zoledronate
- NSAIDs and paracetamol for pain relief

Surgical

Surgical procedures include **fracture fixation** (pathological fracture), **joint replacement** (secondary OA) and **osteotomy** (deformity)

Symptoms

- Paget's disease is usually asymptomatic (70–90%) and therefore diagnosed on incidental abnormal X-ray or biochemical findings (↑alkaline phosphatase)
- Bone pain and deformity
- Pathological fractures
- ↑Skin temperature over affected bone

Signs

- Head signs: ↑skull size, frontal bossing, deep-set eyes, large maxilla with prominent arches
- Bowing of long bones and kyphosis (see *Fig. 1*)
- Increased temperature over affected bone

- Weber's and Rinne's test: to elicit possible sensorineural hearing loss
- Signs of other complications such as OA and spinal cord compression

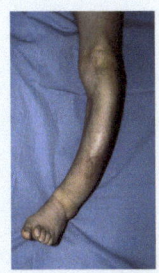

Fig. 1 Clinical bowing of the tibia in Paget's disease

Clinical features

Investigations

- **Blood tests** ↑ALP; bone-specific ALP (if known liver disease), phosphate and calcium are normal (see *Table 1*)

Table 1 Blood test results in conditions affecting bone

Condition	Ca^{2+}	PO_4^{3-}	ALP	PTH
Osteoporosis	→	→	→	→
Osteomalacia	↓	↓	↑	↑
Paget's disease	→	→	↑	→
Hypoparathyroidism	↓	↑	→	↓
Pseudohypoparathyroidism	↓	→	→	→↑

- **X-ray** Localised enlargement, patchy cortical thickening with sclerosis, osteolysis and deformity, advancing lytic lesion in the long bones (see *Fig. 2*)
- **MRI** For suspected spinal stenosis and cord compression

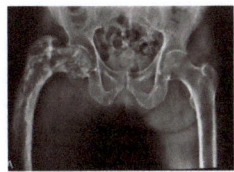

Fig. 2 X-ray of Paget's disease of the femur

Definition

Polymyalgia rheumatica (PMR) is an inflammatory condition of unknown cause which is characterised by severe bilateral pain and morning stiffness of the shoulder, neck and pelvic girdle. Giant cell arteritis (GCA) is a more serious condition that often co-exists with PMR.

Pathophysiology

- The cause of PMR is unknown
- Given the association of PMR with GCA, it is thought that mechanisms similar to those contributing to GCA may be involved
- Both PMR and GCA are associated with specific alleles of HLA-DR4
- ↑IL-6 in serum and temporal artery biopsy specimens has been observed in both PMR and GCA patients, suggesting an inflammatory role for IL-6
- The muscles in PMR are histopathologically normal; proximal upper-extremity symptoms in PMR essentially result from glenohumeral synovitis, subacromial bursitis and biceps tenosynovitis, while pelvic girdle symptoms arise from hip synovitis and bursitis

Risk factors

- **Age** Almost exclusively in people aged >50 years; mean age of onset is approx. 73
- **Gender** Female: male is approximately 3:1
- **GCA** Approx. 40–60% of patients with GCA have PMR
- **Ethnicity** Mainly in people of north European ancestry, although it can occur in any ethnic group

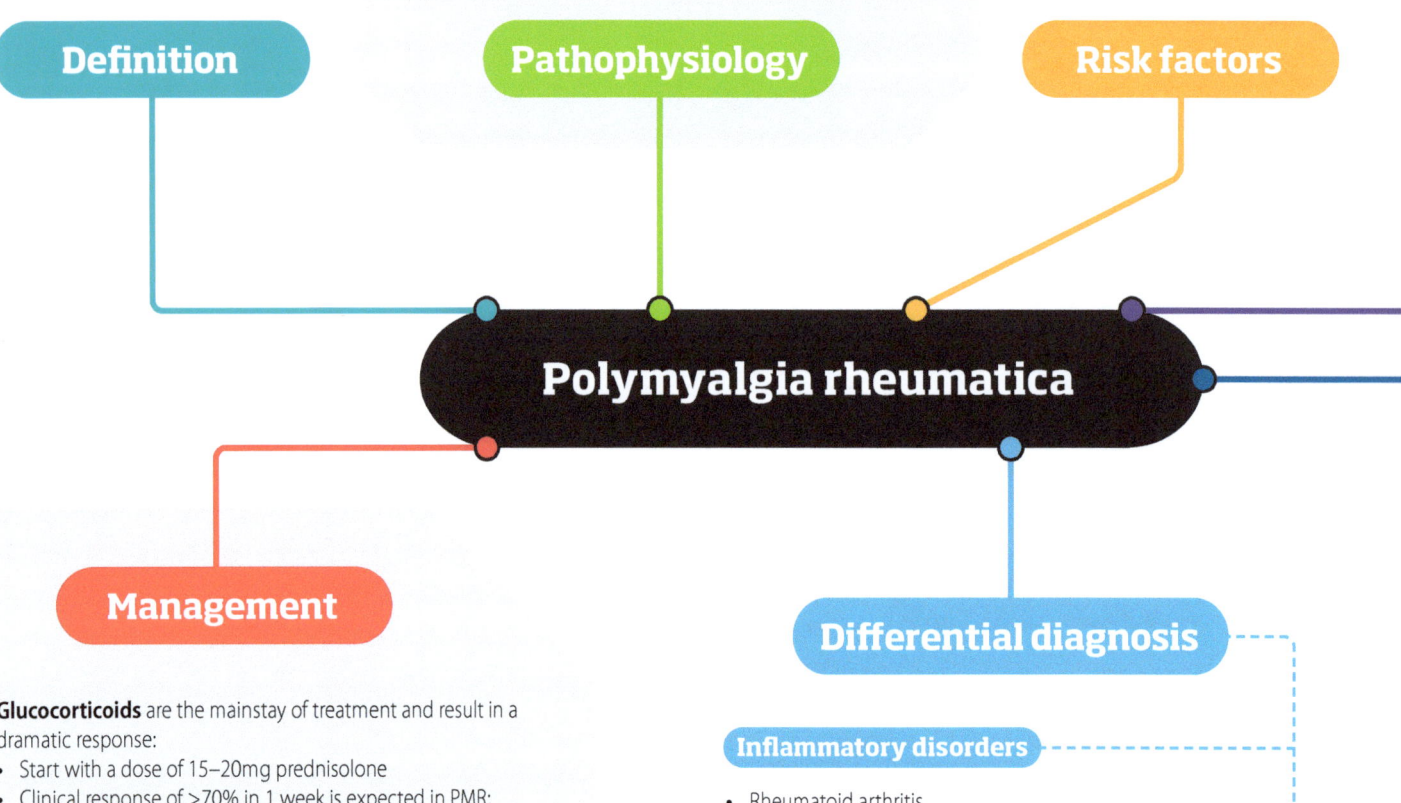

Polymyalgia rheumatica

Management

Glucocorticoids are the mainstay of treatment and result in a dramatic response:

- Start with a dose of 15–20mg prednisolone
- Clinical response of >70% in 1 week is expected in PMR; inflammatory markers should normalise within 4 weeks
- The dose of prednisolone should be tapered down slowly for 3–6 months to a low maintenance level which is sustained for a further 6–12 months then gradually reduced over the next 6 months with the aim of stopping altogether
- Due to long-term use of steroids, bone-protective agents, e.g. bisphosphonates, and gastroprotective agents, e.g. PPIs, should be co-prescribed
- Steroid-sparing agents such as methotrexate and azathioprine may be used
- Patients should be monitored for the emergence of GCA

Differential diagnosis

Inflammatory disorders

- Rheumatoid arthritis
- Spondyloarthropathy
- SLE
- Scleroderma
- Sjögren syndrome
- GCA
- Dermatomyositis, polymyositis

Non-inflammatory disorders

- Degenerative disease: OA, spinal spondylosis
- Rotator cuff disease
- Drug-induced myalgia e.g. statins
- Infections, including viral syndromes, osteomyelitis, tuberculosis
- Paraneoplastic syndromes
- Amyloidosis
- Chronic pain syndromes, fibromyalgia, depression
- Endocrinopathy and metabolic bone disease: hyper/hypothyroidism, hyper/hypoparathyroidism, osteomalacia

- Bilateral shoulder or thigh muscle aching pain for ≥1 month (see *Fig. 1*)
- Morning stiffness >45 min
- Systemic features:
  - Loss of appetite
  - Weight loss
  - Low-grade malaise
  - Signs and symptoms of GCA
  - Depression
- Prompt response to corticosteroids

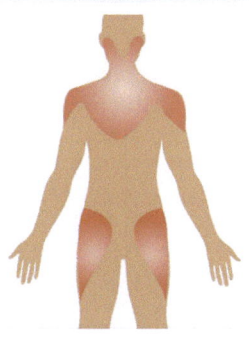

Fig. 1 Typical distribution of pain in patients with PMR

Investigations are essential to support the diagnosis of PMR but also to rule out any other possible diagnosis:
- **Bloods** ESR/plasma viscosity/CRP (usually raised but may be normal), FBC, U&Es, LFTs, bone profile (exclude metabolic bone disease), TFTs (exclude thyroid diseases), protein electrophoresis (exclude myeloma), CK normal (exclude polymyositis and dermatomyositis), ANA (exclude SLE), RF, anti-CCP (exclude RA)
- **Urinalysis**
- **EMG** Normal
- **US** Scan of shoulders and/or hips if diagnosis is unclear; typical findings include subacromial bursitis and biceps tendon tenosynovitis and, less frequently, synovitis of the glenohumeral joint or trochanteric bursitis

Clinical features

Investigations

Notes

Polymyalgia rheumatica

Polymyositis (PM) is a rare autoimmune connective tissue disease characterised by inflammation and weakness primarily of the skeletal muscle. It may however affect other parts of the body such as the joints, the oesophagus, the lungs and heart. When PM pathology extends to the skin, the condition is termed **dermatomyositis (DM)**. DM may co-exist with other connective tissue disorders.

- Remains largely unclear but both environmental and genetic factors are likely to play a part in the disease process
- Involvement of immune mechanisms is supported by the presence of T cells, macrophages and dendritic cells in the muscle biopsy of these patients and by the presence of autoantibodies, and by HLA-B8 and HLA-DR3 being a strong genetic risk factor
- It is thought to be a T-cell-mediated cytotoxic process directed against muscle fibres which may be triggered by viruses; this results in capillary obliteration and consequent muscle infarction leading to weakness of the skeletal muscle
- It may be idiopathic or associated with connective tissue disorders such as SLE
- DM in patients over the age of 60 years may be suggestive of an underlying systemic malignancy (typically ovarian, breast and lung cancer)

- Family history
- Female sex (2.5:1)
- Age: DM has a bimodal distribution with peaks at 5–15 and 40–60 years; PM mainly occurs at 40–60 and is rare in children
- Black people: PM and DM are 3× more common in Black people than in Caucasians
- Underlying malignancy
- UV light: the rashes in DM often occur in sun-exposed areas
- Infections: viral infections e.g. HIV, simian retroviruses, Coxsackie B

Definition

Pathophysiology

Risk factors

Polymyositis and dermatomyositis

Management

Investigations

Non-pharmacological

- Sun-blocking agents should be used for DM
- Encourage regular exercise
- Physiotherapist and occupational therapist involvement
- Speech and language therapist involvement to help with dysphonia and dysphagia
- Monitor CK levels
- Screen thoroughly for malignancy in DM and treat

Pharmacological

- **Steroids** High-dose prednisolone 1st line; dose should be gradually reduced according to clinical response and CK levels

- **DMARDs** If steroids fail, azathioprine, cyclophosphamide, methotrexate can be used; for lung disease, an aggressive combination regimen including ciclosporin A or tacrolimus + cyclophosphamide is recommended to be added to corticosteroids
- **Biological agents** TNF-alpha antagonists, IV immunoglobulin and rituximab can be used for treatment of cutaneous DM

- **Bloods:**
  - **Enzymes** CK can be up to 50× higher than upper limit of normal; rarely normal in active disease and the level is usually a good indicator of disease activity; levels of other enzymes may also be raised: ALT, AST, LDH and aldolase
  - **Inflammatory markers** ESR, CRP (may be raised)
  - **Autoantibodies** ANA (+ve in 60%), anti-Mi-2 antibodies (highly specific for DM, but are only seen in around 25% of patients), anti-Jo-1 antibodies (not commonly seen in DM – they are more common in PM where they are seen in a pattern of disease associated with lung involvement, Raynaud's and fever)
  - **Tumour markers** To screen for malignancy in older patients with DM e.g. CA-125 (ovarian), CA-15-3 (breast cancer) and CA-19-9 (pancreatic malignancy)
- **EMG** Myopathic changes (reduced duration, amplitude and number of action potentials)
- **Muscle biopsy** Confirms diagnosis, shows evidence of myositis (muscle necrosis, phagocytosis of muscle fibres and inflammatory infiltrate)
- **MRI** May show areas of inflammation in muscle

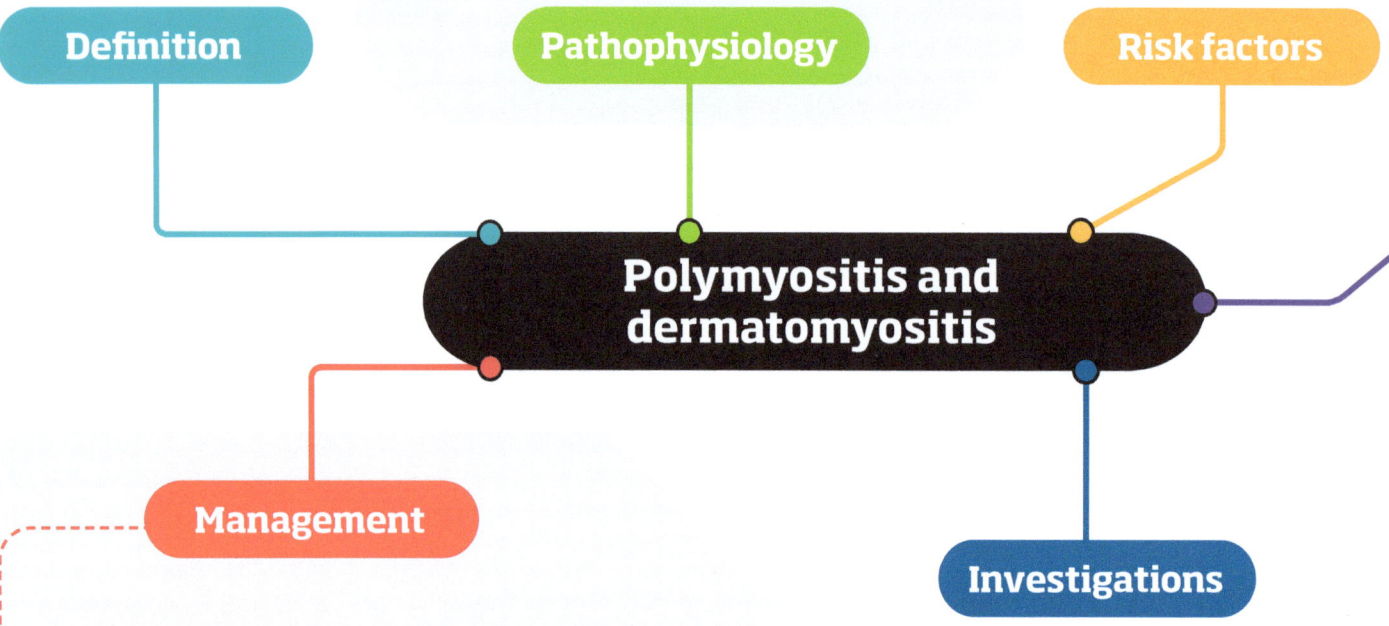

Polymyositis

- Proximal symmetrical muscle weakness
- Muscle pain
- Respiratory muscle weakness
- Raynaud's
- Dysphagia
- Dysphonia
- Interstitial lung disease e.g. fibrosing alveolitis or organising pneumonia
- Systemic features: fever, fatigue and weight loss (due to oesophageal dysmotility)

Dermatomyositis

Presents with above features plus:
- **Gottron's papules** (see *Fig. 1*): scaly, erythematous eruptions particularly over the extensor surfaces of the MCP, PIP and DIP joints
- **Heliotrope rash:** violet discolouration of the eyelids, occasionally accompanied by periorbital oedema (see *Fig. 2*)
- Photosensitivity
- Nail-fold erythema
- Macular rash over back and shoulder

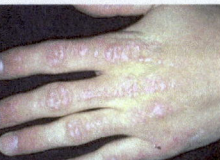

Fig. 1 Gottron's papules

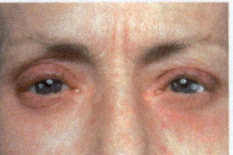

Fig. 2 Heliotrope rash

Clinical features

Notes

Polymyositis and dermatomyositis

Psoriatic arthritis is a **seronegative inflammatory arthritis** affecting the joints and connective tissue and is associated with psoriasis of the skin or nails. A variety of joint patterns are recognised in psoriatic arthritis, although these may overlap.

- The pathophysiology of psoriatic arthritis is poorly understood
- Like other autoimmune conditions, genetically susceptible individuals are exposed to an environmental trigger (bacteria, stress or entheseal-related peptide) which in turn activates the immune system
- This results in T-cell infiltration and chemokine/cytokine release
- HLA and other genes may determine the exact pattern of tissue involvement

- Psoriasis is the strongest risk factor; may occur before (70%), after (25%) or at the same time as joint symptoms (5%)
- Western White population
- Middle age (35–55 years)
- Family history: approximately 40% of individuals with psoriasis or psoriatic arthritis have relatives with psoriasis or psoriatic arthritis; there is an association between HLA-B27 and psoriatic arthritis

Definition

Pathophysiology

Risk factors

Psoriatic arthritis

Management

Non-pharmacological

- **Physical exercise** Helps to maintain mobility and reduce stiffness
- **Physiotherapy** Helps to improve range of motion and pain, as well as muscle strengthening of joints
- **Surgery** Synovectomy and rarely joint replacement

Pharmacological

- **NSAIDs** 1st line for pain relief and soft tissue inflammation
- **DMARDs** 1st line in active disease and should be given at an early stage e.g. methotrexate, sulfasalazine or leflunomide

- **Intra-articular steroids** Adjunctive therapy; systemic steroids at the lowest effective dose may be used but with caution
- **Anti-TNF-alpha** e.g. Adalimumab, etanercept, golimumab and infliximab should be considered in patients with active arthritis and an inadequate response to at least one synthetic DMARD, such as methotrexate
- **Ustekinumab** Monoclonal antibody directed against interleukin (IL)-12/23; it can be used alone or in combination with methotrexate for active disease; treatment with TNF-alpha inhibitors is contraindicated

Investigations

Bloods

- **ESR/CRP** Normal or raised (in active disease)
- **RF/anti-CCP** Negative
- **ANA** Negative
- **Serum IgA** Increase in about two-thirds of sufferers
- **HLA-B27** May aid in diagnosis but needs to be interpreted with care

Imaging

- **X-ray** Soft tissue swelling in early disease; erosion of the DIP joint and periarticular new bone formation, osteolysis and 'pencil-in-cup deformity' (see *Fig. 5*).
- **MRI/CT** May be more specific and sensitive in picking up subtle signs

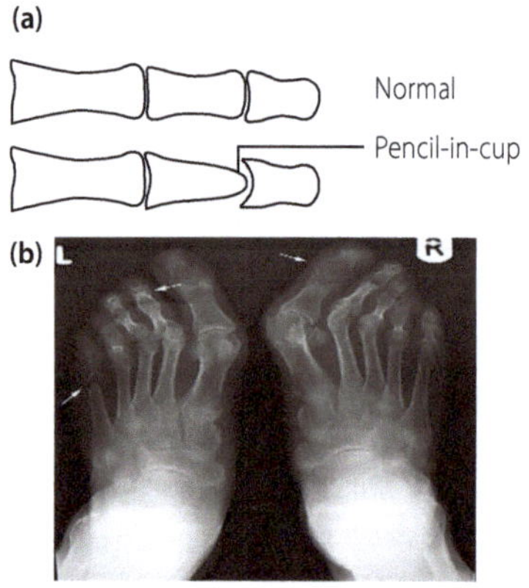

(a) Normal / Pencil-in-cup

(b)

Fig. 5 (a) Diagrammatic representation and **(b)** X-ray (arrows) showing pencil-in-cup deformity caused by underlying osteolysis

General signs and symptoms

- **Joint pain and stiffness**
  Typically prolonged morning stiffness (>30min), improvement with use and recurrence with prolonged rest
- **Dactylitis** or **'sausage digits'** (see *Fig. 1*)
- **Enthesitis** Pain, stiffness and tenderness of insertions into bone e.g. the Achilles tendon
- Extra-articular features:
  - **Psoriatic skin rash** (see *Fig. 2*)
  - **Nail changes** Pitting, onycholysis, hyperkeratosis
  - **Uveitis**

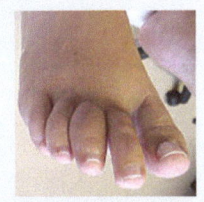

Fig. 1 Dactylitis of the toes

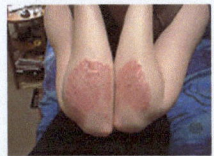

Fig. 2 Psoriatic skin rash

Clinical features

Characteristic patterns of psoriatic arthritis (DR SAM)

- **D**IP joint disease (5–10%) Predominantly DIP joint involvement (see *Fig. 3*); affects men more than women; strongly associated with onycholysis
- **R**heumatoid pattern (25%) Presentation very similar to RA with symmetrical small joint arthritis affecting the MCP, wrist and PIP joints; distinguishing features are lack of rheumatoid nodules, RF negative and often presence of psoriasis
- **S**pondyloarthritis (20%) May present with isolated sacroiliitis, typical or atypical AS
- **A**symmetrical oligoarthritis (50%) Large joint inflammatory arthritis often with ankle, knee, wrist or shoulder involvement
- **M**utilans arthritis (1–5%) Most rare but severe form (see *Fig. 4*); osteolysis results in destruction of the small joints of the digits with shortening

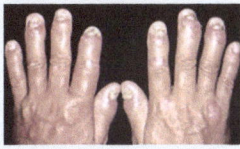

Fig. 3 DIP involvement in psoriatic arthritis – highly characteristic

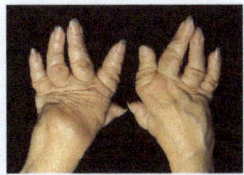

Fig. 4 Hands showing psoriatic arthritis mutilans

Notes

Psoriatic arthritis

Reactive arthritis is a form of **seronegative spondyloarthritis** that develops in response to an extra-articular infection, typically originating from the gastrointestinal (GI) or genitourinary (GU) tract. It encompasses **Reiter syndrome**, a term which describes a classic triad of urethritis, conjunctivitis and arthritis.

- Reactive arthritis is thought to be caused by an infectious trigger, usually a bacterial GI or GU infection (see *Fig. 1*) in genetically susceptible individuals
- This leads to immune activation and cross-reactivity with self-antigens causing acute inflammation in the affected joint and other tissues e.g. enthesis, skin, mucous membranes and eyes approx. 2–6 weeks after the initial infection
- **HLA-B27** is positive in most patients and not only confers strong risk of reactive arthritis but also predicts the severity and chronicity of the disease

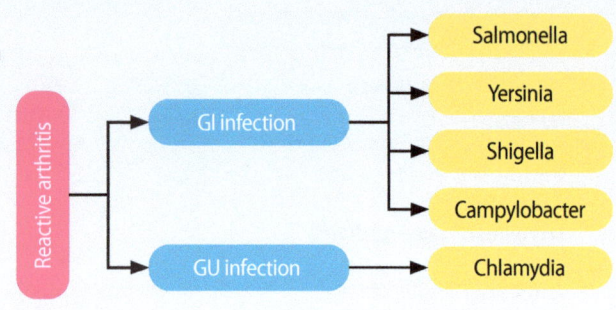

Fig. 1 The key GI and GU bacteria implicated in reactive arthritis

Definition

Pathophysiology

Reactive arthritis

Management

Non-pharmacological

- Rest and splint affected joint(s)
- Physiotherapy

Pharmacological

- **NSAIDs** For pain relief and soft tissue inflammation
- **Corticosteroids** Intra-articular, for instance sacroiliac joints can be injected; a short course of oral corticosteroids can be considered for patients who are unresponsive to NSAIDs or who develop adverse effects; topical corticosteroids can be used to treat skin involvement
- **Antibiotics** To treat an identified causative organism; tetracyclines may be useful for chlamydia urethritis
- **DMARDs** e.g. Sulfasalazine, methotrexate and ciclosporin may be used in patients unresponsive to standard treatments

Investigations

- **Bloods** Raised CRP, ESR, leucocytosis and thrombocytosis (acute phase), ANA, RF and anti-CCP negative, HLA-B27 positive in 75%, serology for chlamydia
- **X-ray** Normal in early stages; marginal erosions, plantar spurs, sacroiliitis and asymmetrical syndesmophytes may occur in chronic cases
- **Joint aspiration** To rule out crystal or septic arthritis; synovial fluid is usually sterile and cloudy with high WCC
- **Throat, stool, urine culture** To identify causative organism
- **MRI** Asymmetrical sacroiliitis and enthesitis (chronic stage)

- **Arthritis** Acute, asymmetrical large joint arthritis (often lower limbs), occurring 2–6 weeks after the infection (most often acute, with malaise, fatigue and fever)
- **Lower back pain** Due to sacroiliitis and spondylitis
- **Enthesitis** Plantar fasciitis and Achilles tendinitis
- **Eyes** Uveitis, episcleritis, keratitis and corneal ulcerations
- **Dactylitis** May occur at one or more toes
- **Urethritis** and **circinate balanitis** (see *Fig. 2*)
- **Mouth ulcers**
- **Nail dystrophy** and **keratoderma blennorrhagica** (see *Fig. 3*)
- **Reiter syndrome** Triad of **conjunctivitis, urethritis** and **reactive arthritis**; although rare, it follows a GU or GI infection; it can be easily remembered using the mnemonic 'can't see, can't wee and can't bend your knee!'

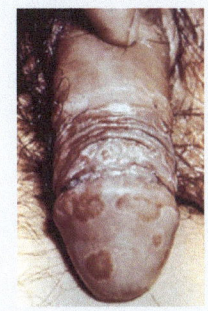

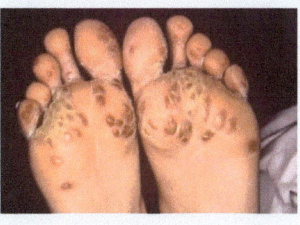

Fig. 3 Keratoderma blennorrhagica

Fig. 2 Circinate balanitis (ulcers and vesicles surrounding the glans penis)

Risk factors

Notes

Reactive arthritis

Definition

Rheumatoid arthritis (RA) is a common chronic inflammatory autoimmune disease characterised by inflammation of the **synovial joints** leading to a typically **symmetrical** and occasionally deforming **peripheral polyarthritis**. It also has a wide variety of extra-articular manifestations.

Pathophysiology

- RA is thought to occur in genetically susceptible individuals who are exposed to an unknown environmental antigen resulting in self-stimulation of the immune system
- T cells seem to be the most important cells in the immune response and release a variety of pro-inflammatory cytokines including TNF-alpha, IL-1 and IL-6
- B cells further the pathogenic process through antigen presentation, and autoantibody and cytokine production
- Joint damage begins at the synovial membrane, where there is an influx and/or local activation of mononuclear cells and the formation of new blood vessels causing synovitis and pannus formation; the pannus destroys bone, whereas enzymes secreted by synoviocytes and chondrocytes degrade cartilage

Risk factors

- **Gender** Women are affected 2–4× more often than men
- **Genetic susceptibility** There are strong associations between HLA-DR4 and HLA-DR1 with RA
- **Cigarette smoking** A strong risk factor for the development of RA
- **Infection** Viral or bacterial infection is a possible trigger for RA
- **Autoantibodies** Rheumatoid factor (RF) and anti-cyclic citrullinated peptide (anti-CCP) may be present in the blood prior to the appearance of arthritis

Rheumatoid arthritis

Prognosis

A number of features have been shown to predict a poor prognosis in patients with RA:
- RF positive
- Poor functional status at presentation
- HLA-DR4
- X-ray: early erosions (e.g. <2 years from onset)
- Extra-articular features
- Insidious onset
- Anti-CCP antibodies

Management

Conservative

- Regular exercise
- Physiotherapy
- Smoking cessation
- Access to multidisciplinary team: including nurse specialist, physiotherapist, rheumatologist, podiatrist and occupational therapist
- Transcutaneous electrical nerve stimulation (TENS)

Medical (see *Table 5*)

- NSAIDs
- Corticosteroids
- DMARDs
- Biological agents

Surgical

- A surgical opinion should be sought in some circumstances if the patient does not respond to non-surgical management
- Surgical procedures include joint prosthesis (e.g. hip and knee), arthroscopy and tendon reconstruction

Articular

- **S**tiffness in joints (particularly in the morning and lasts >1h)
- **S**ymmetrical joint pain
- **S**wollen joints
- **S**mall joints of the hand, feet and wrist mainly affected
- **S**ex Female : male ratio 3:1
- **S**peed Relatively quick onset over weeks to months
- **S**pecific hand signs:
  - Early: swollen MCP, PIP, MTP joints
  - Later: Boutonnière deformity, swan neck deformity, Z-thumb, ulnar deviation (see *Fig. 1*)

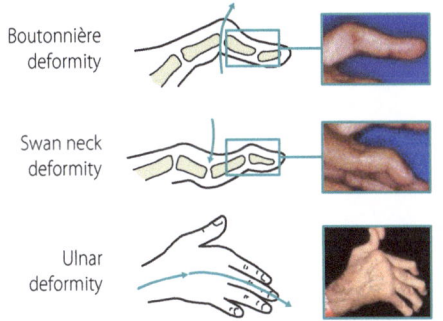

Boutonnière deformity

Swan neck deformity

Ulnar deformity

Fig. 1 Late specific hand signs of RA

Extra-articular (see *Fig. 2*)

- **Eyes** Secondary Sjögren syndrome, scleritis and episcleritis, corneal ulceration, keratitis
- **Skin** Leg ulcers especially in Felty syndrome (triad of RF-positive RA, neutropenia and splenomegaly), vasculitis rash, nail fold infarcts
- **Rheumatoid nodules** Common and may occur in the eyes, subcutaneously, in the lung(s), heart, and less commonly in the vocal cords
- **Neurological** Peripheral nerve entrapment, atlanto-axial subluxation, polyneuropathy, mononeuritis multiplex
- **Respiratory system** Pleural involvement (pleurisy, pleural effusion), pulmonary fibrosis, obliterative bronchiolitis, Caplan syndrome (large fibrotic nodules with occupational coal dust exposure)
- **Cardiovascular system** Pericardial involvement, valvulitis and myocardial fibrosis, immune complex vasculitis, increased risk of myocardial infarction
- **Kidney** Rare but includes analgesic nephropathy, amyloidosis
- **Liver** Mild hepatomegaly and abnormal transaminases are common
- Other: thyroid disorders, osteoporosis, depression, splenomegaly

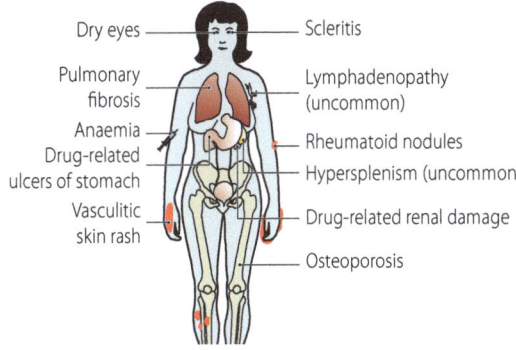

Dry eyes — Scleritis
Pulmonary fibrosis — Lymphadenopathy (uncommon)
Anaemia — Rheumatoid nodules
Drug-related ulcers of stomach — Hypersplenism (uncommon)
Vasculitic skin rash — Drug-related renal damage
— Osteoporosis

Fig. 2 Extra-articular manifestations of RA

Clinical features

Investigations

Non-specific

- **Bloods** FBC (normochromic, normocytic anaemia and reactive thrombocytosis are common in active disease), CRP/ESR (usually raised but may be normal), U&Es, LFTs (may have mild elevation of ALP and gamma-GT, also useful as a baseline prior to starting DMARDs), urate, ANA (positive in SLE and related conditions; also in up to 30% of RA)
- **X-ray joint(s)** Soft tissue swelling, periarticular osteopenia, loss of joint space, bony erosions, deformity (*Fig. 3*)
- **Urinalysis** Microscopic haematuria/proteinuria may suggest connective tissue disease
- **CXR** To exclude lung involvement and as a baseline before starting methotrexate
- **Synovial fluid analysis** Exclude septic arthritis or gout if diagnosis unclear

Specific

- **RF** Positive in 60–70% of patients
- **Anti-CCP** Better specificity than RF
- **X-ray affected joints** (see *Fig. 3*): soft tissue swelling, periarticular osteopenia, loss of joint space, bony erosions and deformity

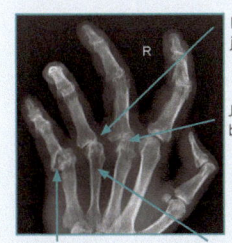

Narrowing of joint space

Juxta-articular bone erosion

Subluxation of proximal phalanx

Periarticular osteopenia

Fig. 3 Late X-ray features of RA

Rheumatoid arthritis notes

Diagnostic criteria for RA

The American College of Rheumatology (ACR) and European League Against Rheumatism (EULAR) criteria are shown in *Tables 1* and *2*.
A comparison of the clinical features of OA and RA is shown in *Table 3*.

Table 1 Joint ACR/EULAR criteria (2010)

Joint involvement	
1 large joint = 0	0
2–10 large joints	1
1–3 small joints	2
4–10 small joints	3
>10 joints (including at least one small joint)	5
Serology	
Negative RF and anti-CCP	0
Low-positive RF or anti-CCP	2
High-positive RF or anti-CCP	3
Duration of symptoms	
<6 weeks	0
≥6 weeks	1
Acute-phase reactants	
Normal CRP and ESR	0
Abnormal CRP or ESR	1
A total score of ≥6 is diagnostic of RA	

Table 2 ACR criteria (1987)

1. Morning stiffness in or around the joints lasting at least 1h	1
2. Arthritis of ≥3 joint areas	1
3. Arthritis of hand joints (at least one area swollen in wrist, MCP or PIP joints	1
4. Symmetrical arthritis	1
5. Rheumatoid nodules	1
6. Positive RF	1
7. Radiographic changes	1

Note: criteria 1–4 must be present for at least 6 weeks
A total score of ≥4 is diagnostic of RA

Table 3 RA vs OA: clinical features

RA	OA
RA usually presents symmetrically	OA usually presents in an asymmetrical joint
RA usually involves multiple small joints	OA more common in larger joint(s)
Pain in RA usually not worsened by movement	OA pain usually worsened by movement
Common age of onset of RA is 20–40	Common age of onset of OA is >50
RA onset is relatively quick (weeks to months)	OA onset is typically years
RA has extra-articular manifestations	OA does not have extra-articular manifestations
RA tends to be worse in the morning	OA tends to be worse after activities

Assessing severity of RA

The **Disease Activity Score 28 (DAS28)** is a tool used to assess the severity of RA based on tenderness and swelling at 28 joints (see *Fig. 4*), ESR and patient's self-reported symptom severity (see *Table 4*).

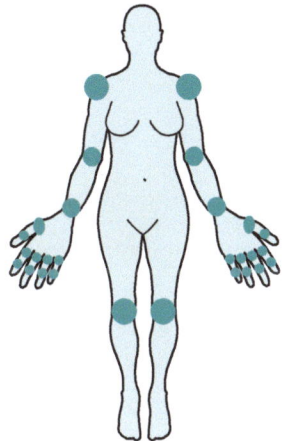

Fig. 4 The 28 joints (MCPs, PIPs, wrists, elbows, shoulders and knees) that are examined to help calculate the DAS28 score

Table 4 Interpretation of DAS28

>5.1	High disease activity
3.2–5.1	Moderate disease activity
<3.2	Low disease activity
<2.6	Remission
A decrease by ≤0.6 points or less	Poor response
A decrease by >1.2 points	Moderate or good response

Table 5 Pharmacological management of RA

NSAIDs	• Examples include ibuprofen, naproxen and diclofenac • Used for symptomatic relief and also reduced inflammation • Side effects: bronchospasm in asthmatics, dyspepsia/peptic ulceration
Corticosteroids	• e.g. Prednisolone • Results in rapid reduction in symptom onset and inflammation • Can be given via intra-muscular, intra-articular and oral routes • Usually given short term in combination with DMARDs for active disease

Table 5 (*continued*)

DMARDs	• 1st-line; it is recommended that patients with newly diagnosed active RA should start a combination of DMARDs (including methotrexate and at least one other DMARD, plus short-term glucocorticoids) • The most commonly used DMARDs are methotrexate, sulfasalazine and hydroxychloroquine; others include azathioprine, ciclosporin, ᴅ-penicillamine, leflunomide and mycophenolate mofetil • Early DMARD treatment is associated with better long-term prognosis (ideally within 3 months of onset)

Biological agents

TNF-alpha inhibitors	• Examples include infliximab, adalimumab and etanercept • Blocks the pivotal action of TNF-alpha, a key cytokine in the pathogenesis of RA • The current indication for a TNF inhibitor is an inadequate response to at least two DMARDs including methotrexate
Rituximab	• An anti-CD20 monoclonal antibody that results in B-cell depletion • Used in treatment of severe active RA in combination with methotrexate for patients whose condition has not responded adequately to other DMARDs (including one or more TNF-alpha inhibitors) or who are intolerant of them
Anakinra	• An IL-1 receptor antagonist • Used for RA (in combination with methotrexate) which has not responded to methotrexate alone • On the balance of its clinical benefits and cost effectiveness, anakinra is not currently recommended by NICE
Tocilizumab	• An anti-IL-6 receptor monoclonal antibody • Indicated for moderate–severe RA (in combination with methotrexate or alone if methotrexate is inappropriate), when response to at least one DMARD or TNF-alpha inhibitor has been inadequate, or in those who are intolerant of these drugs
Abatacept	• Fusion protein that modulates a key signal required for activation of T lymphocytes which leads to decreased T-cell proliferation and cytokine production • It is given via an infusion or SC injection • Not currently recommended by NICE

Definition

Scleroderma is an autoimmune connective tissue disorder that affects the skin and other organs. There are two main types: **localised** and **systemic sclerosis**. **Localised scleroderma** is more common in children and is confined to the skin and subcutaneous tissue. **Systemic scleroderma** (SSc) may be **limited** (also known as **CREST syndrome**), which accounts for 70% of SSc cases; the remaining 30% of cases are **diffuse**.

Pathophysiology

- Clinical and pathological manifestations of SSc are the result of innate/adaptive immune system abnormalities leading to production of autoantibodies and cell-mediated autoimmunity
- This results in upregulation of certain cytokines, e.g. IL-1, 4 and 6, which causes connective tissue producing cells (namely fibroblasts/myofibroblasts) to produce excessive collagen leading to hardening of the tissue
- Systemic sclerosis pathology and inflammation extends to small blood vessels which results in clinical manifestations of vasculopathy such as Raynaud's phenomenon, digit ulcers, renal crisis and pulmonary hypertension

Risk factors

- Positive ANA
- Family history
- Female gender (4:1)

Scleroderma

Management

- **Skin** Skin hygiene and use of emollients for dry skin; low-dose prednisolone or methotrexate if there is associated synovitis
- **Raynaud's** 1st-line treatment is a calcium-channel blocker such as nifedipine, or an angiotensin II receptor antagonist e.g. losartan; other options include SSRIs, alpha blockers, statins and phosphodiesterase type 5 inhibitors
- **GI** For GORD see *Ch3: Gastro-oesophageal reflux* disease; for constipation: dietary fibre and good fluid intake, softening laxatives e.g. lactulose and/or soluble fibre e.g. ispaghula
- **Renal disease** Treatment of renal crisis is with ACE inhibitors and dialysis if necessary
- **Cardiac** For systolic heart failure: immunosuppression with or without a pacemaker, implantable cardioverter defibrillator; ACE inhibitors and carvedilol; for diastolic heart failure with preserved LV: diuretics and calcium-channel blockers
- **Respiratory** For pulmonary fibrosis: IV cyclophosphamide with or without mycophenolate mofetil; supportive treatment e.g. oxygen and antibiotics (if infection); for pulmonary arterial hypertension: endothelin receptor antagonists e.g. bosentan, phosphodiesterase type 5 inhibitors e.g. sildenafil, prostaglandin derivatives e.g. iloprost; supportive measures include oxygen and diuretics

Investigations

- **Bloods** FBC (WCC may be raised, anaemia of chronic disease), ESR and CRP (may be raised), LFTs (baseline) and renal function (scleroderma can cause renal disease)
- **Antibodies** ANA positive (90%), RF positive (30%), anti-topoisomerase-1 (scl-70) antibodies associated with diffuse cutaneous systemic sclerosis, anti-centromere antibodies (ACA) associated with limited cutaneous systemic sclerosis, anti-RNA polymerase 1 and 3 antibodies associated with diffuse sclerosis (especially with kidney involvement)
- **Respiratory** Complete pulmonary function tests, CXR, high-resolution CT chest for suspected interstitial lung disease
- **Cardiovascular** ECHO may show raised pulmonary arterial pressure / hypertension and right ventricular failure
- **GI** Barium swallow test for oesophageal dysmotility

►Limited/CREST syndrome:

Limited scleroderma affects face and distal limbs predominantly (see *Fig. 1*); **CREST** syndrome is a subtype of limited systemic sclerosis:

- **C**alcinosis: typically under fingertips
- **R**aynaud's phenomenon: usually first sign to show up (see *Fig. 2*)
- **OE**sophageal dysmotility: may present as dysphagia or GORD
- **S**clerodactyly (stiff fingers) (see *Fig. 3*)
- **T**elangiectasia (dilated small vessels)

►Diffuse:

- Scleroderma affects trunk and proximal limbs predominantly (see *Fig. 1*)
- Sudden and aggressive onset
- Raynaud's may not present initially
- Telangiectasia
- Hypertension, lung fibrosis and renal involvement seen
- Poor prognosis

►Morphea

- Oval itchy skin patches; waxy and red in appearance
- Does not involve fingers
- Raynaud's phenomenon is uncommon
- Dilated nailbed capillaries

►Linear

- Thickened line of skin; 'knife-like scar'
- Develops in childhood
- Occurs on arm, leg and forehead
- Raynaud's phenomenon is uncommon

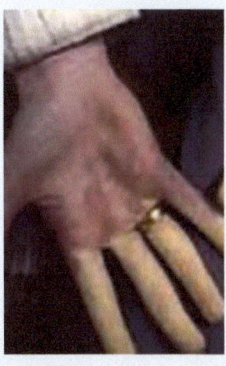

Fig. 2 Raynaud's phenomenon: transient vasospasm leading to digital hypoxia resulting in digits changing colour from white → blue → red; stress and cold are classic triggers

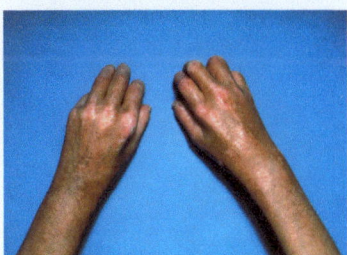

Fig. 3 Build-up of fibrous tissue in the skin can cause the skin to tighten to cause the fingers to curl and reduce their mobility in scleroderma

Clinical features

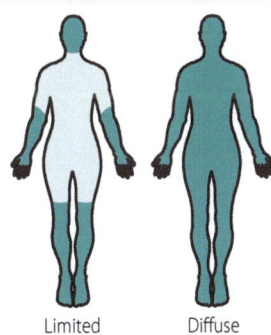

Limited   Diffuse

Fig. 1 Skin involvement distribution in systemic scleroderma

Notes

Scleroderma

Definition

Septic arthritis is an acute infection (usually bacterial) of a native or prosthetic joint. Since septic arthritis can lead to rapid joint destruction, immediate accurate diagnosis and treatment are essential. Any joint can be affected, particularly the lower limb joints (most commonly hip and knee).

Pathophysiology

- Septic arthritis usually occurs due to the spread of bacteria from another site in the body to the affected joint(s)
- The commonest route of spread is via the bloodstream (e.g. respiratory or urinary tract infections)
- It can also occur from direct inoculation e.g. penetrating trauma or local tissue infection e.g. cellulitis and osteomyelitis
- The normal joint has several protective components; healthy synovial cells possess significant phagocytic activity, and synovial fluid normally has significant bactericidal activity; septic arthritis is more likely if these defence mechanisms are disrupted e.g. by pre-existing joint disease, joint surgery or immunodeficiency
- Bacteria are the most common causative pathogens, with viruses and fungi rarely causing septic arthritis

Causative agents

Gram-positive cocci

- *Staphylococcus aureus* (most common)
- Coagulase-negative staphylococci (more common in prosthetic joints)

Gram-negative cocci

- *Neisseria gonorrhoeae* (more common in young adults who are sexually active)

Gram-negative bacilli

- For example *E. coli* (more common in diabetics, the elderly and IV drug users)

Septic arthritis

Complications

- Sepsis
- Avascular necrosis
- Septic dislocation
- Chondrolysis
- Shortening of limb
- Late degenerative change

Management

- Empirical IV antibiotics, e.g. flucloxacillin, while waiting for synovial fluid joint analysis – refer to local guidelines and consultant microbiologist; antibiotics are usually later switched to oral antibiotics and given for several weeks
- Orthopaedic review for consideration of arthrocentesis, lavage and debridement of joint
- Joint immobilisation with splinting may be required

Investigations

Bloods

- FBC (↑WCC)
- CRP/ESR (↑)
- Blood culture: may reveal presence of microorganisms, organism type and sensitivities to antibiotics

Imaging

- X-ray affected joint(s): usually normal but may reveal underlying joint disease
- US affected joint: may show presence of effusion
- CT and MRI affected joint: the most sensitive methods for diagnosing periarticular abscesses, joint effusions and osteomyelitis

Joint aspiration and synovial fluid analysis

- Gram stain (may show presence of organisms)
- WCC (often raised)
- Culture (reveals organism type and sensitivities to antibiotics)
- Polarised light microscopy (rule out gout/pseudogout)

- Prosthetic joint
- Prior joint damage e.g. RA, gout, systemic connective tissue disorders
- Diabetes mellitus
- Joint surgery
- Penetrating injury
- Low socioeconomic status
- Extremes of age (<15 and >55 years)
- IV drug use
- Immunodeficiency e.g. HIV
- Immunosuppression e.g. on corticosteroids

Risk factors

Joint distribution

- Usually one joint is affected only; however less often more than one can be affected
- Any joint can be affected but the knee is the most common site affected overall with the hip most common in children; this is followed by the shoulder, wrist, elbow and ankle

Symptoms/signs (see *Fig. 1*)

- Acutely painful joint(s): worse on movement
- Swollen joint
- ↓Mobility of joint
- Tender, erythematous and warm joint
- Effusion around joint
- Systemic features: fever, tachycardia, rash, malaise
- Unable to weight bear on affected side (if lower limb joint affected)
- Loosening of implant (chronic infection in prosthetic joint)

Clinical features

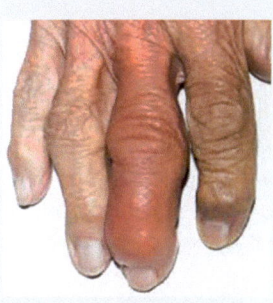

Fig. 1 Septic arthritis of the metacarpophalangeal joints

Notes

Septic arthritis

Sjögren syndrome (SS) is an autoimmune condition in which there is lymphocytic infiltration of exocrine glands, producing the main symptoms of **xerophthalmia** (dry eyes), **xerostomia** (dry mouth) and enlargement of the parotid glands. The disease is referred to as **primary** if it develops in isolation and **secondary** if it occurs with other autoimmune diseases, usually RA, SLE, scleroderma.

- Environmental or endogenous antigens trigger an innate and adaptive immune-induced inflammatory response in genetically susceptible individuals
- Biopsies of glandular and extraglandular sites are characterised by lymphocytic infiltration
- Cellular adhesive molecules, metalloproteinases and neural transmitters show alterations in the affected target organs causing fibrosis
- The overlapping clinical features between primary SS and SLE have led to the suggestion primary SS is likely to share similar features to the pathogenesis of SLE

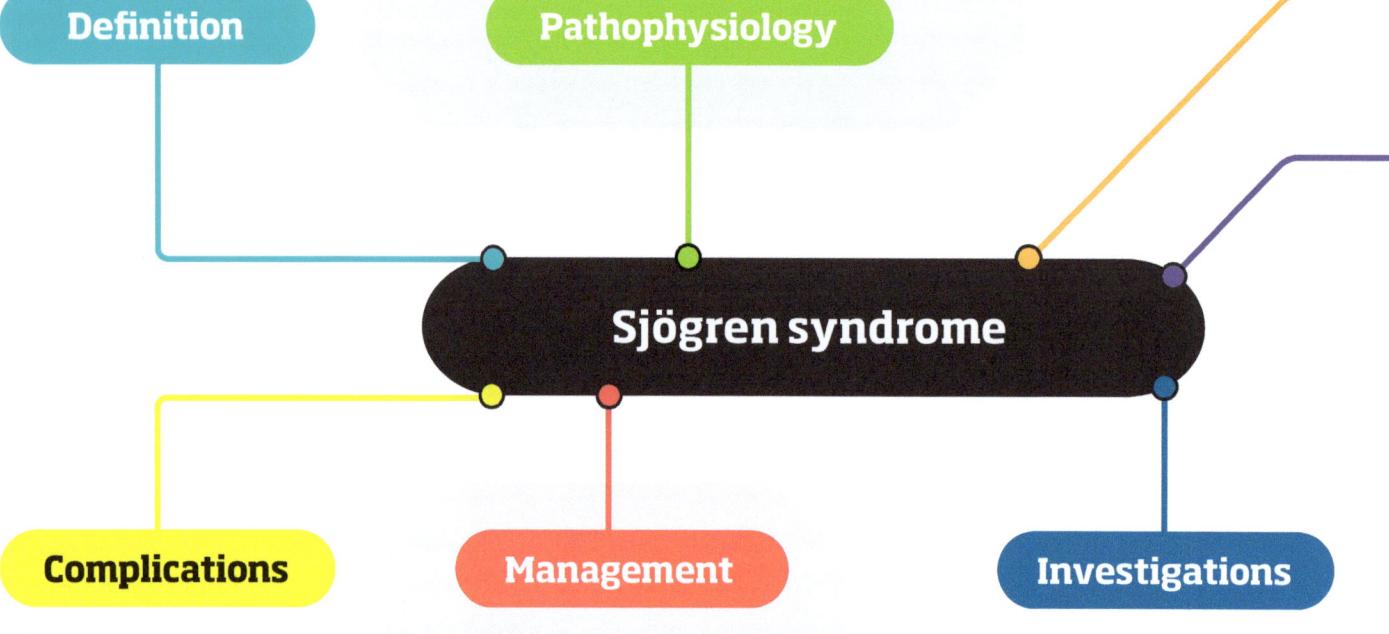

Definition

Pathophysiology

Sjögren syndrome

Complications

- ↑Risk of infection around the eyes, mouth, the parotid gland and vaginal candidiasis
- Parotid tumours
- ↑Risk of developing non-Hodgkin's lymphoma

Management

- **Dry eyes:**
  - Artificial tears (1st line)
  - Ciclosporin eye drops
  - Spectacle eye shields
  - Humidifiers
- **Dry mouth:**
  - Encourage oral fluid intake
  - Salivary substitutes
  - Cholinergic drugs to stimulate secretion of exocrine glands e.g. pilocarpine
- **Dry skin** Emollients
- **Dry vagina/dyspareunia** Vaginal lubricants
- **Arthralgia** Hydroxychloroquine may be useful

Investigations

- **Schirmer's test** Filter paper near conjunctival sac to measure tear formation (see *Fig. 2*)
- **Bloods** FBC, CRP/ESR (may be raised), U&Es, LFTs, anti-Ro (positive in approx. 70% of patients), anti-La antibodies (positive in approx. 30%), ANA (positive in 70%), RF (positive in nearly 100%), immunoglobulins (hypergammaglobulinaemia), C4 (low)
- **Salivary gland** or **lip biopsy** Shows lymphocyte infiltration
- **Lissamine green test** and **rose bengal eye staining** May show keratitis
- **Salivary gland scintigraphy** Shows decreased salivary gland function
- **MRI salivary glands** May show chronic sialadenitis

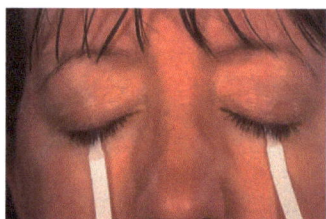

Fig. 2 Schirmer's test

- SS is much more common in females than males (9:1)
- SS peaks at age 30–50 years and after menopause
- There is a significant overlap between SLE, RA, scleroderma and SS
- HLA class markers: HLA-DR3, B8, DQ2 and C4 allele found in about 50% of Caucasian patients with SS
- Family history confers susceptibility
- A role for viruses, e.g. EBV as an environmental trigger, has been suggested but the evidence is mixed

Epidemiology and risk factors

- **D**ry eyes (keratoconjunctivitis sicca)
- **D**ry mouth
- Paroti**D** swelling (see *Fig. 1*)
- Vaginal **D**ryness and **D**yspareunia
- **D**ry cough
- **D**ysphagia
- Systemic features: polyarthritis, arthralgia, Raynaud's, lymphadenopathy, vasculitis, lung, kidney and liver involvement, peripheral neuropathy, myositis, fatigue

Clinical features

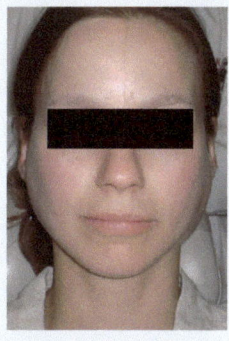

Fig. 1 Bilateral parotid swelling in Sjögren syndrome

Notes

Sjögren syndrome

- The exact cause of SLE is unknown but multiple factors are associated with the development of the disease, including genetic and environmental factors (see *Fig. 1*)

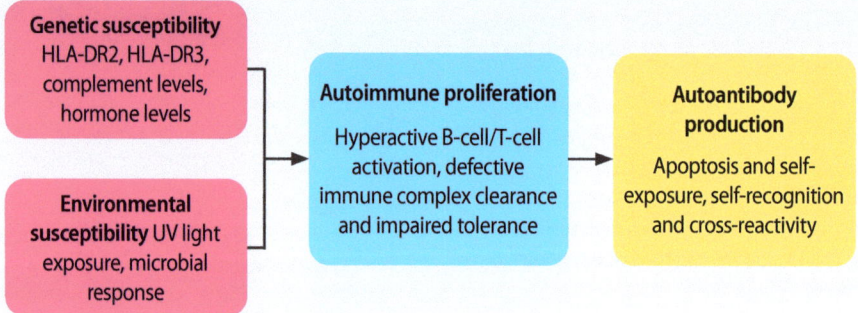

Systemic lupus erythematosus (SLE) is a heterogeneous, inflammatory, **multisystem autoimmune disease** of unknown cause in which **antinuclear antibodies (ANA)** are found (often years preceding clinical symptoms).

Fig. 1 Summary of the pathogenesis of SLE

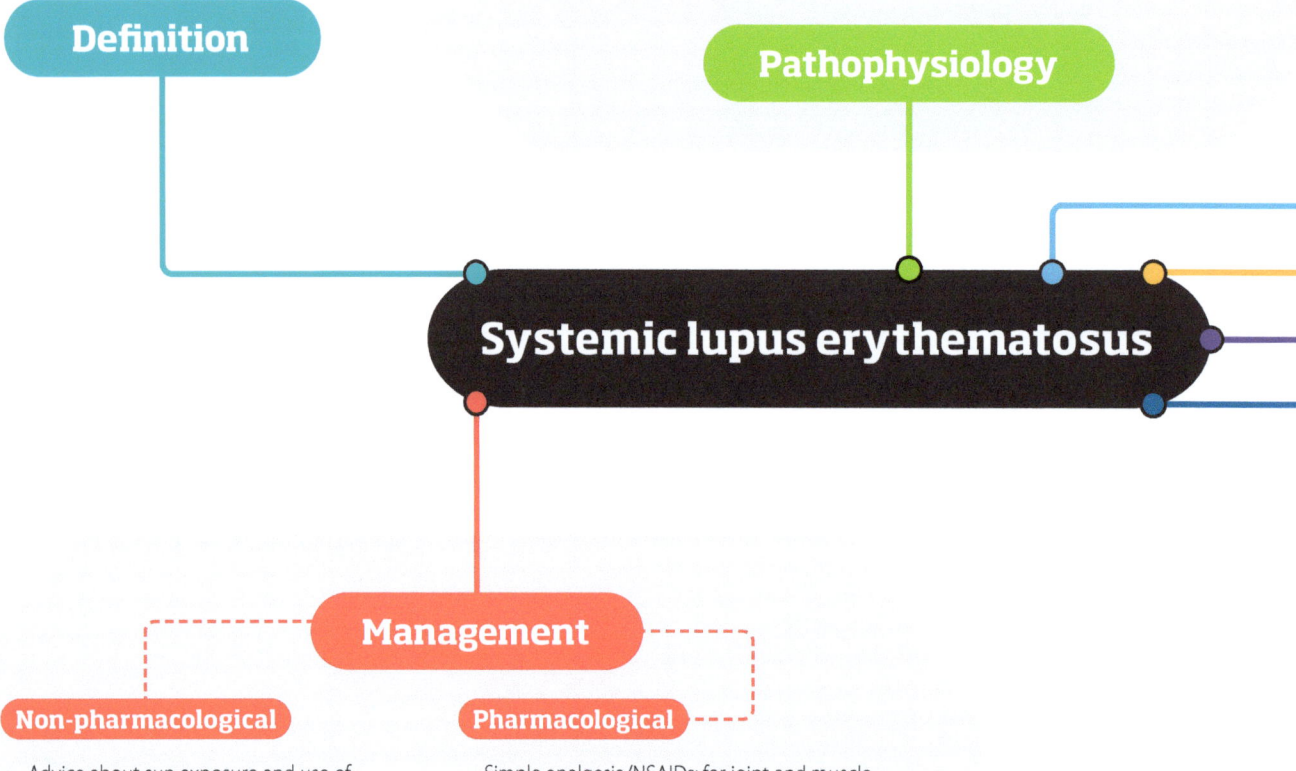

Definition

Pathophysiology

Systemic lupus erythematosus

Management

Non-pharmacological

- Advice about sun exposure and use of sunscreen
- Smoking cessation
- Pregnancy and contraception: pregnancy should be planned; risk of problems with pregnancy is greatly reduced if disease is well controlled prior to conception; drug therapy should be reviewed before pregnancy; pills that contain oestrogen may exacerbate lupus disease or thrombosis and should be used with caution (barrier methods or progesterone-only contraception is preferred)
- Monitoring disease activity: anti-dsDNA antibody titres, complement levels (↓C3, C4 and ↑C3d and C4d suggest increased activity) ESR, CRP

Pharmacological

- Simple analgesia/NSAIDs: for joint and muscle pains
- Corticosteroids: when simple analgesia and NSAIDs are insufficient to control symptoms or disease
- Hydroxychloroquine: useful for skin lesions, arthralgia, myalgia and malaise
- Cyclophosphamide: reserved for treatment of life-threatening disease, particularly lupus nephritis, vasculitis and cerebral disease
- Mycophenolate mofetil: can be used to induce remission or as maintenance therapy
- Azathioprine: used as a steroid-sparing agent
- IV high-dose pooled gammaglobulin and granulocyte-colony stimulating factor: have a role in autoimmune thrombocytopenia and neutropenia
- Belimumab (cytokine modulator): monoclonal antibody used as adjunctive therapy in patients with active autoantibody-positive SLE with a high degree of disease activity despite standard therapy

Epidemiology

- SLE affects approx. 1 in 1000 people in the UK
- SLE is more common in women than men: 10:1 in the age range 18–65 years
- SLE is more common in those of Chinese, Southeast Asian and African–Caribbean origin
- The usual age of onset is 16–55 years

Risk factors

- **HLA markers:** HLA-DR2 and HLA-DR3 are more common in patients with SLE
- **Defective C4 complement gene:** these patients are more likely to develop a lupus-like illness
- **Sunlight exposure** due to UV light is thought to be an important environmental factor
- **Viruses:** e.g. Epstein–Barr virus has been linked
- **Drugs:** chlorpromazine, methyldopa, hydralazine, isoniazid, D-penicillamine and minocycline are known to cause drug-induced lupus
- **Tobacco smoking:** smoking is linked to the development of SLE and also the prognosis

Clinical features

- Non-specific symptoms: malaise, fatigue, fever, myalgia, lymphadenopathy, weight loss
- Arthralgia: joints and muscle pain, joint swelling, Jaccoud's arthropathy (non-erosive arthropathy characterised by ulnar deviation of the 2nd to 5th fingers with metacarpophalangeal joint subluxation)
- Skin rashes: photosensitive rash, malar (butterfly) rash (see *Fig. 2*), discoid rash (see *Fig. 3*), livedo reticularis (see *Fig. 4*)
- Serositis: pleuritic, pericarditis
- Raynaud's phenomenon
- Non-scarring alopecia
- Mouth ulcers
- Renal: proteinuria, haematuria, hypertension or a raised serum urea or creatinine
- Neuropsychiatric: psychosis, seizures, anxiety/depression

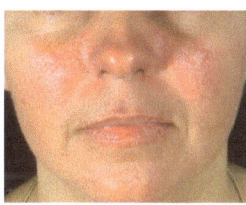

Fig. 2 Malar rash

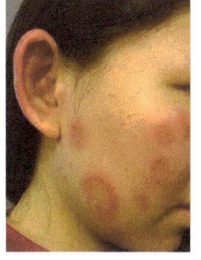

Fig. 3 Discoid lupus: can occur in the absence of any systemic features

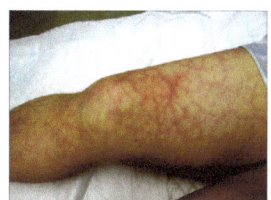

Fig. 4 Livedo reticularis

Investigations

Bloods

- **FBC** Anaemia, leucopenia, thrombocytopenia and rarely pancytopenia
- **Activated prothrombin time** May be prolonged in patients with antiphospholipids
- **ESR** Often elevated
- **CRP** Often normal unless there is intercurrent infection or serositis
- **Immunology** ANA (99% positive), anti-dsDNA (highly specific), anti-Smith (highly specific) positive, RF (positive in 20%), complement C3 and C4 (low during active disease) and C3d (a degradation product)
- **U&Es** May be abnormal in renal disease

Urinalysis

- Haematuria, casts (red cell, granular, tubular or mixed) or proteinuria

CXR

- To check for pleural effusion, infiltrates and cardiomegaly (if symptomatic)

X-ray affected joint

- Periarticular osteopenia may be present

MRI

- In suspected CNS lupus

ECG

- For all patients with cardiopulmonary symptoms

ECHO

- To investigate pericardial involvement

SLE diagnostic criteria

Patients can be classified as having SLE if they satisfy 4 of the clinical or immunological criteria (including at least 1 clinical criterion and 1 immunological criterion):

Clinical criteria

- **Acute cutaneous lupus (≥1 of the following)** Malar rash, bullous lupus, maculopapular rash, photosensitive rash
- **Chronic cutaneous lupus (≥1 of the following)** Classic discoid rash (localised or generalised), hypertrophic lupus, lupus panniculitis, mucosal lupus, lupus erythematosus tumidus, chilblains lupus, discoid lupus/lichen planus overlap
- **Oral ulcers** Palate, buccal, tongue or nasal ulcers
- **Non-scarring alopecia**
- **Synovitis** ≥2 joints, characterised by swelling or effusion *or* tenderness in ≥2 joints and ≥30min morning stiffness
- **Serositis** Pleurisy or pleural effusions or pleural rub
- **Renal** Persistent proteinuria or red cell casts; characteristic pericardial pain or pericardial effusion or pericardial rub or pericarditis on ECG
- **Neurological** Seizures or psychosis
- **Haemolytic anaemia**

Immunological criteria

- **ANA** Above laboratory reference range
- **Anti-dsDNA** Above laboratory reference range
- **Anti-Smith antibodies**
- **Antiphospholipid antibody**
- **Low complement levels**
- **Positive direct Coombs test** (in the absence of haemolytic anaemia)

Antiphospholipid syndrome

Definition

Antiphospholipid syndrome is an autoimmune disorder which may be associated with SLE but mainly exists as a primary disease. It is an important cause of recurrent arterial or venous thrombosis and miscarriages. It is associated with the presence of antiphospholipid antibodies.

Clinical features (CLOT)

- **C**oagulation defects
- **L**ivedo reticularis (see *Fig. 4*)
- **O**bstetric (recurrent miscarriage)
- **T**hrombocytopenia

Diagnosis (1 clinical and 1 lab finding)

- **Clinical** 1 episode of arterial and/or venous thrombosis or morbidity in pregnancy
- **Lab** Anticardiolipin antibodies or lupus anticoagulant in plasma

Management

Give low-dose aspirin or warfarin for recurrent thromboses. Expert advice should be sought for pregnancy.

Definition

Vitamin D deficiency or hypovitaminosis D remains one of the most common vitamin deficiencies. It results in inadequate mineralisation of bone and clinically manifests as **rickets** in children and **osteomalacia** in adults.

Causes

- Lack of sunlight
- Renal disease: due to impairment of C-1 hydroxylation of 25(OH)D
- GI malabsorption: coeliac disease, short bowel syndrome and cystic fibrosis
- Liver disease: due to impaired C-25 hydroxylation of vitamin D
- Drugs including anticonvulsants, rifampicin, cholestyramine, highly active antiretroviral treatment (HAART) and glucocorticoids
- Genetic causes: hypophosphataemic rickets, type 1 (impaired C-1 hydroxylation) and type 2 vitamin D resistance rickets (target organ resistance)

Risk factors

- Darker skin: African–Caribbean, Middle Eastern and South Asian
- Age: children and elderly
- Breastfeeding: mums that are breastfeeding and infants who are exclusively breastfed
- Obesity
- Routine covering of face and hands: common in Muslim women who wear veils
- Housebound: particularly elderly
- Sunscreen: skin-concealing garments or strict sunscreen use
- Pregnancy
- Family history of vitamin D deficiency

Complications

Apart from osteomalacia and rickets, vitamin D deficiency is also associated with increased risk of the following:
- Osteoporosis
- Diabetes mellitus
- Cardiovascular disease
- Cancers such as prostate cancer

Vitamin D deficiency

Investigations

Bloods

- Vitamin D: low
- Calcium: normal or low
- PTH: usually raised
- Phosphate: low
- ALP: normal or raised

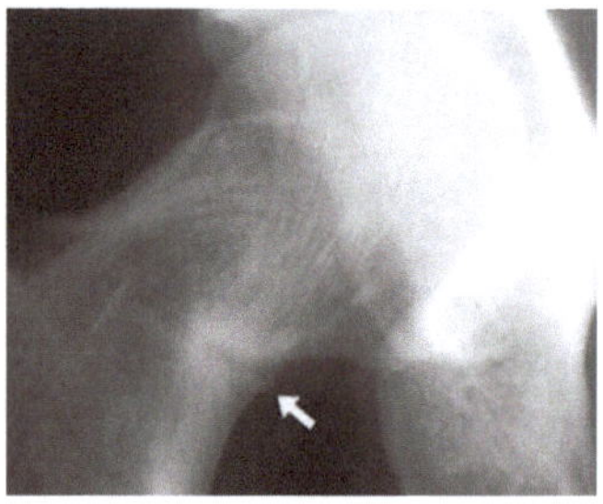

X-rays

Osteomalacia:
- Pseudofractures or Looser zones: pathognomonic of osteomalacia; they are low-density bands extending from the cortex inwards in the shafts of long bones (see Fig. 3)
- Coarse trabeculae
- Osteopenia

Rickets:
- Metaphyseal cupping and flaring
- Epiphyseal irregularities
- Widening of the epiphyseal plates

Fig. 3 Looser zone (arrow) seen in the femoral neck of a patient with osteomalacia

Management

General measures and prevention

- Treat underlying cause of vitamin D deficiency
- Adequate sun exposure
- Adequate dietary intake of vitamin D: foods such as oily fish/cod liver oil, egg yolk and milk are rich in vitamin D; some foods are supplemented with vitamin D, such as breakfast cereals
- The following groups are advised to take daily vitamin D tablets e.g. Adcal-D3:
  - All pregnant and breastfeeding women
  - All children aged 6 months to 5 years (unless babies are formula milk fed more than 500ml/day)
  - Adults >65 years
  - People who are not exposed to much sun
- Manage pain symptoms

Treatment

- Vitamin D deficiency requires high-dose replacement; e.g. in adults, a daily dose of cholecalciferol 10 000IU or a weekly dose of 60 000IU will lead to restoration of body stores of vitamin D over 8–12 weeks
- Serum vitamin D and calcium levels should be monitored in patients with vitamin D deficiency after treatment

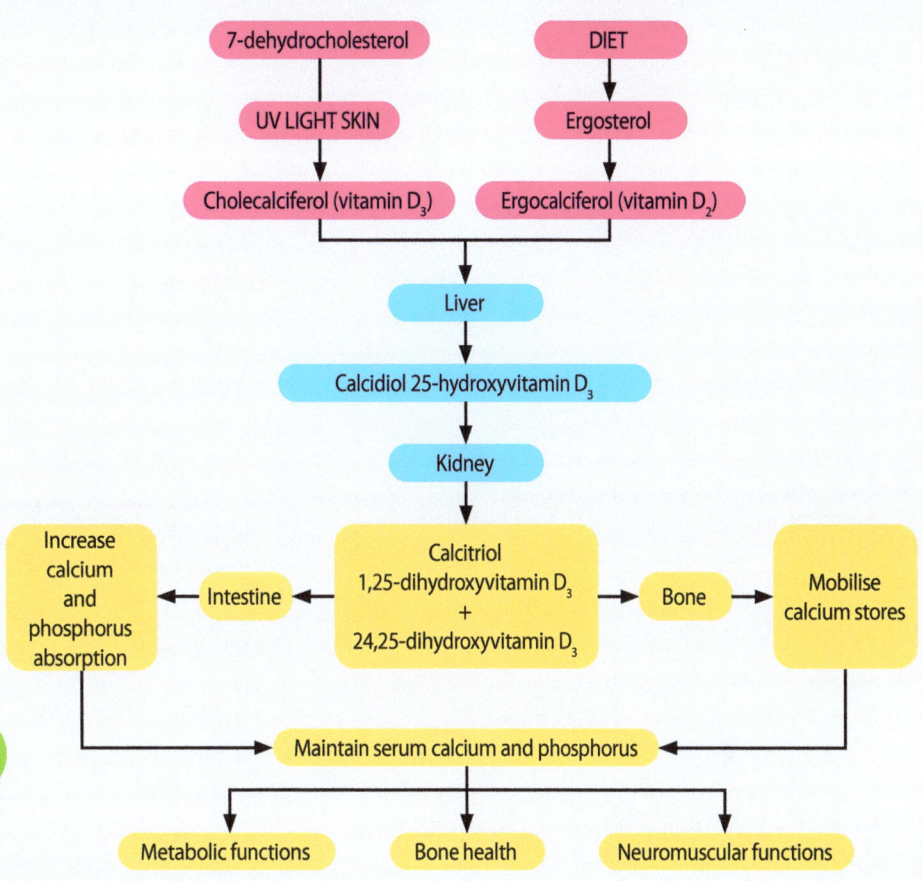

Fig. 1 Vitamin D physiology

- Normal bone mineralisation depends on adequate calcium and phosphate which is maintained by vitamin D (see *Fig. 1*)
- Vitamin D deficiency is most commonly caused by failure of the kidneys to hydroxylate 25-hydroxyvitamin D (25(OH)D) to 1,25-dihydroxyvitamin D (1,25(OH)$_2$D) due to chronic kidney disease and from inadequate UVB sunlight exposure for the formation of vitamin D$_3$ in the skin
- This results in reduced mineralisation of bone due to increased PTH in response to low circulating levels of phosphate and calcium

Pathophysiology

Clinical features

Rickets

- Infants: growth retardation, hypotonia and apathy (infants)
- Once walking: knock-kneed or genu valgum, bow-Legged or genu varum, bone deformities (see *Fig. 2*)
- Features of hypocalcaemia (severe vitamin D deficiency): paraesthesia, tetany, cramps, seizures

Osteomalacia

- Bone pain and tenderness
- Pathological fractures (particularly femoral neck)
- Proximal myopathy causing proximal weakness and potentially a waddling gait

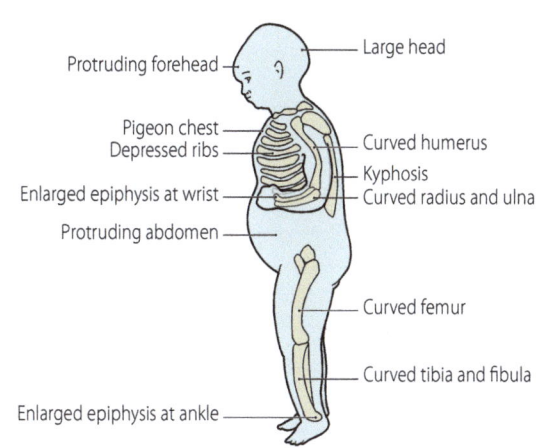

Fig. 2 Bone deformities in children with rickets

Chapter 8

Infectious diseases

Hepatitis A refers to inflammation of the liver caused by infection with the hepatitis A virus (HAV). It is the most common type of viral hepatitis.

- Worldwide, approximately 1.4 million cases of HAV are reported every year, but the true incidence is likely to be much higher
- HAV is uncommon in the UK and other high-income countries
- HAV is endemic in many developing countries where standards of sanitation and food hygiene may be poor e.g. the Indian subcontinent, sub-Saharan Africa and North Africa, and parts of the Far East, South and Central America and the Middle East

Transmission of HAV is by the faecal–oral route

Around 85% of people with HAV infection make a complete recovery within 3 months; almost all people with HAV recover fully within 6 months.

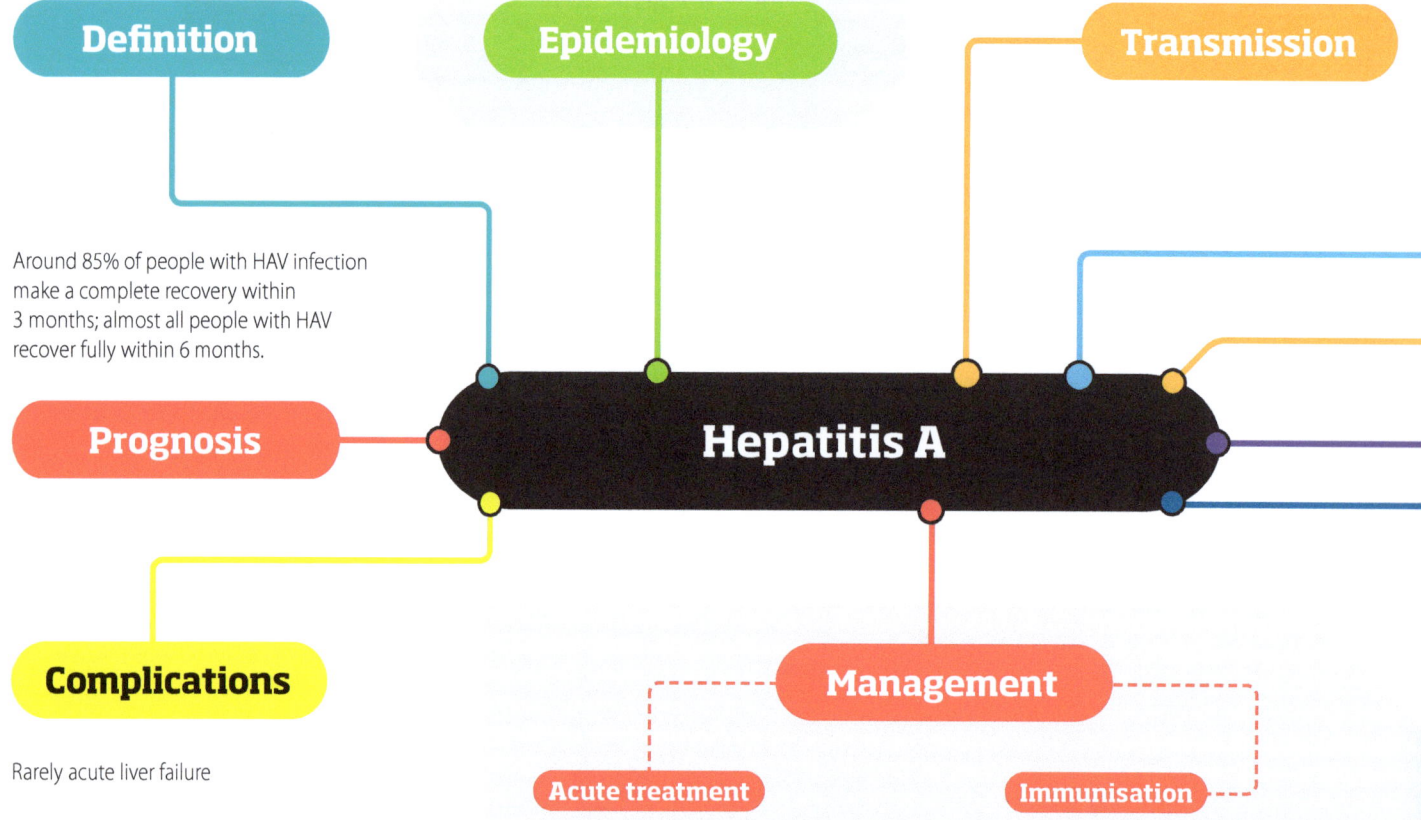

Definition

Epidemiology

Transmission

Hepatitis A

Prognosis

Complications

Rarely acute liver failure

Management

Acute treatment

- Mainly supportive e.g. rest, fluids and anti-emetics
- Avoid alcohol until LFTs normalise
- Admit patients with severe systemic upset or intractable vomiting for rehydration and observation
- Advise pregnant women of increased risk of miscarriage and premature labour and need to seek medical advice if symptoms develop
- Employment history should be sought so patient can be advised appropriately; until patients become non-infectious, they should avoid food handling and unprotected sexual intercourse
- Advice on managing outbreaks should be sought from UK regional public health organisations

Immunisation

- An effective vaccine is available; after initial dose, give booster 6–12 months later
- Indications for vaccination include:
  - People travelling to or going to reside in areas of high or intermediate prevalence (if aged >1 year)
  - People with chronic liver disease
  - Patients with haemophilia
  - Men who have sex with men
  - Injecting drug users
  - Individuals at occupational risk: laboratory worker; staff of large residential institutions; sewage workers; people who work with primates
  - People infected with HIV

Incubation period

The mean incubation period is 28–30 days, with a range of 15–50 days

Risk factors

- Travellers to areas with a high prevalence
- People with clotting factor disorders (Factor VIII and Factor IX concentrates have been identified as rare sources of HAV infection)
- Men who have sex with men (MSM), and people with risky sexual behaviours
- Injecting drug users and their close contacts (at risk of poor standards of personal hygiene, with possible faecal contamination of shared drug equipment and other paraphernalia)
- People at occupational risk e.g. laboratory workers, staff of large residential institutions, sewage workers, and people who work with primates

Clinical features

Prodromal phase

- Usually lasts 3–10 days
- Flu-like symptoms e.g. general fatigue, malaise, joint and muscle pain, low-grade fever up to 39°C
- GI symptoms including anorexia, nausea, vomiting, and right upper quadrant abdominal pain
- May also be headache, cough, sore throat, constipation, diarrhoea, itch or urticaria

Icteric phase

- Usually lasts 1–3 weeks, but can persist >12 weeks
- Jaundice, pale stools and dark urine if cholestasis
- Pruritus
- Fatigue, anorexia and nausea/vomiting
- Hepatomegaly, splenomegaly, lymphadenopathy and hepatic tenderness are often present on examination

Convalescent phase

- May take up to 6 months
- Malaise, anorexia, muscle weakness and hepatic tenderness

Investigations

Specific antibody tests

- **IgM antibody to HAV** Positive with onset of symptoms (it is sensitive and specific); it usually remains positive for between 3 and 6 months (up to 12 months) and remains positive in relapsing hepatitis
- **IgG antibody to HAV** Appears soon after IgM; in the absence of IgM it indicates past infection or vaccination rather than acute infection; IgG remains detectable for life

LFTs and other tests

- Alanine transaminase (ALT) rises more than aspartate transaminase (AST) with onset of symptoms; levels usually return to reference ranges over several weeks but can remain elevated for months
- Alkaline phosphatase (ALP) rises with ALT and AST
- Bilirubin rises soon after increase in ALT/AST levels and may remain very high for several months
- Serum albumin levels may fall
- Prothrombin time (PT) usually remains normal but prolongation is a sign of severe infection
- FBC: mild lymphocytosis is common; pure red cell aplasia and pancytopenia are very rare
- Liver imaging, e.g. ultrasound, may rarely be required to exclude other diseases

Hepatitis D and E notes

Hepatitis D

- Hepatitis D (HDV) is a single-stranded RNA virus; it is an incomplete virus that requires hepatitis B (HBV) surface antigen (HBsAg) to complete its replication and transmission cycle
- **Co-infection** Refers to hepatitis B and HDV infection at the same time
- **Superinfection** A HBsAg-positive patient who subsequently develops HDV infection; this is associated with high risk of fulminant hepatitis, chronic hepatitis status and cirrhosis
- **Epidemiology** Approx. 15–20 million people infected with HBV worldwide are also infected with HDV
- **Transmission** Transmitted parenterally in a similar fashion to HBV (exchange of bodily fluids) and patients may be infected with HBV and HDV at the same time
- **Diagnosis** Via reverse polymerase chain reaction of HDV RNA
- **Management** Specific treatments include pegylated interferon-alpha and liver transplantation (which can be curative); management is otherwise supportive

Hepatitis E

- Hepatitis E is a liver disease caused by infection with the hepatitis E virus (HEV, a non-enveloped RNA virus)
- **Epidemiology** It is common in Central and South-East Asia, North and West Africa, and Mexico
- **Transmission** Spread by the faecal–oral route (usually by contaminated sewage water)
- **Clinical features** Incubation period is around 3–8 weeks; it causes a similar disease to HAV and is usually self-limiting; fulminant disease occurs in about 10% of individuals, however, and in pregnancy it carries a significant mortality (about 20%)
- **Diagnosis** Serum IgM and IgG anti-HEV can be detected by enzyme-linked immunosorbent assay (ELISA)
- **Management** Mainly supportive; a promising vaccine has shown a high degree of efficacy against HEV but is not yet in widespread use

Notes

Hepatitis B is an infectious disease of the liver caused by the hepatitis B virus (HBV). It can be acute or chronic.

- The prevalence of chronic HBV infection in the UK is approx. 0.3%
- In regions with high prevalence, more than 8% of the population have chronic HBV infection (e.g. in Southeast Asia (excluding Japan), China and sub-Saharan Africa)

- Accidental inoculation of minute amounts of blood or fluid
- Sexual transmission
- Vertical transmission

75 days on average, but can vary from 30 to 180 days

Definition

Epidemiology

Transmission

Incubation period

Hepatitis B

Complications

- Fulminant liver failure (1%)
- Hepatocellular carcinoma
- Glomerulonephritis
- Polyarteritis nodosa
- Cryoglobulinaemia

Management

Acute hepatitis B

- There is no specific treatment for *acute* hepatitis B
- Admission to hospital should be arranged if very unwell; treatment is aimed at maintaining comfort and adequate nutritional balance, including replacement of fluids lost from vomiting and diarrhoea
- It is vital to avoid unnecessary medications including paracetamol and anti-emetics; alcohol should be avoided until liver enzymes are within normal range
- The local health protection team should be notified of suspected cases of acute viral hepatitis

Chronic hepatitis B

- **Pegylated interferon-alpha** Reduces viral replication in up to 30% of chronic carriers; a better response is predicted for the following: females, <50 years, low HBV DNA levels, non-Asian, HIV negative, high degree of inflammation on liver biopsy
- Other antiviral medications aimed at suppressing viral replication include tenofovir, entecavir and telbivudine (a synthetic thymidine nucleoside analogue)

Vaccination

Passive immunity

Specific hepatitis immunoglobulin provides passive immunity which can give immediate but temporary protection in the event of exposure.

Active immunity

Preparation

The HBV vaccine in the UK contains HBsAg adsorbed onto aluminium hydroxide adjuvant and is prepared from yeast cells using recombinant DNA technology.

Indications

- Children born in the UK as part of the routine immunisation schedule given at 2, 3 and 4 months of age
- At-risk groups: healthcare workers, IV drug users, sex workers, close family contacts

- Injecting drug users and their close contacts
- People who change sexual partners frequently, MSM, and sex workers and their clients
- Travellers to high-prevalence areas (common via sexual exposure or invasive medical procedures)
- People from a country with a high prevalence
- Household contacts of people with HBV, including close family and carers
- Families adopting a child from a country with a high prevalence of HBV
- People receiving regular blood/blood products (e.g. those with haemophilia) and their carers
- People with chronic renal failure or chronic liver disease
- People with an occupational risk e.g. healthcare workers, laboratory staff and morticians
- Looked-after children and young people, including those living in care homes
- Prison inmates and staff
- Infants born to women with HBV infection
- Hajj and Umrah pilgrims with shaved heads (using unlicensed barbers)

Risk factors

Acute infection

- Fever, arthralgia, or a rash (may appear 2 weeks prior to the onset of jaundice, then resolves)
- Non-specific malaise, fatigue, fever, nausea and poor appetite
- Right upper quadrant abdominal pain
- Jaundice (with dark urine and/or pale stools if cholestasis)

Note: Acute HBV infection is asymptomatic in almost all infants and children, 10–50% of adults, and is especially likely in people with HIV

Chronic infection

Often there are no physical signs but, depending on the severity and duration, there may be:
- Spider naevi
- Finger clubbing
- Jaundice
- Hepatosplenomegaly
- Skin thinning, bruising, ascites, liver flap and encephalopathy (severe cases)

Clinical features

Investigations

of an individual with HBV, individuals receiving blood transfusions regularly, end-stage CKD patients, prisoners, chronic liver disease patients

Testing for anti-HBs following immunisation
- Around 10–15% of adults fail to respond or respond poorly to 3 doses of the vaccine
- Testing for anti-HBs is only recommended for those at risk of occupational exposure and patients with CKD; in these patients anti-HBs levels should be checked 1–4 months after primary immunisation
- Interpretation of **anti-HBs levels**:
  - **>100 (adequate response)** No further testing required; should still receive booster at 5 years
  - **10–100 (suboptimal response)** 1 additional vaccine dose should be given
  - **<10 (non-responder)** A further vaccine course (i.e. 3 doses again) followed by testing

Hepatitis B serology

- **Surface antigen (HBsAg)** 1st marker to appear and causes the production of anti-HBs. It usually implies acute disease (if present for 1–6 months) and chronic disease if present for >6 months (i.e. infective)
- **Anti-HBs** Implies immunity (either exposure or immunisation); negative in chronic disease
- **Anti-HBc** Implies previous (or current) infection; IgM anti-HBc appears during acute or recent HBV infection and is present for about 6 months; IgG anti-HBc persists
- **HbeAg** Results from breakdown of core antigen from infected liver cells thus a marker of infectivity

Other investigations

- Baseline FBC, U&Es, LFTs, clotting screen, HbA1c, TFTs, ferritin
- Screening for HCV, HDV, HIV (high co-infection rates)
- Screening for hepatocellular carcinoma through ultrasound scans of liver and alpha-fetoprotein
- Transient elastography (less invasive) or liver biopsy can be used to diagnose cirrhosis

Definition

Hepatitis C infection is a disease of the liver caused by infection with the blood-borne hepatitis C virus (HCV). It can cause both acute and chronic hepatitis and is a major cause of liver cancer.

Epidemiology

- Around 214 000 individuals are chronically infected with HCV in the UK
- It is estimated that around 3% (170 million) of the world's population are infected; in parts of Europe and the Indian subcontinent the prevalence might be as high as 5%

Transmission

- Inoculation of minute amounts of blood or fluid (most common)
- Sexual transmission
- Vertical transmission

Hepatitis C

Complications

Acute hepatitis C

- Mortality (very low and estimated to be 0.1% or less)
- Acute fulminant hepatitis (rare), affecting <1% of all people with HCV infection

Chronic hepatitis C

- Symptoms such as fatigue, anxiety and depression can negatively impact on the person's quality of life
- Cirrhosis
- Hepatocellular cancer
- Effects of decompensated liver disease include oesophageal varices, ascites, bleeding problems, hepatic encephalopathy and death

Management

Acute infection

- If acute hepatitis C is suspected a same-day assessment should be arranged or immediate specialist advice should be sought
- The local health protection team of suspected cases should be notified immediately

Chronic infection

- The management of hepatitis C has advanced rapidly in recent years resulting in clearance rates of around 95% (interferon-based treatments are no longer recommended)
- The aim of treatment is sustained virological response (defined as undetectable serum HCV RNA 6 months after the end of therapy)
- A combination of protease inhibitors (e.g. daclatasvir + sofosbuvir, or sofosbuvir + simeprevir) ± ribavirin is used

Prevention

There is no effective vaccine against hepatitis C, therefore prevention of HCV infection depends upon reducing the risk of exposure which includes the following:
- Safe and appropriate use of healthcare injections
- Safe handling and disposal of sharps and waste
- Provision of comprehensive harm-reduction services to people who inject drugs e.g. needle exchange programme
- Testing of donated blood for HBV and HCV (as well as HIV and syphilis)
- Training of health personnel
- Prevention of exposure to blood during sex
- Hand hygiene, including surgical hand preparation, hand washing and use of gloves
- Promotion of correct and consistent use of condoms

Ranges from 2 weeks to 6 months

Incubation period

Risk factors

- Drug misuse: injecting drug use is the single most important reported risk factor
- Blood transfusions: receiving a blood transfusion before September 1991 in the UK
- Pregnancy and breastfeeding: transmission rate from mother to child is about 6% (breastfeeding is considered safe)
- Sexual transmission of HCV is possible but uncommon
- Needle stick injury: a significant occupational risk factor, e.g. healthcare workers, police, prison staff etc.
- Use of poorly sterilised medical and dental equipment as well as infected blood products
- Tattooing, ear piercing, body piercing or acupuncture when performed with unsterile equipment
- Sharing razors or toothbrushes which are contaminated with blood

Clinical features

- Approximately 80% of people do not exhibit any symptoms
- Clinical features of acutely symptomatic patients may include fever, fatigue, decreased appetite, nausea, vomiting, abdominal pain, dark urine, grey-coloured faeces, joint pain and jaundice

Investigations

Testing for HCV

- Testing for **anti-HCV antibodies** identifies people who have been infected with the virus
- If the test is positive for anti-HCV antibodies, a nucleic acid test for **HCV ribonucleic acid (RNA)** is needed to confirm chronic infection (as approx. 30% of people infected with HCV spontaneously clear the infection without the need for treatment and though no longer infected they will still test positive for anti-HCV antibodies)

Other investigations

- Baseline FBC, U&Es, LFTs, clotting screen, HbA1c, TFTs, ferritin
- Screening for HAV, HBV and HIV
- Liver ultrasound is used in people with advanced fibrosis or cirrhosis to screen for hepatocellular cancer
- Transient elastography can be offered to diagnose cirrhosis
- Liver biopsy considered in individual cases e.g. to assess the extent of liver damage from inflammation and cirrhosis, identify iron overload and exclude other causes of liver damage

Notes

Hepatitis C

Definition

Human immunodeficiency virus (HIV) is a retrovirus that infects and destroys cells of the immune system, in particular the CD4 cells (a class of T lymphocyte, also known as T-helper cells).

Pathophysiology

- HIV binds to CD4 receptors on helper T lymphocytes, monocytes, macrophages and neural cells
- CD4 cells migrate to the lymphoid tissue where the virus replicates and then infects new CD4-positive cells; as the infection progresses, depletion or impaired function of CD4 cells predisposes to the development of immune dysfunction
- AIDS is the advanced stage of HIV infection when the number of CD4 cells is very low (<200cells/μl); when the immune system is impaired to this extent certain opportunistic infections and malignancies can develop, such as pneumocystis pneumonia and Kaposi's sarcoma, respectively

Transmission

- **Sexual activity** Through vaginal, anal or oral sex
- **Vertically** From mother to child during pregnancy or childbirth, or with breastfeeding
- **By inoculation** Via a contaminated needle, instrument, blood/blood product; through direct exposure of mucous membranes or an open wound to infected bodily fluids; or by a human bite

Human immunodeficiency virus

Complications

Increased risk of opportunistic infections

- Toxoplasmosis
- *Pneumocystis jirovecii* pneumonia
- CMV infection
- Cryptococcal meningitis
- Candidiasis
- Aspergillosis
- *Mycobacterium* spp. infection

Increased risk of malignancies

- Kaposi's sarcoma
- Anal cancer
- Non-Hodgkin's lymphoma
- Cervical cancer

Management

Conservative

- Patient education including transmission reduction advice and psychological support
- Contact tracing
- General health promotion advice on smoking cessation, alcohol, diet and exercise, particularly due to cardiovascular, metabolic and hepatotoxic risk associated with HAART

Highly active antiretroviral therapy (HAART) (see *Notes*)

It is recommended that patients start HAART as soon as they have been diagnosed with HIV

Prevention of spread

- Promote lifelong safer sex, barrier contraception and reduction in the number of partners
- Warn heterosexuals about the dangers of sexual tourism/multiple sexual partners
- Tell drug users not to share needles; use needle-exchange schemes
- Vigorous control of other STIs can reduce HIV incidence by 40%
- Strengthen awareness of clinics for STIs
- Reduce unnecessary blood transfusions
- HIV testing in pregnant women; in women with HIV, maternal antiretroviral therapy, C-section (instead of vaginal), neonatal antiretroviral therapy and bottle feeding (instead of breastfeeding)
- Post-exposure prophylaxis after occupational and sexual exposure also helps to limit HIV spread

- HIV continues to be a major global public health issue, having claimed over 32 million lives so far
- However, with better access to effective HIV prevention, diagnosis, treatment and care, it has become a manageable chronic health condition, enabling people living with HIV to lead long and healthy lives
- There are 2 main types of HIV:
  - **HIV-1** (the predominant type in the UK) is highly virulent and found worldwide
  - **HIV-2** is found mainly in West Africa but has also been reported in Portugal, France and increasingly in India and South America

Epidemiology

- Have a current or former partner who is infected with HIV
- Men who have sex with men (MSM)
- Female sexual contacts of MSM
- From an area of high prevalence of HIV including many parts of Africa
- Have had multiple sexual partners
- Have a history of sexually transmitted infections (STIs), hepatitis B or hepatitis C infection
- Have a history of injecting drug use
- Have been raped
- Have had blood transfusions, transplants, or other risk-prone procedures in countries without rigorous procedures for HIV screening
- Occupational exposure such as a needle stick injury

Risk factors

Stages of HIV and clinical features

1. Seroconversion illness

- Occurs between 1 and 6 weeks after infection
- Common symptoms are fever, malaise, myalgia, pharyngitis, headaches, diarrhoea, neuralgia or neuropathy, lymphadenopathy and/or a maculopapular rash; acute infection may be asymptomatic
- Although antibody tests are negative, viral p24 antigen and HIV RNA levels are raised in early infection

2. Asymptomatic infection

After seroconversion, virus levels are low (although gradual replication continues); CD4 and CD8 lymphocyte levels are normal; this situation may persist for many years

3. Persistent generalised lymphadenopathy (PGL)

- Nodes >1cm in diameter at 2 extra-inguinal sites persisting for ≥3 months not due to any other cause
- Biopsy is not advised unless an alternative diagnosis must be excluded as features are non-specific

4. Symptomatic infection

- Non-specific constitutional symptoms develop: fever, night sweats, diarrhoea and weight loss
- Minor opportunistic infections may be present e.g. oral candida, oral hairy leucoplakia, herpes zoster, recurrent herpes simplex, seborrhoeic dermatitis, tinea infections
- The collective name for the above is the AIDS-related complex (ARC), a prodrome to AIDS

5. AIDS

Severe immunodeficiency and evidence of life-threatening infections and unusual tumours

Investigations

- **HIV antibody** Usually with both a screening ELISA and a confirmatory western blot assay; most people develop antibodies to HIV at 4–6 weeks (99% by 3 months), thus asymptomatic patients should be tested 4 weeks post-exposure after an initial negative result, and a repeat test at 12 weeks
- **P24 antigen test** Usually positive from about 1–4 weeks after infection with HIV
- **HIV viral load** HIV RNA or branched DNA assay
- **FBC** May show anaemia, thrombocytopenia, ↓WCC with ↓CD4 cell count
- **CRP/ESR** May be ↑
- Screening for other infections if clinically appropriate: e.g. TB, hepatitis B, toxoplasma, other STIs
- Baseline CXR and cervical smear

Human immunodeficiency virus notes

Monitoring in HIV

Monitoring of HIV will usually be done in specialist clinics using the CD4 lymphocyte cell (CD4) count and viral load.

CD4 count

- In a healthy person not infected with HIV, the CD4 count is usually >500cells/μl
- CD4 counts are variable and can be reduced by common infections, so overall trends are more important than single values
- People with CD4 counts <200cells/μl are most at risk of HIV-related opportunistic infections and cancers, but some may not have significant symptoms
- CD4 counts are the main determinant of when prophylaxis for opportunistic infections and antiretroviral therapy (ART) is started

Viral load

- Viral load reflects rates of viral replication and is measured using a polymerase chain reaction (PCR) test
- A rising viral load may indicate non-adherence to ART or resistance to one or more antiretroviral drugs
- Viral load ranges from undetectable (<50 copies of viral genome/ml blood) to over 1 million copies/ml
- The degree of viral replication is linked to the rate of CD4 decline and therefore disease progression—when viral load is suppressed through ART, CD4 counts recover and risk of HIV-related opportunistic infections and cancers declines

Highly active antiretroviral therapy (HAART)

- HAART involves a combination of at least 3 drugs, typically 2 nucleoside reverse transcriptase inhibitors (NRTIs) and either a protease inhibitor (PI) or a non-nucleoside reverse transcriptase inhibitor (NNRTI)
- This combination reduces viral replication and the risk of viral resistance emerging

Table 1 Highly active anti-retroviral therapy

Nucleoside reverse transcriptase inhibitors		
Examples	**Mechanism of action**	**Side effects**
Zidovudine (AZT), abacavir, emtricitabine, didanosine, lamivudine, tenofovir	Inhibits synthesis of DNA by reverse transcription and also acts as DNA terminator	General side effects: peripheral neuropathy Tenofovir: renal impairment and osteoporosis Zidovudine: anaemia, myopathy, black nails Didanosine: pancreatitis
Non-nucleoside reverse transcriptase inhibitors		
Nevirapine, efavirenz	Binds directly to and inhibits HIV reverse transcriptase, which prevents HIV from replicating	P450 enzyme interaction (nevirapine induces), hepatic disorders, abdominal pain, rashes
Protease inhibitors		
Indinavir, nelfinavir, ritonavir, saquinavir	Acts competitively on HIV protease enzyme, which is involved in production of functional viral proteins and enzymes	Diabetes, hyperlipidaemia, buffalo hump, central obesity, P450 enzyme inhibition
Entry inhibitors		
Maraviroc, enfuvirtide	Maraviroc binds to CCR5, preventing an interaction with gp41; enfuvirtide binds to gp41, also known as a 'fusion inhibitor' and prevents HIV-1 from entering and infecting immune cells	Alopecia, arthralgia, diabetes, diarrhoea, dizziness, dyslipidaemia, dyspnoea, fever, headache, neutropenia, oral ulceration, pancreatitis, peripheral neuropathy
Integrase inhibitors		
Raltegravir, elvitegravir, dolutegravir	Prevents insertion of HIV DNA into the human genome	GI side effects, headaches, myopathy, rhabdomyolysis

Species of plasmodium that are known to cause malaria in humans include:
- **P. falciparum** Most prevalent malaria parasite on the African continent and responsible for the majority of malaria deaths
- **P. vivax** Most common form of malaria parasite outside sub-Saharan Africa; it has dormant liver stages which can cause 'relapses' of malaria months or years after the initial infection
- **P. ovale** Found mostly in Africa and the islands of the western Pacific; it has dormant liver stages which can cause 'relapses' of malaria months or years after the initial infection
- **P. malariae** Found in South America, Asia and Africa; if untreated it can cause lifelong chronic infection
- **P. knowlesi** A malaria parasite of monkeys in Southeast Asia which can cause severe and sometimes fatal illness in humans
- **Mixed infections** Infection with more than one species of plasmodium can occur

Malaria is a life-threatening illness caused by infection of red blood cells by *Plasmodium* **spp. parasites**.

Definition

Causes

Malaria

Complications

- **Brain** Cerebral malaria (due to *P. falciparum*) resulting in reduced consciousness, confusion, convulsions, coma and eventually death
- **Lungs** Acute respiratory distress syndrome
- **Blood** Severe anaemia, spontaneous bleeding and coagulopathy, septicaemia
- **Kidneys** Nephrotic syndrome, AKI, haemoglobinuria ('black water fever')
- **Metabolic** Hypoglycaemia, metabolic acidosis
- **Gastrointestinal** Jaundice, splenic rupture

Management

General

- Immediate hospital admission should be considered in any of the following:
  - Suspected of having severe or complicated malaria
  - Suspected of having falciparum malaria
  - Is a child, pregnant or older than 65 years
- All others suspected of having malaria should be discussed with an infectious disease specialist urgently
- Public health should be notified of all suspected cases

Antimalarial drugs

- **Artesunate** Parenteral artesunate is used to treat severe or complicated malaria
- **Quinine** Used initially to treat severe or complicated malaria if artesunate is unavailable
- **Artemisinin-based combination therapy (ACT)** Is used to treat uncomplicated malaria and is the preferred treatment for mixed infection
- **Atovaquone-proguanil (Malarone)** Is used to treat uncomplicated falciparum malaria

- **Quinine and doxycycline** Quinine + doxycycline or doxycycline alone may be used to treat uncomplicated falciparum malaria; doxycycline should not be given to children <12 years
- **Chloroquine** Is used to treat uncomplicated *P. malariae*, *P. ovale* and *P. knowlesi* and most cases of *P. vivax* malaria but use depends upon patterns of resistance and tolerance
- **Primaquine** Only current effective drug for the eradication of hypnozoites (dormant parasites which persist in the liver after treatment of *P. vivax* and *P. ovale*); screening for G6PD deficiency is essential before treatment (as can cause haemolysis and be fatal in G6PD-deficient individuals); it is also contraindicated in pregnancy and breastfeeding

Prevention (ABCD)

- **A**wareness of risk Travellers should be aware of malaria risk areas
- **B**ite avoidance Use mosquito repellent, e.g. *N,N*-diethyl-meta-toluamide (DEET), covering arms and legs, sleep under an insecticide-treated net
- **C**hemoprophylaxis Malarone, chloroquine, doxycycline, mefloquine or proguanil
- **D**iagnosis Be aware of symptoms and seek immediate medical advice if develop malaria symptoms, including up to a year after return from travelling

- Humans, who are the intermediate hosts, become infected by the bite of an infected **female Anopheles mosquito**
- The mosquito injects sporozoites (the infecting agent of the parasite) into the blood circulation which circulates and enters liver cells
- The sporozoites divide inside liver cells into a schizont containing approx. 30 000 offspring (merozoites) which are released into the bloodstream when the schizont ruptures
- Vivax and ovale malaria also have a dormant (hypnozoite) stage in the liver which may 'awaken' and become schizont (months or even years after exposure)
- Red cells infected with *P. falciparum* adhere to the endothelium of small vessels and cause vascular occlusion resulting in severe organ damage (mainly gut, kidney, liver and brain)
- The parasite can also be transmitted by blood transfusion, transplacentally, organ transplantation and via the use of improperly cleaned syringes

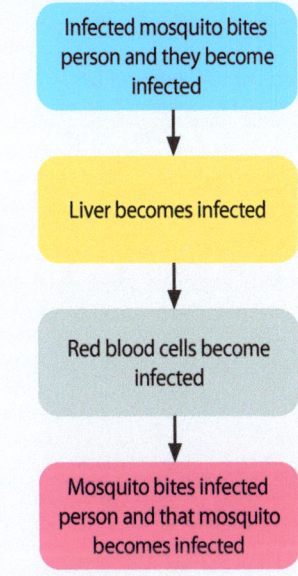

Infected mosquito bites person and they become infected

↓

Liver becomes infected

↓

Red blood cells become infected

↓

Mosquito bites infected person and that mosquito becomes infected

Fig. 1 Malaria transmission cycle

- In 2018, there were an estimated 228 million cases of malaria worldwide
- Most malaria cases and deaths occur in sub-Saharan Africa; however Southeast Asia, eastern Mediterranean, western Pacific and the Americas are areas also affected
- Children aged under 5 years are the most vulnerable group affected by malaria

Pathophysiology (see *Fig. 1*)

Epidemiology

Investigations

Diagnostic

►Thick and thin blood films:
- Thick and thin blood films: repeat bloods should be done after 12–24h and again after a further 24h in patients with initial negative blood film
- In patients with 3 negative slides over a period of 48–72h, the disease is unlikely

►Rapid diagnostic test (RDT):
- Another frequently used diagnostic test which detects malaria antigen or enzymes
- Slightly less sensitive and not reliable to detect non-falciparum malaria when compared with good-quality blood films; therefore should not be used as an alternative to blood films

Other
- FBC: typically reveals thrombocytopenia and anaemia, ↑WCC may also be present
- Glucose (low in severe disease), U&Es (may show ↓Na⁺ and AKI), LFTs (often abnormal)
- G6PD activity: prior to giving primaquine
- In severe cases may also need blood gases, blood cultures, clotting, urine/stool culture, CXR and lumbar puncture

Clinical features

Most patients with *P. falciparum* infection present in the 1st month or within 6 months of infection. *P. vivax* or *P. ovale* infections commonly present >6 months after exposure (sometimes after years).

Symptoms
- Fever (often recurring), chills and rigors
- Headache
- Cough
- Myalgia
- Gastrointestinal upset

Signs
- Fever
- Splenomegaly, hepatomegaly
- Jaundice
- ± Abdominal tenderness

Primary TB

- The initial infection with **M. tuberculosis** usually occurs in the upper zone of the lung producing a lesion called the **Ghon focus**
- The Ghon focus comprises macrophages which have engulfed the bacilli resulting in the typical **granulomatous lesions with caseating central necrosis** surrounded by epithelioid cells and Langerhans giant cells
- The Ghon focus is almost always accompanied by caseous lesions in the hilar lymph nodes and the combination of these is known as a **Ghon complex**
- In immunocompetent people the initial lesion usually heals by fibrosis; those who are immunocompromised may develop disseminated disease (**miliary TB**)

Secondary (post-primary) TB

- If the host becomes immunocompromised the initial infection may become reactivated; reactivation generally occurs in the apex of the lungs and may spread locally or to more distant sites
- The lungs remain the most common site for secondary TB; extrapulmonary infection may occur in the following areas:
  - Central nervous system (tuberculous meningitis, the most serious complication)
  - Vertebral bodies (Pott's disease)
  - Cervical lymph nodes (scrofuloderma)
  - Renal
  - GI tract

Tuberculosis (TB) is an infection caused by bacteria of the **Mycobacterium** genus that most commonly affect the lungs.

Definition

Pathophysiology

Tuberculosis

Complications

- Reduced quality of life
- Transmission to others
- Drug resistance
- Post-TB bronchiectasis, COPD and aspergilloma (occur in residual lung cavities)
- Post-TB cor pulmonale/respiratory failure may result from lung cavitation, scarring and fibrosis following pulmonary TB
- Death

Management

Non-pharmacological

- Care should be coordinated through the local multidisciplinary TB team
- For all TB cases in the UK, the local public health authority should be notified so that screening and contact tracing (see *Notes*) can be arranged
- Patient education, particularly the importance of complying with medical therapy

Pharmacological

Anti-TB drugs (see *Notes, Side effects of anti-TB drugs*)
Active TB standard treatment (**RIPE**):
- **R**ifampicin For 6 months (2 months initiation phase + 4 months continuation phase)
- **I**soniazid For 6 months (2 months initiation phase + 4 months continuation phase)
- **P**yrazinamide For initial 2 months (2 months initiation phase)
- **E**thambutol For initial 2 months (2 months initiation phase)

Latent TB:
The treatment for **latent TB** is 3 months of isoniazid with pyridoxine and rifampicin *or* 6 months of isoniazid (with pyridoxine).

Meningeal TB:
Patients with **meningeal TB** are treated for a prolonged period (at least 12 months) with the addition of steroids.

- Close contact of TB patient
- Ethnic minority groups: predominantly from South Asia and sub-Saharan Africa
- Homeless patients, those with alcohol dependency and other drug misusers
- HIV-positive and other immunocompromised patients; patients on immunosuppressant drugs are particularly at risk (e.g. infliximab and etanercept, azathioprine, ciclosporin)
- Children and elderly patients
- Other conditions: haematological and some solid cancers, long-term steroids, diabetes, end-stage renal disease, silicosis and gastrectomy/jejunoileal bypass

Risk factors

- Worldwide, TB is one of the top 10 causes of death and the leading cause from a single infectious agent (above HIV/AIDS)
- In 2018, an estimated 10 million people fell ill with TB worldwide

Epidemiology

Clinical features

Systemic features

- May be asymptomatic
- Night sweats
- Weight loss
- Malaise
- Fever
- Anorexia

Local features

- **Lung/pleura** Cough, sputum, haemoptysis, breathlessness, lobar collapse, bronchopneumonia, hoarseness, chest pain, effusion
- **Heart/pericardium** Pain, arrhythmias, cardiac failure, pericarditis
- **Intestine** Malabsorption, diarrhoea, obstruction
- **GU tract** Haematuria, renal failure, epididymitis, salpingitis, infertility
- **Adrenals** Adrenal insufficiency
- **Skin** Erythema nodosum, erythema induratum, lupus vulgaris
- **Eyes** Iritis, choroiditis, phlyctenular keratoconjunctivitis
- **Bones/joints** Arthritis, osteomyelitis
- **Lymphatics** Lymphadenopathy, cold abscesses, sinuses
- **Brain** Tuberculoma, meningitis

Investigations

- **CXR** Typically shows patchy or nodular shadows in the upper zone (see *Fig. 1*); with miliary TB the CXR may be normal or show miliary shadows throughout the lung (see *Fig. 2*)
- **Sputum** (at least 3 samples) Ziehl–Neelsen or auramine staining of a sputum smear may demonstrate the presence of acid-fast bacilli; *in vitro* culture of the sputum (e.g. Löwenstein–Jensen medium) may take 4–7 weeks to provide a result and a further 3 weeks is required to identify drug sensitivity
- **Whole blood interferon-gamma** Aids diagnosis of TB
- **Bronchoscopy** with washings of the affected lobes; useful if there is no sputum available
- **Biopsy** Diagnosis can sometimes be made based on the histological demonstration of a caseating granuloma)
- **HIV screening** HIV is a big risk factor for TB (see *Ch8: Human immunodeficiency virus*)
- **Tuberculin test** Hypersensitivity to the tubercle bacillus develops about 3 weeks after initial infection; the Mantoux test is usually used

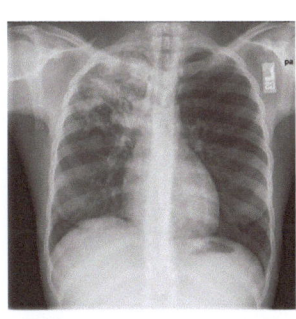

Fig. 1 Pulmonary TB

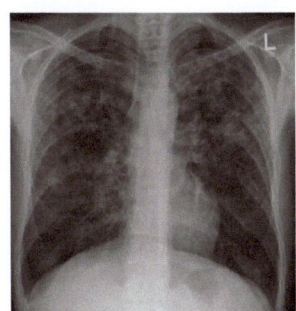

Fig. 2 Miliary TB

Side effects of anti-TB drugs (see *Table 1*)

Table 1 Side effects of the main anti-TB drugs

Rifampicin	• Discolours body secretions and urine pink • Induces liver enzymes • Flu-like symptoms • Elevation of liver transferases and hepatitis
Isoniazid	• Peripheral neuropathy: prevent with pyridoxine (vitamin B$_6$) • Hepatitis • Allergic reactions: skin rash and fever • Agranulocytosis • Inhibits liver enzymes
Pyrazinamide	• Hyperuricaemia • Arthralgia and myalgia • Gout • Hepatitis (rare)
Ethambutol	Eyes: optic neuritis (visual acuity and red-green colour perception should be done before treatment)

The Bacille Calmette-Guérin (BCG) vaccination

The BCG vaccine contains live attenuated *M. bovis*. It offers limited protection against TB and leprosy.

Administration

- Any person being considered for the BCG vaccine must first be given a tuberculin skin test; the only exceptions are children <6 years who have had no contact with tuberculosis
- Given intradermally, normally to the lateral aspect of the left upper arm
- BCG can be given at the same time as other live vaccines, but if not administered simultaneously there should be a 4-week interval

Indications

- All infants (aged 0–12 months) living in areas of the UK where the annual incidence of TB is 40/100 000 or greater
- All infants (aged 0–12 months) with a parent or grandparent who was born in a country where the annual incidence of TB is 40/100 000 or greater; the same applies to older children but if they are 6 years or older they require a tuberculin skin test first
- Previously unvaccinated tuberculin-negative contacts of cases of respiratory TB

- Previously unvaccinated, tuberculin-negative new entrants under 16 years who were born in or who have lived for a prolonged period (at least 3 months) in a country with an annual TB incidence of 40/100 000 or greater
- Healthcare workers
- Prison staff
- Staff of care homes for the elderly
- Those who work with homeless people

Contraindications

- Previous BCG vaccination or a past history of TB
- Positive tuberculin test (Heaf or Mantoux)
- HIV
- Pregnancy

Contact tracing

- The **Mantoux test** should be used to diagnose latent TB in people who are either household contacts or close work or school contacts (aged ≥5 years) of all patients diagnosed with active TB
- As the Mantoux test may be positive in patients who have had the bacillus (BCG vaccine) interferon-gamma testing is the recommended 2nd-line test for people whose Mantoux testing shows positive results, or instead of Mantoux test in people for whom Mantoux testing may be less reliable

Observed therapy

- Individualised supportive care may be required for people with clinically or socially complex needs considered to be at high risk of poor adherence to treatment
- Examples of these individuals include the homeless, history of drug misuse; previous TB treatment; multiple drug resistance TB; prisoners; significant mental health, memory or cognitive problems
- This may include 'directly observed therapy' (**DOT**), where drug treatment is given under the observation of a key worker and the person is observed to swallow each dose of medication, or 'video observed therapy' (**VOT**) to improve adherence, reduce the risk of stopping treatment early and reduce drug resistance

Appendix: Figure acknowledgements

Chapter 1: Cardiology

Acute coronary syndrome

- **Fig. 1** – Adapted from http://medicalnotesonline.blogspot. com/2011/01/cardiology-myocardial-infarction-and.html
- **Fig. 2** – Reproduced from *Cardiology in a Heartbeat* (Vaswani *et al.*) under the Creative Commons Attribution-ShareAlike 4.0 International Licence; reproduced with permission from **Life In The Fast Lane** (http://lifeinthefastlane.com).
- **Fig. 3** – Reproduced from *Cardiology in a Heartbeat* (Vaswani *et al.*) under the Creative Commons Attribution-ShareAlike 4.0 International Licence; reproduced with permission from **Life In The Fast Lane** (http://lifeinthefastlane.com).

Acute pericarditis

- **Fig. 1** – Reproduced from *Cardiology in a Heartbeat* (Vaswani *et al.*) under the Creative Commons Attribution-ShareAlike 4.0 International Licence; reproduced with permission from **Life In The Fast Lane** (http://lifeinthefastlane.com).
- **Fig. 2** – author's own

Atrial fibrillation

- **Fig. 1** – basic trace

Heart failure

- **Fig. 1** – author's own
- **Fig. 2** – Reproduced from *Anatomy and Physiology: an introduction for nursing and healthcare* (Minett & Ginesi)
- **Fig. 3** – Reproduced from https://meded.ucsd.edu/clinicalmed/ heart.html with permission
- **Fig. 4** – Adapted from https://medmnemonics.wordpress. com/2011/03/04/heart-failure-chest-x-ray-signs-2/

Hypertension

- **Fig. 1** – Reproduced from *Medicine in a Minute* (Vaswani & Khaw).
- **Fig. 2** – Reproduced from *Medicine in a Minute* (Vaswani & Khaw).

Infective endocarditis

- **Fig. 1** – Reproduced from www.slideserve.com/derry/ infective-endocarditis

- **Fig. 2** – Reproduced from *Cardiology in a Heartbeat* (Vaswani *et al.*); Licensed under: Public Domain; available at: http://commons.wikimedia.org/wiki/File:Splinter_ hemorrhage.jpg
- **Fig. 3** – Reproduced from *Cardiology in a Heartbeat* (Vaswani *et al.*); Licensed under: Creative Commons Attribution-Share Alike 4.0 International; additional attribution: Wikimedia Commons, Gonzalo M. Garcia; available at: http://commons. wikimedia.org/wiki/File:Acopaquia.jpg
- **Fig. 4** – Reproduced from http://simple-cardio.blogspot. com/2012/06/peripheral-signs-of-infective.html with permission from Professor Sanjay Sharma

Valvular heart disease

- **Fig. 1** – Reproduced from https://ecg.utah.edu with permission
- **Fig. 2** – Reproduced from http://learningradiology.com/index. htm with permission
- **Fig. 3** – Reproduced from *Cardiology in a Heartbeat* (Vaswani *et al.*) under the Creative Commons Attribution-ShareAlike 4.0 International Licence; reproduced with permission from **Life In The Fast Lane** (http://lifeinthefastlane.com).

Chapter 2: Respiratory

Acute respiratory distress syndrome

- **Fig. 1** – Reproduced from *Medicine in a Minute* (Vaswani & Khaw).

Asthma

- **Fig. 1** – Reproduced from *Anatomy and Physiology: an introduction for nursing and healthcare* (Minett & Ginesi).
- **Fig. 2** – Reproduced from https://radiopaedia.org/articles/lung-hyperinflation-1?lang=us (Case courtesy of Assoc Prof Frank Gaillard, Radiopaedia.org, rID: 10550) with permission.

Bronchiectasis

- **Fig. 1** – Licensed under: Creative Commons Attribution-Share Alike 4.0 International; additional attribution: Wikimedia Commons, Gonzalo M. Garcia; available at: http://commons. wikimedia.org/wiki/File:Acopaquia.jpg
- **Fig. 2** – Reproduced from image https://radiopaedia.org/cases/ cystic-bronchiectasis-3 (Case courtesy of Dr Bruno Di Muzio, Radiopaedia.org, rID: 18289) with permission.

Chronic obstructive pulmonary disease
- **Fig. 1** – Reproduced from *Interpreting Chest X-Rays* (Ellis).

Interstitial lung disease
- **Fig. 1** – Reproduced from *Interpreting Chest X-Rays* (Ellis).

Lung cancer
- **Fig. 1** – Reproduced from *Medicine in a Minute* (Vaswani & Khaw). Licensed under Creative Commons Attribution-Share Alike 3.0 Unported; additional attribution: James Heilman, MD; available at: https://commons.wikimedia.org/wiki/File:LungCACXR.PNG

Pleural effusion
- **Fig. 1** – Reproduced from *Interpreting Chest X-Rays* (Ellis).

Pneumonia
- **Fig. 1** – Reproduced from *Medicine in a Minute* (Vaswani & Khaw). Licensed under Creative Commons Attribution-Share Alike 3.0 Unported; additional attribution: Hellerhoff; available at: https://commons.wikimedia.org/wiki/File:03-01-Infiltrat_Ausgang.png

Pneumothorax
- **Fig. 1** – Reproduced from *Medicine in a Minute* (Vaswani & Khaw). Licensed under Creative Commons Attribution-Share Alike 3.0 Unported; additional attribution: Karthik Easvur; available at: https://commons.wikimedia.org/wiki/File:Pneumothorax_gif_1.gif
- **Fig. 2** – Reproduced from *Interpreting Chest X-Rays* (Ellis).
- **Notes Fig.** (Flowchart of management of spontaneous pneumothorax) – Reproduced from *Thorax* (2010) 65: 18 with permission from BMJ Publishing Group Ltd.

Pulmonary embolism
- **Fig. 2** – Reproduced from *Medicine in a Minute* (Vaswani & Khaw). Licensed under the Creative Commons Attribution-ShareAlike 4.0 International Licence; reproduced with permission from **Life In The Fast Lane** (http://lifeinthefastlane.com).
- **Fig. 3** – Reproduced from *Medicine in a Minute* (Vaswani & Khaw). Licensed under Creative Commons Attributions-Share Alike 4.0 International; additional attribution: Rvahudson; available at: https://commons.wikimedia.org/wiki/File:CTA_Chest_With_Massive_Pulmonary_Embolism_and_Complete_Occlusion.jpg

Respiratory failure
- **Fig. 1** – Reproduced from www.indiamart.com/proddetail/venturi-mask-3663147912.html.

Sarcoidosis
- **Fig. 1** – Reproduced from *Medicine in a Minute* (Vaswani & Khaw). Licensed under Creative Commons Attribution-Share Alike 3.0 Unported; additional attribution: James Heilman, MD; available at: https://commons.wikimedia.org/wiki/index.php?curid=11520780
- **Fig. 2** – Reproduced from *Current Clinical Medicine*; Sarcoidosis (DA Culver) (© 2009, 2010 The Cleveland Clinic Foundation, all rights reserved) with permission.

Chapter 3: Gastroenterology

Acute pancreatitis
- **Fig. 1** – reproduced from Chauhan, *et al.* (2008) *Clinical Picture*, **372**: 54 (DOI: https://doi.org/10.1016/S0140-6736(08)60993-9) with permission from Elsevier.

Chronic pancreatitis
- **Fig. 1** – Reproduced from https://radiopaedia.org/cases/pancreatic-calcifications-chronic-pancreatitis (Case courtesy of Dr Domenico Nicoletti, Radiopaedia.org, rID: 67773) with permission.

Cirrhosis
- **Fig. 1** – Reproduced from www.luxeclinic.co.uk/what-is-spider-naevus-and-how-to-treat-it/
- **Fig. 2** – Licensed under Creative Commons Attributions-Share Alike 3.0; available at: https://commons.wikimedia.org/wiki/File:Gynecomastia_001.jpg

Coeliac disease
- **Fig. 1** – Adapted from www.glutenfreetherapeutics.com/living-gluten-free/medicine-research/chronic-inflammation
- **Fig. 2** – Reproduced from *Medicine in a Minute* (Vaswani & Khaw). Licensed under Creative Commons Attribution-Share Alike 3.0 Unported; additional attribution: BallenaBlanca; available at: https://commons.wikimedia.org/wiki/File%3ADiapositiva_1.jpg
- **Fig. 3** – Reproduced from www.passmedicine.com/review/textbook.php?s= with permission.

Gastric cancer
- **Fig. 1** – Reproduced from www.nguyenthienhung.com
- **Fig. 2** – Reproduced from *Medicine in a Minute* (Vaswani & Khaw). Licensed under Creative Commons Attributions-Share Alike 3.0 Unported; additional attribution: Thomas Habif; available at: https://commons.wikimedia.org/wiki/File:Acanthosis-nigricans4.jpg

Gastro-oesophageal reflux disease
- **Fig. 1** – Adapted from https://herniagallbladderwa.com.au/conditions/hiatal-hernia-treatment-perth

Hereditary haemochromatosis
- **Fig. 1** – Reprinted by permission from Springer Nature; Brissot *et al.* (2018) Haemochromatosis. *Nat Rev Dis Primers* **4**, 18016 (https://doi.org/10.1038/nrdp.2018.16)

Jaundice
- **Fig. 1** – Reproduced from https://imannooor.wordpress.com
- **Fig. 2** – Adapted from https://medical-dictionary.thefreedictionary.com/Bilirubin+metabolism

Oesophageal cancer and other causes of dysphagia
- **Fig. 2** – reproduced from *The Lancet*, **290**: 2383, Lagergren, *et al.* (2017) (DOI: https://doi.org/10.1016/S0140-6736(17)31462-9) with permission from Elsevier.

Wilson's disease

- **Fig. 1** – Reproduced from *Medicine in a Minute* (Vaswani & Khaw). Licensed under Creative Commons Attribution-Share Alike 3.0 Unported; additional attribution: Herbert L. Fred, MD, Hendrik A. van Dijk; available at: https://commons.wikimedia.org/wiki/File:Kayser-Fleischer_ring.jpg

Chapter 4: Renal

Nephritic syndrome

- **Fig. 1** – Reproduced under the Open Government Licence v3.0 from www.nhs.uk/conditions/henoch-schonlein-purpura-hsp/
- **Fig. 2** – Reproduced from *Journal of Intensive Care* (2017) **5**: 57 (DOI 10.1186/s40560-017-0251-y) under a CC Attribution 4.0 International License.

Nephrotic syndrome

- **Fig. 1** – Reproduced under a CC Attribution License 3.0 Germany; additional attribution: Klaus D. Peter; available at: https://en.wikipedia.org/wiki/Periorbital_puffiness#/media/File:Oedema.jpg
- **Fig. 2** – Reproduced under the Open Government Licence v3.0 from www.nhs.uk/conditions/nail-problems/
- **Fig. 3** – Reproduced from *Medicine in a Minute* (Vaswani & Khaw). Licensed under CC Attribution License 3.0 Germany; additional attribution: Klaus D. Peter; available at: https://commons.wikimedia.org/wiki/File:Xanthelasma.jpg

Chapter 5: Endocrinology

Acromegaly

- **Fig. 1** – Adapted from www.endotext.org.
- **Fig. 2** – Reproduced from *Medicine in a Minute* (Vaswani & Khaw). Licensed under CC Attribution 2.0 Generic; additional attributions: Philippe Chanson and Sylvie Salenave; available at: https://commons.wikimedia.org/wiki/File:Acromegaly_prognathism.JPEG
- **Fig. 3** – Licensed under CC Attribution 3.0 Unported; additional attributions: Deshpande P1, Guledgud MV1, Patil K1, Hegde U2, Sahni A1, Huchanahalli Sheshanna S2; available from https://en.wikipedia.org/wiki/Macroglossia#/media/File:Macroglossia_with_crenations_along_the_margins_and_loss_of_papillae_on_dorsum_surface_of_the_tongue.png
- **Fig. 4** – Reproduced from *Clinical Endocrinology* (Whitehead & Miell).

Adrenal insufficiency

- **Fig. 1** – Reproduced from *Clinical Endocrinology* (Whitehead & Miell).

Cushing syndrome

- **Fig. 2** – Reproduced from https://commons.wikimedia.org/wiki/File:CushingsFace.jpg under a CC Attribution 2.5 Generic license.
- **Fig. 3** – Reproduced from www.reddit.com/r/Pathognomonic/comments/1sxyig/purple_abdominal_striae_1cm_cushings_syndrome/

Hyperthyroidism

- **Fig. 1** – Reproduced from *Medicine in a Minute* (Vaswani & Khaw). Licensed under Creative Commons Attribution-Share Alike 4.0 International; additional attribution: OpenStax; available at: https://cnx.org/contents/FPtK1zmh@8.108:YhivaL0u@4/The-Thyroid-Gland
- **Fig. 2** – Reproduced from *Medicine in a Minute* (Vaswani & Khaw). Licensed under Creative Commons Attribution 2.0 Generic; additional attributions: Herbert L. Fred, MD and Hendrik A. van Dijk; available at: https://commons.wikimedia.org/wiki/File:Myxedema.jpg
- **Fig. 3** – Reproduced from *Medicine in a Minute* (Vaswani & Khaw). Licensed under Creative Commons Attributions-Share Alike 3.0 Unported; additional attributions: Jonathan Trobe, M.D. – University of Michigan Kellogg Eye Center; available at: https://commons.wikimedia.org/wiki/File:Proptosis_and_lid_retraction_from_Graves%27_Disease.jpg

Hypocalcaemia

- **Fig. 2** – Reproduced from https://what-when-how.com/nursing/endocrine-disorders-adult-care-nursing-part-3/

Hypothyroidism

- **Fig. 1** – Reproduced from *Anatomy and Physiology: an introduction for nursing and healthcare* (Minett & Ginesi).

Polycystic ovary syndrome

- **Fig. 1** – Reproduced from Science Photo Library with permission.
- **Fig. 2** – Reproduced from *Clinical Endocrinology* (Whitehead & Miell).

Chapter 6: Neurology

Bell's palsy

- **Fig. 1** – Reproduced from *Medicine in a Minute* (Vaswani & Khaw). Licensed under CC Attribution-Share Alike 3.0 Unported; additional attribution: James Heilman, MD; available at: https://commons.wikimedia.org/wiki/File:Bellspalsy.JPG
- **Fig. 2** – Reproduced from www.pinterest.co.uk/pin/773985885937936621/
- **Fig. 3** – Reproduced from Mortada et al. (2009) *Transplant Infectious Disease,* **11**: 72 (https://doi.org/10.1111/j.1399-3062.2008.00353.x) with permission from John Wiley and Sons.

Extradural haematoma

- **Fig. 2** – Reproduced from *Anatomy and Physiology in Healthcare* (Marshall *et al.*).
- **Fig. 3** – Reproduced from *Eureka: Neurology and Neurosurgery* (Collins *et al.*).

Multiple sclerosis

- **Fig. 1** – Adapted from *Anatomy and Physiology in Healthcare* (Marshall *et al.*).
- **Fig. 2** – Reproduced from *Eureka: Neurology and Neurosurgery* (Collins *et al.*).

Myasthenia gravis

- **Fig. 1** – Reproduced from www.epainassist.com/images/Article-Images/Myasthenia-Gravis.jpg with permission.

Neurofibromatosis

- **Fig. 1** – Reproduced from *Medicine in a Minute* (Vaswani & Khaw). Licensed under CC Attribution-Share Alike 3.0 Unported; additional attribution: Accrochoc; available at: https://commons.wikimedia.org/wiki/File:NF-1-Tache_cafe-au-lait.jpg
- **Fig. 2** – Reproduced from *Medicine in a Minute* (Vaswani & Khaw). Licensed under CC Attribution-Share Alike 4.0 International; available at: https://commons.wikimedia.org/wiki/File:Cutaneous_neurofibroma_(MedMedicine).jpg
- **Fig. 3** – Reproduced from *Medicine in a Minute* (Vaswani & Khaw). Licensed under Public Domain

Stroke

- **Fig. 1** – Reproduced from *Eureka: Neurology and Neurosurgery* (Collins *et al.*).

Subarachnoid haemorrhage

- **Fig. 2** – Reproduced from *Medicine in a Minute* (Vaswani & Khaw). Licensed under CC Attribution-Share Alike 3.0 Unported; additional attribution: James Heilman, MD; available at: https://commons.wikimedia.org/wiki/File:Subarach.png

Subdural haematoma

- **Fig. 1** – Reproduced from *Eureka: Neurology and Neurosurgery* (Collins *et al.*).
- **Fig. 2** – Reproduced from *Eureka: Neurology and Neurosurgery* (Collins *et al.*).

Chapter 7: Rheumatology

Ankylosing spondylitis

- **Fig. 1** – Reproduced from *Rheumatology: a clinical handbook* (Al-Sukaini *et al.*).
- **Fig. 2** – Reproduced from *Rheumatology: a clinical handbook* (Al-Sukaini *et al.*).
- **Fig. 3** – Reproduced from *Rheumatology: a clinical handbook* (Al-Sukaini *et al.*).

Fibromyalgia

- **Fig. 1** – Reproduced from *Rheumatology: a clinical handbook* (Al-Sukaini *et al.*).

Giant cell arteritis

- **Fig. 1** – Reproduced from *Rheumatology: a clinical handbook* (Al-Sukaini *et al.*).

Gout

- **Fig. 1** – Reproduced from *Rheumatology: a clinical handbook* (Al-Sukaini *et al.*).

- **Fig. 2** – Reproduced from *Medicine in a Minute* (Vaswani & Khaw). Licensed under CC Attribution 2.0 Generic; additional attribution: Arthritis Research UK Primary Care Centre, Primary Care Sciences, Keele University, Keele, UK; available at: https://commons.wikimedia.org/wiki/File:Tophaceous_gout.jpg

Osteoarthritis

- **Fig. 1** – Reproduced from *Medicine in a Minute* (Vaswani & Khaw). Licensed under CC Attribution-Share Alike 3.0 Unported; additional attribution: Drahreg01; available at: https://commons.wikimedia.org/wiki/File:Heberden-Arthrose.JPG
- **Fig. 2** – Reproduced from *Medicine in a Minute* (Vaswani & Khaw). Licensed under CC Attribution-Share Alike 3.0 Unported; additional attribution: James Heilman, MD; available at: https://commons.wikimedia.org/wiki/File:Osteoarthritis_left_knee.jpg

Paget's disease

- **Fig. 1** – Reproduced from *Rheumatology: a clinical handbook* (Al-Sukaini *et al.*).
- **Fig. 2** – Reproduced from *Rheumatology: a clinical handbook* (Al-Sukaini *et al.*).

Polymyositis and dermatomyositis

- **Fig. 1** – Reproduced from *Rheumatology: a clinical handbook* (Al-Sukaini *et al.*).
- **Fig. 2** – Reproduced from *Rheumatology: a clinical handbook* (Al-Sukaini *et al.*).

Psoriatic arthritis

- **Fig. 1** – Reproduced from *Rheumatology: a clinical handbook* (Al-Sukaini *et al.*).
- **Fig. 2** – Reproduced from *Rheumatology: a clinical handbook* (Al-Sukaini *et al.*).
- **Fig. 3** – Reproduced from *Rheumatology: a clinical handbook* (Al-Sukaini *et al.*).
- **Fig. 4** – Reproduced from *Rheumatology: a clinical handbook* (Al-Sukaini *et al.*).
- **Fig. 5** – Reproduced from *Rheumatology: a clinical handbook* (Al-Sukaini *et al.*).

Reactive arthritis

- **Fig. 1** – Reproduced from *Rheumatology: a clinical handbook* (Al-Sukaini *et al.*).
- **Fig. 2** – Reproduced from *Rheumatology: a clinical handbook* (Al-Sukaini *et al.*).
- **Fig. 3** – Reproduced from *Rheumatology: a clinical handbook* (Al-Sukaini *et al.*).

Rheumatoid arthritis

- **Fig. 1** – Reproduced from *Rheumatology: a clinical handbook* (Al-Sukaini *et al.*).
- **Fig. 2** – Reproduced from *Rheumatology: a clinical handbook* (Al-Sukaini *et al.*).

- **Fig. 3** – Reproduced from *Rheumatology: a clinical handbook* (Al-Sukaini *et al.*).
- **Fig. 4** – Reproduced from *Rheumatology: a clinical handbook* (Al-Sukaini *et al.*).

Scleroderma

- **Fig. 1** – Reproduced from *Rheumatology: a clinical handbook* (Al-Sukaini *et al.*).
- **Fig. 2** – Reproduced from *Rheumatology: a clinical handbook* (Al-Sukaini *et al.*).
- **Fig. 3** – Reproduced from Science Photo Library with permission.

Septic arthritis

- **Fig. 1** – Reproduced from www.omicsonline.org/mexico/septic-arthritis-peer-reviewed-pdf-ppt-articles/ under a CC Attribution 4.0 license.

Sjögren syndrome

- **Fig. 1** – Reproduced from *Rheumatology: a clinical handbook* (Al-Sukaini *et al.*).
- **Fig. 2** – Reproduced from *Rheumatology: a clinical handbook* (Al-Sukaini *et al.*).

Systemic lupus erythematosus

- **Fig. 1** – Reproduced from *Rheumatology: a clinical handbook* (Al-Sukaini *et al.*).
- **Fig. 2** – Reproduced from *Rheumatology: a clinical handbook* (Al-Sukaini *et al.*).

- **Fig. 3** – Reproduced from *Rheumatology: a clinical handbook* (Al-Sukaini *et al.*).
- **Fig. 4** – Reproduced from *Rheumatology: a clinical handbook* (Al-Sukaini *et al.*).

Vitamin D deficiency

- **Fig. 1** – Adapted from *Clinical Endocrinology* (Whitehead & Miell).
- **Fig. 2** – Reproduced from *Rheumatology: a clinical handbook* (Al-Sukaini *et al.*).
- **Fig. 3** – Reproduced from *Rheumatology: a clinical handbook* (Al-Sukaini *et al.*).

Chapter 8: Infectious diseases

Tuberculosis

- **Fig. 1** – Reproduced from https://radiopaedia.org/cases/pulmonary-tuberculosis-29 (Case courtesy of Assoc Prof Frank Gaillard, Radiopaedia.or g, rID: 8632) with permission.
- **Fig. 2** – Licensed under CC Share Alike 4.0; additional attribution: James Heilman, MD; available at: https://en.wikipedia.org/wiki/Miliary_tuberculosis#/media/File:PulmonaryTBCXR.png

Index